Clinics in Developmental Medicine No. 168

COGNITIVE AND BEHAVIOURAL DISORDERS OF EPILEPTIC ORIGIN IN CHILDREN

30 Furnival Street, London EC4A 1JQ

Editor: Hilary M. Hart
Managing Editor: Michael Pountney
Project Manager: Sarah Pearsall

First published in this edition 2005

British Library Cataloguing-in-Publication data
A catalogue record for this book is available from the British Library

ISSN: 0069 4835
ISBN: 1 898683 43 3

Typeset by Keystroke, Jacaranda Lodge, Wolverhampton
Printed by The Lavenham Press Ltd, Water Street, Lavenham, Suffolk
Mac Keith Press is supported by Scope

Clinics in Developmental Medicine No. 168

Cognitive and Behavioural Disorders of Epileptic Origin in Children

THIERRY DEONNA
University Children's Hospital, CHUV, Lausanne, Switzerland

ELIANE ROULET-PEREZ
University Children's Hospital, CHUV, Lausanne, Switzerland

Foreword by
JEAN AICARDI

2005
Mac Keith Press

Distributed by 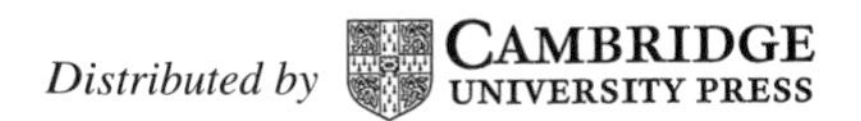

CONTENTS

AUTHORS' APPOINTMENTS

Thierry Deonna	Honorary Professor and Former Head of Neuropaediatric Unit, University Children's Hospital, CHUV, Lausanne, Switzerland
Eliane Roulet-Perez	Head of Neuropaediatric Unit, University Children's Hospital, CHUV, Lausanne, Switzerland
Claire Mayor-Dubois	Neuropsychologist, Neuropaediatric Unit, University Children's Hospital, CHUV, Lausanne, Switzerland

ACKNOWLEDGEMENTS

The opportunity to obtain so much data on the children reported in this book (which we believe is one of its main justifications) was offered to us over many years by colleagues from different areas of expertise. Had any of them been uninterested or unavailable, a crucial piece of the puzzle of the child's epilepsy would have been missing and the overall meaning of his/her unique history would have been lost. One particular piece of luck was the continuous and enthusiastic presence of the same people throughout the years, with newer and younger forces joining us along the way. The difficult task of giving credit to all of them may be made easier if we follow the order of their appearance over the years.

Dr Anne-Lise Ziegler, who entered into paediatric neurology after a long career in general paediatrics, has been involved on all fronts of our longitudinal studies in epilepsy, starting with adult follow-up studies of acquired epileptic aphasia and moving on to prospective follow-up of infants with severe epilepsies, pioneering the practice of infant testing at home and the use of questionnaires in these situations. She has been an efficient, faithful and critical help whose too frequent but self-imposed non-appearance in the list of authors of many of our papers (and of this book) must be recognized and admired.

Professor Paul-André Despland, Chief of the Neurophysiology Department at our hospital (CHUV: Centre Hospitalier Universitaire Vaudois), and his excellent team (especially Mrs Colette Gander who has saved, filed and retrieved hundreds of EEGs dating back to the earliest days) have always given us free access to their EEG lab and files, and for decades have been happy to perform EEGs day or night, as necessitated by clinical inquiries. The EEG records (and later systematic videoEEG recordings) have been faithfully kept and read by Professor Despland or his collaborators (mainly Dr Malin Maeder), who were always ready to do the extra work that made the clinical study significant. We are very grateful to them.

Véronique Davidoff, a clinical psychologist, was the first to systematically evaluate and regularly follow the children. She showed that no child was 'untestable' because they were too disturbed, and she was both firm and kind enough to encourage children and families to come back.

Pascal Zesiger, a neuropsychologist from the University of Geneva, helped us with the development of new tests and participated in several of our studies. In more recent years, we have been able to have working with us on a permanent basis Claire Mayor-Dubois and later Stephanie Cronel-Ohayon, two excellent neuropsychologists. Claire Mayor-Dubois has examined many of the children reported in the book and her systematic data collection and analysis have contributed to taking our clinical observations beyond the realm of simple anecdotes. Chapters 7 and 13 have been written in collaboration with her.

A special tribute should be given to Dr Claude Chevrie-Müller in Paris, a physician and speech pathologist who developed many of the now currently used tests of children's normal language development in French. She recognized very early on the importance of studying the possible role of some epilepsies in childhood language disorders, and created in the 1990s the 'Reseau INSERM Epilepsie-Language', in which professionals from various disciplines regularly met to share methods and ideas.

The authors' personal knowledge of children's language and communication and its disorders owes a lot to our early encounter and regular contacts with Professor Isabelle Rapin; and our education in the field of developmental neuropsychology in general was fostered by Professor Dorothy Bishop's contributions to the field, by the excellent contacts and advice she has given us, and the discussions that we have had with her over many years.

In the last 10 years, childhood epilepsy surgery has developed in the Suisse Romande, especially since the arrival of Professor Jean-Guy Villemure, a pioneer in epilepsy surgery in Montreal and now Head of the Neurosurgery Department at our centre (CHUV), and the creation of the Laboratory of Presurgical Epilepsy Evaluation in Geneva (Dr Margitta Seek). Our close clinical and research involvement with this team has opened up a new avenue for us in the study of the cognitive-behavioural aspects of epilepsy.

We are very grateful and fortunate to have had several expert and critical colleagues read the manuscript: Isabelle Rapin, Mary Coleman, Stuart Green, Walter Boas van Emde, Juan Narbona, Marie-Odile Livet and Jean-Guy Villemure. We owe special gratitude to Jean Aicardi, both for warmly encouraging us in the idea of writing this book and providing useful comments on it, and also for his thoughtful appraisal of our single case approach, and his caveats (see his Foreword).

On the editorial side, Martin Bax welcomed the idea of a whole book on such a subject, and along with Hilary Hart made very useful criticisms and also encouraged us to make the book larger, clearer and more detailed, so that it might be useful outside pediatric neurology and epileptology circles. We thank them a lot for their efforts.

Professor Emile Gautier, former Head of the University Department of Pediatrics in Lausanne, in which our work started, and Sergio Fanconi, its present Head, must also be warmly mentioned. Emile Gautier was always enthusiastic and supportive of our unconventional approach, and Sergio Fanconi has allowed Thierry Deonna to take sabbatical and other leave to write the book.

It is a pleasure to thank the families and children for their cooperation and efforts to help us obtain the data we needed for our studies (tests, questionnaires, videos, EEGs, etc.). We are happy to acknowledge the cooperation of the families in helping us in the study of difficult and rarely examined conditions – something that never ceases to surprise us. They always understood that our studies would help to increase knowledge and improve the care of other children, even if it was not always to their own child's immediate benefit.

During all these years, we have received financial support from the Swiss Ligue against Epilepsy, the Fondation pour le 350ème Anniversaire de l'Université de Lausanne, la Société Académique Vaudoise and la Fondation Charles Leopold Mayer pour le Progrès de l'Homme. Finally, the Swiss National Fund for Scientific Research has been a regular source of support since the beginning of our studies in the 1990s, first to Thierry Deonna, and more recently to Eliane Roulet-Perez for the study of the impact of epilepsy on the development of young children, especially those undergoing early epilepsy surgery (grants 3200-52991.97 and 3200-68105.02).

FOREWORD

Jean Aicardi

For centuries, medicine has been built on collecting case histories and observations on patients whom physicians have tried to help and cure, though often with moderate success. The collected observations were later interpreted and integrated into general systems, many of which were proved to be erroneous as the modern scientific method developed. The introduction of the clinico-pathologic method, complemented by the development of radiology, histology, biochemistry, electrophysiology and later genetics and molecular pathology, led to novel theories based on the new scientific evidence. These developments led to the reinterpretation of many previously known diseases and to the understanding of physiopathological mechanisms, as well as to a revolution in therapy. In the field of epilepsy, the introduction of the EEG brought major progress in clinical diagnosis, even though understanding of the pathophysiology and the mechanisms involved remained limited. As a result of these conceptual and technical developments, a new nosography, with much more precise descriptions of many new syndromes with well-defined clinical and EEG characteristics, was established, and treatment was also given considerable attention. A considerable amount of work was dedicated to the psychological study of epilepsy and its impact on the life of affected children, especially the consequences of epilepsy on school attendance and quality of life. However, relatively little attention was given to the neuropsychological study of epilepsy and its possible effects on brain function, cognition and behaviour, and to the causal role of epilepsy itself. During the same period a vast number of basic neurophysiological studies drew attention to the effects of normal and abnormal neural activity on brain development, especially on the formation of neuronal circuits and synaptogenesis.

The introduction of the scientific method in all fields of medicine has led to such spectacular progress over the past two centuries that the traditional method of collecting histories and facts has tended to be neglected. The emphasis has been, predominantly, on large case series amenable to statistical treatment, so that evidence from single case histories has come to be dismissed as 'anecdotal'. The current age is one of evidence-based medicine, which, in itself, represents progress and is a desirable objective. However, every doctor knows that many diagnostic and especially therapeutic decisions still have to be made on less than optimal objective evidence, and they have to rely on 'clinical experience' gained mostly from the slow accumulation of single cases.

Clearly, an approach based on the observation and reporting of single cases has many limitations. The construction of a nosological system, which is the necessary base for the process of diagnosis and therefore of prognosis and treatment, requires generalizations that must be founded on repeated, and carefully controlled, observations. A major, inevitable consequence of the process of generalization is a loss of information, as many isolated data are lost in the global analysis. Among these individual observations, some may be highly significant, or even fundamental, not only for the interpretation of single cases but also sometimes for a more general understanding of certain essential phenomena. Therefore, an individual approach is a necessary complement to classic studies of series of cases. It may be the only way to recognize new previously undetected important characteristic signs and symptoms, peculiar etiological circumstances, and evolutive peculiarities, which would remain undetected because of their very singularity in large series of cases. This is especially true in the case of epilepsy and its neuropsychological manifestations, as the number and heterogeneity of possible manifestations is enormous and their variable and unpredictable combinations and time course make the classic series approach of heterogeneous series of cases particularly difficult or even impossible. Single case studies, on the other hand, are well suited to delineate correlations between multiple sets of data (clinical, EEG, selected neuropsychological tests) collected over sufficiently long periods of time. In a number of cases, they may be the only possible method of study, as studies of large series are very difficult to perform or even impractical because of the multiple constraints (in terms of number of cases required, homogeneity of patients, duration of study, etc.), and also because the time and skills required are often not available or are too costly.

In this book, Deonna and Roulet-Perez have undertaken, in my opinion successfully, to rehabilitate the 'anecdote' by showing how powerful the study of carefully selected cases (which are followed up for a sufficiently long time) can be, and how such an approach can usefully complement the more traditional methods of large group statistical studies. Clearly, the 'anecdote', as understood here, has little in common with what is usually meant by this term. The cases reported in this book have been studied in depth and submitted to strict criticism according to the norms of the scientific method. This book illustrates, with a series of fascinating cases drawn from the vast experience of the authors, the actual application of this approach to the clinical and neuropsychological study of children with multiple types of epilepsy. Many of these case reports are presented in a graphic way that makes the significance of the cases easy to grasp at a glance. These examples nicely show how, even with single cases, the astute observations of an alert mind may open up new perspectives from both a clinical and a theoretical point of view – even though such perspectives clearly have to be confirmed and validated by larger studies.

The approach to clinical problems outlined in this book – the detailed study of individual cases or observations from small series – has another merit: it reminds physicians that any single patient may represent the 'fugitive opportunity' that Hippocrates' first aphorism underlined 2500 years ago, which, if recognized and correctly interpreted, can be the source of important developments and can be of great teaching value. This should remind doctors of the vital importance, all too often forgotten, of giving continuous personal attention to each individual patient – which is imperative not only from a humane point of view but also from a scientific perspective. Giving personal care and attention to the individual patient thus not only conforms to the traditional practice of medicine but is also scientifically important as a major source of new information that constantly adds new elements to the general body of medical knowledge.

In the pages of this book the reader will find not only a record of the authors' unique experience, but also a thorough and thoughtful review of the recent literature on neuropsychology as it applies to its relationship with epilepsy. Deonna and Roulet-Perez are particularly suited for this task as they have over the years given special attention to the harmful effects of epilepsy on cognitive and behavioural processes in children, a domain in which they are pioneers and have contributed so much.

The basic argument is that such harmful effects are not entirely, or even mainly, the result of the cause of the epilepsy condition, or of the psychosocial consequences, but mostly the result of interference of chronic epileptic activity with neuronal function, with maturation, with post-synaptic structure and organization that may be sufficient, at the behavioural level, to preclude, transiently or permanently, a child's ability to normally interact with his/her environment and with learning. This represents a major departure from previously held opinions that epilepsy was essentially a paroxysmal intermittent disorder, whose consequences were due to the practical and social disadvantages from such factors as overprotection, low self-esteem, low parental expectations, or interference of seizures with schooling, or due to the effect of causal lesions, or due to pathological damage incurred during prolonged or repeated attacks. These changes, which were largely initiated by the authors, have profoundly modified the approach to the clinical study and the therapeutic perspectives of cognitive/behavioural problems in epilepsy, and have redirected the attention of neurologists, epileptologists and neurophysiologists towards the study of the hidden neurophysiological dysfunction that directly results from epilepsy itself and should not necessarily be interpreted solely as a drug effect or as due to sociopsychological problems. Importantly, this dysfunction can only take place during the interictal period which is now considered to be of central importance as the source of the neuropsychological problems so often encountered in children with epilepsy. The interictal period is no longer regarded as just a silent interval separating two seizures but one during which profound consequences result from the continuous paroxysmal epileptic activity. It is now accepted that epilepsy is much more than having seizures. The concept applies especially to children, in whom epilepsy can interfere in multiple ways with the ongoing process of neurological development and learning.

The new views have both practical and theoretical consequences. From a practical viewpoint, they radically change the therapeutic approach to these children as they clearly suggest that even in the absence of seizures (or with only rare mild and/or atypical attacks) attempts to control interictal manifestations (EEG) are indicated. From a theoretical point of view, they may open up new avenues of investigation, as the clinical knowledge thus gained may contribute to the discovery, and possibly to some understanding, of the factors that can influence neuropsychological development and its deviation. Such views may also shed light on some basic processes such as brain plasticity and its role in normal and abnormal brain development and learning. This reappraisal of epilepsy has been a major revolution in thinking. However, the very nature and mechanisms of action of 'epileptic activity' remain unclear and much more basic work needs to be done to unravel some of its mysteries.

The noxious influence of epileptic activity on cognition and/or behavioural development had long been known in the case of infantile spasms with hyspsarrhythmia, although initially it had been misinterpreted as a result of the underlying pathological cause of the syndrome. The authors have shown, and nicely illustrate in this book, that the effects of epilepsy on cognition, behaviour or learning can also be observed in many other epilepsy syndromes and can be expressed in a subtle manner. They may be transient or lasting, probably depending on the duration of uncontrolled epilepsy. Such minor behavioural or intellectual difficulties can be difficult to recognize and, especially, to attribute to epilepsy because of the apparent 'benignity' of the classic epilepsy manifestations, or even the absence of clinical seizures. It is of note that this absence of seizures, as emphasized in several chapters, may only be apparent when seizures are so unusual that they are not recognized as such. The concept of 'cognitive epilepsy' introduced by Deonna and Roulet-Perez is important in this regard because it allows the attribution of unexplained behavioural/cognitive manifestations to epilepsy, thus making effective treatment possible in some cases.

Especially interesting is the view that the epileptic activity, especially as expressed by EEG paroxysms, might have a long-lasting, even permanent, influence on brain function and structure as a result of the plasticity of the young brain. Because of the demonstrated importance of neural activity on synaptic functions and circuit formation, the abnormal epileptic activity could result in an abnormal connectivity leading to lasting aberrant function. This view is of fundamental importance because early successful medical or surgical control of epilepsy, if feasible, might result in prevention of long-lasting brain sequelae.

However important the contribution of 'anecdotal' evidence, it is clear that it represents only one way of acquiring medical knowledge. Deonna and Roulet-Perez's book should not be mistaken as – and is clearly not intended as – a substitute for evidence-based and other currently accepted forms of scientific clinical investigation. It is clearly an important adjunct to our clinical armoury, uniquely suited for the detection of new facts destined to become the source of new hypotheses and new ideas. These in turn need to be validated in large series by conventional methods including statistical techniques and comparison with appropriate controls. The latter are indispensable in assessing the validity of evidence drawn from single cases or small series. For example, the real long-term practical significance of subtle neuropsychological or learning problems such as are observed in some types of childhood epilepsy, e.g. rolandic epilepsy, will be appreciated fully only by following large enough groups of unselected patients and comparing them with the general population or adequate control samples. This ideal validation may not be attainable in many situations because of the nature of the problems or because the numbers of available patients are not sufficient. In such cases, individual studies of 'privileged' cases will remain the only possible way of approaching the problem scientifically. With its limitations, the method is valid and the lesson to be drawn applies to many a field of medicine.

1 INTRODUCTION

Several textbooks have been written on epilepsy in children and new ones keep appearing (O'Donohue 1981, Dreifuss 1983, Fröscher and Vassella 1993, Aicardi 1994, Pellock et al 2001, Arzimanoglou et al 2004, Wallace and Farrell 2004). The frequent cognitive and behavioural problems encountered in children with epilepsy are usually acknowledged under the general heading of 'psychosocial aspects' of epilepsy. However, because of the intricacy of all the variables which need to be studied over prolonged periods of time and by several disciplines, special recognition of and systematic research on the direct effects of epilepsy on behaviour and cognition have not been given the attention which now appears so critically important. The often fluctuating character of the cognitive problems and the great diversity of associated brain pathology and seizure manifestations, amidst many other reasons, make it a difficult situation to study. Developmental neuropsychologists have an increasing interest in childhood brain disorders in which certain hypotheses about cerebral organization and brain plasticity can be tested, but epilepsy is usually treated as any other chronic childhood brain disorder without taking into account its unique characteristics.

The authors of this book suggest that the bioelectric disorder itself, especially in a developing brain, can lead to specific original neuroanatomical-neurophysiological consequences which reflect on the clinical and existential level in a way quite different from those seen in chronic static brain pathologies.

Our aim is to present an overview of these problems and our personal experience over several years. Some of our work has appeared in individual articles or book chapters, but a significant part of the data presented here has not been published previously.

Note that the term 'cognitive', at this broad level, also includes behavioural manifestations of epilepsy, in addition to general intelligence, specific cognitive skills, learning abilities and school performance.

1.1 Epilepsy, intelligence and the importance of psychological factors

It may seem paradoxical or counterproductive that one should focus on those apparently rare situations in which epilepsy has direct and sometimes severe consequences on cognition and behaviour when many years of careful work have shown that most children with epilepsy are intellectually normal and do not deteriorate with time (Bourgeois et al 1983, Ellenberg et al 1986). We have indeed spent an important part of our working lives reassuring parents about this.

The purpose of this book is to show that these situations are in fact not so rare, and that they can be analysed and should be better recognized and studied. The subject is both of major practical importance and also offers a remarkable opportunity to study a unique and complex form of brain dysfunction during development. Besides paediatric neurology, it should be of interest and concern to several other disciplines, such as child psychology and psychiatry, education and the developmental neurosciences.

From the psychological point of view, it should be said from the beginning that many children with epilepsy suffer more from the consequences of being 'an epileptic', rather than from the disorder itself. After all, the time spent in a seizure or in a postictal state is minimal in most childhood epilepsies, and even in the more severe ones, the child is most of the time asymptomatic. However, because of its unpredictable occurrence, social impact, frequent associated learning difficulties and need for medical treatment, the diagnosis of epilepsy carries many secondary negative psychological consequences for the child and his or her family. In the most common forms of epilepsy affecting otherwise normal children, these may be far more important than the direct effect of epilepsy on cognition, if any, which is the main topic of this book. In this respect, the recent surge of clinical research on the 'quality of life' of children with epilepsy, which focuses on the scientific study of the various factors that negatively influence their overall welfare, is fully acknowledged here. This is a very important target for secondary prevention (Voeller and Rothenberg 1973, Deonna 2003, 2005).

One must recognize the fact that some children with epilepsy have low cognitive abilities and that epilepsy itself is only an additional disability. In such cases, antiepileptic therapy will not contribute at all or only in a minor degree to improve cognitive function. This is often the great hope of the parents who are naturally inclined to believe that it is only the epilepsy which is to blame for their child's low performance. This book would be doing the parents a disservice if it encouraged their sometimes unrealistic hopes, and it could make the clinician's life even more difficult.

1.2 A change of perspective

We have grown up in a period of exciting progress in epileptology. New epileptic syndromes were being discovered, more effective antiepileptic drugs came on the market, and revolutionary methods of brain imaging became available. Better descriptions and follow-up studies of different childhood epilepsies allowed more precise diagnosis with earlier, often good prognosis (in some situations even at the time of the first epileptic seizure), such as in idiopathic partial epilepsy with rolandic spikes. This was an era of intense optimism. The aphorisms of Lennox (1960) – 'time is on the side of the epileptic', and 'epilepsy is, in truth, the hopeful disorder' – were our motto. We knew that most normal children with 'epilepsy only' and without history of brain damage would recover before adolescence, and we spent long hours demystifying epilepsy, calling it an ordinary childhood disease. We knew that the psychological consequences of the disease, even given the most reassuring attitude, were very important (Deonna et al 2002). Studies of this chronic myth-laden disease in children and the effects of the child's epilepsy on the family attracted attention.

We tended to believe that when a normally intelligent child with epilepsy had learning difficulties or behaviour problems, it was a psychological reaction to the disease, or the result of unrecognized underlying brain damage, or drug side-effects. As it was generally impossible or very difficult to sort out these different possibilities, it was suggested and generally accepted that the child's problems were 'multifactorial', the easy 'oreiller de paresse' of clinicians. We lived with a simple dichotomy between symptomatic epilepsies with 'organic' cognitive and psychiatric problems and idiopathic epilepsies with normal intelligence.

We were inclined to dismiss interictal paroxysmal EEG abnormalities which we knew could be observed in perfectly normal children, and another motto was 'treat the child and not the EEG'. The older publications on paroxysmal EEG abnormalities in children with learning disabilities or behavioural disturbance were considered with scepticism (Green 1961).

We considered with irritation (and still do) the numerous publications comparing intelligence quotients and school results of children with epilepsy and controls, which invariably found that the latter were doing a little better or much better as a group!

This was reminiscent of the common-sense 'adage' which says 'it is better to be healthy and rich than poor and sick'. These studies, however, did have the merit of pointing out that epilepsy was not only a succession of paroxysmal events and that one should pay attention to other and often more important aspects of the condition. This was useful in a period when severity or benignity of an epilepsy was judged exclusively on frequency of seizures and likelihood of remission.

In fact, child neurologists and epileptologists were so busy at the time with semiology, nosology, electrophysiology, delineation of discrete epileptic syndromes, drug treatment and prognosis of seizures that the cognitive dimension was overshadowed. It took many years for a leader in childhood epilepsy research, Jean Aicardi, to publish on 'the hidden part of the iceberg', referring to cognitive and psychiatric disturbances as possible direct consequences of the epileptic process (Aicardi 1999).

In the first modern book by a paediatric neurologist on disorders of higher cortical function in children (Rapin 1982), the chapter on epilepsy dealt only marginally with what is now perceived as its most important aspect, although it was fully recognized: 'chronic epileptic activity may thus interfere with neuronal function and metabolism, with neuronal maturation, with postsynaptic structure and organization, and at the behavioural level, preclude transiently or permanently a child's ability to interact with his environment, and to learn'.

This change in perspective was also prompted by several circumstances (Deonna et al 1993a). First, it was realized that some children whose epilepsy was controlled with minimal medication or who had no more seizures and were off therapy still had persistent cognitive problems, and that this should be looked at more closely. Second, the fact that transient isolated cognitive dysfunction could occasionally be either very prolonged (the so-called 'non-convulsive status epilepticus') or so short that only special tests could detect it (the transient cognitive impairment, or TCI, during apparently 'subclinical' EEG epileptic discharges) made one realize the existence of potentially important and relatively hidden cognitive dysfunctions directly related to epilepsy. Along the same line of thinking came the hypothesis that an acquired and persistent loss of language (or other acquired cognitive functions) could be the direct consequence of a bioelectrical disturbance on the EEG, the historical prototype being acquired epileptic aphasia or Landau–Kleffner syndrome. This hypothesis raised a lot of discussion, because it was against the prevalent idea that epileptic symptoms are by definition paroxysmal and short-lived. Clinicians had long been sceptical that the cause of the disorder was bioelectrical and not due to an underlying rare or new smouldering brain disease affecting crucial brain areas and also causing paroxysmal EEG abnormalities.

The increasing development of epilepsy surgery for intractable epilepsies showed that cessation of seizures not only brought about a better quality of life but that some children rapidly improved in their cognitive functioning after long periods of stagnation. This could not simply be explained by a decrease of drug treatment or better psychosocial functioning, and strongly suggested a more direct effect of seizures on cognitive function.

On the experimental side, it could be demonstrated that a focally induced epilepsy in very young animals could alter the development of cortical networks and create abnormal local synaptic circuits, another way in which epilepsy can directly interfere with brain structure.

The acknowledgement that some epilepsies and even epileptic EEG discharges without clinical epilepsy could have a direct impact on cognition and behaviour raised many hopes but was also the source of much frustration. It turned out to be very difficult in most instances to distinguish this impact from other variables and to be sure that seizures or epileptic EEG discharges were in fact the major factor in a given individual case. The absence of improvement or even worsening of symptoms with antiepileptic drugs seen in many of these situations often led to diverse and probably equally unjustified conclusions.

On the one hand, the causal role of epilepsy was excluded and, on the other, drug trials were abandoned since in the absence of better evidence it was more reasonable to have an attitude of 'primum non nocere'.

It was also not fully realized that the monitoring of clinical changes under therapy in the cognitive and behavioural domain required totally different tools from the simple classical approach of just counting the number of seizures and measuring the percentage change with a drug. It involved the quantitative approach of measuring cognitive and behavioural changes. This posed methodological problems. One first had to have *ad hoc*, standardized neuropsychological tools and the availability and competence of specialists in developmental cognitive neuropsychology. These specialists had to be present at the precise moment when the clinical changes were important to evaluate and correlate these with EEG findings. Second, one needed to monitor changes over time, with the inherent difficulties of repeated assessments such as test-retest effects.

Most neuropaediatric centres did not have the time or means to embark on such difficult tasks, or were doubtful that the pursuit of individual case studies was a scientifically valid enterprise. In fact, when we first asked for research funds, we were advised to do multicentric studies, which we felt at the time was unrealistic and probably fruitless.

In a climate of profound scepticism, we tried to find out whether specific cognitive or behavioural dysfunctions could be a direct and reversible effect of epilepsy, when so many other explanations were possible, and evaluate how this could be demonstrated. This has been the basic 'philosophy' of our group in Lausanne and the line that we have pursued for the last 20 years. The longitudinal approach has also made us aware of what can be learned from prolonged follow-up of children with early brain dysfunction. In this respect, epilepsy is a very special situation. A cortical brain region which has suffered from local abnormal electrical activity during development cannot be compared to a focally malformed or destroyed brain. The functional 'lesion' due to epilepsy, and the new organization which takes place in these circumstances, is probably unique, with late consequences and potential for prolonged recovery that we are only beginning to appreciate.

1.3 Personal studies, source of cases and classification of epilepsies

Our Neuropaediatric Unit at the Centre Hospitalier Universitaire Vaudois (CHUV) in Lausanne, which is the source of practically all the cases presented in this book, is providing care for most, if not all, children with epilepsy in the area, so that we see both common and benign epilepsies and, of course, the more severe ones, from the newborn period to adulthood. Furthermore, our interest in childhood neuropsychology and developmental disorders and close association with our colleagues in child psychiatry has given us the opportunity to evaluate children with recent or past epilepsy or in whom epilepsy was unexpectedly discovered. This has helped us to document the sometimes hidden cognitive effects of epilepsy.

We are fully aware that our approach of using single cases – an approach upon which most of the conclusions proposed in this book are based – differs from the classical approach of group studies with controls. It carries several risks of overinterpretation which should be clearly spelled out. 'We', as used throughout this book, refers to the two authors, Deonna and Roulet-Perez, whose studies have been conducted with the help of several co-workers whose contributions are discussed in the acknowledgements section and who have been regular co-authors of many of our publications.

Note on classification of the epilepsies and synonyms used in the book (Table 1.1)

Epilepsies can be classified according to: (1) seizure types (classification of epileptic seizures, e.g. partial vs generalized with many subdivisions between these); (2) presumed localization (i.e. frontal, occipital); and in recent years and most usefully, when possible, into (3) epileptic syndromes (i.e. a complex of signs and symptoms which defines a unique epileptic condition and which also includes EEG characteristics). The same syndrome may have different etiologies (e.g. West syndrome), genetic and non-genetic.

An epileptic disease is a pathological condition with a unique etiology and only a few are defined at the present time (e.g. Unverricht–Lundborg disease). No single classification is fully adequate for a given case or can take into account all facets of a given epilepsy, so that several may be used for different purposes or to define one important clinical aspect. Furthermore, they are likely to change as new knowledge, especially about the genetics and physiopathology of the epilepsies, emerges. Cognitive symptoms as such do not correspond to any recognized existing clinical seizure description, although they of course occur in many different epileptic situations. Some epileptic syndromes have a special impact on cognitive functions, and personal case descriptions included in this book are classified mainly under epileptic syndromes (see Tables 3.2, 6.1 and 8.1) when possible. When this is not possible, a seizure-type or localization-related classification is given. What is important to the reader is to know the different synonyms used for the same epileptic disorder, regardless of whether it belongs to a syndrome or whether it is classified according to seizure phenomenology.

Some terms are no longer in use and imprecise, but still deeply rooted, and can sometimes be found in our personal case studies or in the relevant literature cited on these epilepsies. These are summarized in the table. With this information, the reader will easily find all the important modern clinical knowledge on these epilepsies in recent textbooks,

TABLE 1.1
Epileptic syndromes and disorders: synonyms used in the book

The epileptic syndromes and other epileptic situations (which cannot be classified into syndromes) which are described in various contexts in the book are given here in alphabetical order, simply for convenience.

Epileptic disorder (commonly used term)	Synonym(s)
Atypical benign partial epilepsy	'Pseudo-Lennox' syndrome
Benign childhood epilepsy with centrotemporal spikes	Rolandic epilepsy Benign epilepsy with rolandic spikes Benign partial epilepsy with rolandic spikes
Childhood absence epilepsy	Petit mal, petit mal absences Pycnolepsy Generalized epilepsy with petit mal absences
Complex partial epilepsy	Temporal lobe epilepsy Psychomotor epilepsy Complex partial epilepsy of temporal or frontal origin
Continuous spike-waves during sleep syndrome (CSWS)	Epilepsy with CSWS Partial epilepsy with CSWS Electrical status epilepticus during slow wave sleep (EEG description)
Landau–Kleffner syndrome	Acquired childhood epileptic aphasia Acquired epileptic aphasia
Myoclonic-astatic epilepsy	Doose syndrome
Non-convulsive status epilepticus	(a) Petit mal status, absence status, status pycnolepticus in primary generalized epilepsy, spike-wave stupor (b) Non-convulsive status epilepticus of frontal or temporal origin
Severe myoclonic epilepsy of infancy	Severe polymorphic epilepsy of infancy Dravet syndrome
Temporal lobe epilepsy	Psychomotor epilepsy Complex partial epilepsy of temporal origin
West syndrome	Infantile spasms with hypsarhythmia Epileptic spasms

including discussions on classification (particularly in *Epilepsy in Children*, by Wallace and Farrell (2004), and *Aicardi's Epilepsy in Children*, by Arzimanoglou et al (2004)).

1.4 Importance and limits of the single case longitudinal study approach

The criterion standard of comparing a group of patients to a normal control group in a complex condition such as epilepsy, on multifaceted variables such as intelligence or learning abilities, is fraught with so many uncontrolled factors that only very general answers can be given. This is especially true when differences are not spectacular, which is often the case. Important individual differences may be hidden in overall group results (Guyatt et al 1992).

When the child is their own control, their individual characteristics will usually remain the same across time, so that one can better isolate the one (cognitive change) which is being measured in relation to the epilepsy (therapy and seizure-EEG activity). If a rapid loss or recovery of an already mastered function can be documented, or if, especially in very young children, the change is significant enough across time and is not part of the normal developmental tempo (for instance, language acquisition or learning curve), it can reasonably be attributed to a single or a limited number of 'epileptic' variables. It should be remembered that many important discoveries in neuropsychology in adults have started with the detailed study of one patient, or a small group of patients, with an extreme pathological condition. In children, before embarking on large studies, the first step is to study single cases in depth and longitudinally.

Of course, generalizing from results obtained in single cases is contrary to the classical scientific method based on statistical significance between groups. A given case may have individual unusual characteristics which are unrepresentative of a population with that same problem. However, when the apparent abnormality differs markedly from any normally occurring known variation, and the changes observed within a narrow time frame are of a degree of magnitude never seen in normal development (or other known pathology) and correlate with epileptic variables (onset of therapy, cessation of seizures or of paroxysmal EEG abnormalities), it offers strong evidence that the two are related. It should also be acknowledged that one important variable, the paroxysmal EEG abnormality, is not a stable one, and that one is measuring a dynamic situation which of course fluctuates and is measured only during a few repeated periods which are not necessarily representative of the brain state at other times.

In practice, another problem is that the clinical and EEG data often cannot be obtained, for different practical reasons, at the exact same period. Finally, when the clinical changes are not drastic and do not occur rapidly, it becomes even more difficult to conclude that they are not part of variations that could occur in normal children or in conditions other than epilepsy. The problem of differentiating normal variations in development from those which are due to pathology is indeed a recurrent one in developmental medicine and child neurology.

Normal children develop different cognitive functions in a certain temporal order, at a certain rhythm, and to a certain level of competence, but can vary significantly along all these dimensions. These variations depend on numerous factors of both genetic and environmental nature. The heterogeneity of these factors is still more marked in children whose 'normal' development has to proceed in the face of some congenital or early acquired brain dysfunction.

The advocate of single case studies notes that although it is feasible to isolate a group of children of a certain age with more or less the same cognitive abilities (the controls), in such a way that this group would indeed constitute a viable point of comparison, no such thing is feasible with regard to the dysfunctional group whose multifaceted underlying neurological impairment is suspected to be at the root of the cognitive deficit.

It is unwise of course to draw from one case study conclusive evidence for the hypothesis that the study purports to establish. It is indeed only one piece of the evidence. Conclusive evidence, if ever achieved, then comes when many single cases exhibit the same kind of similarity and difference from the normal population. In this sense, there is no a priori reason for thinking that, in the long run, single case studies cannot replicate the feature of group studies that rightly makes it a scientific standard.

We strongly object to published single case studies claiming a favourable cognitive effect of an antiepileptic therapy, for example when results are based on clinical impression only and without clinical and EEG follow-up of sufficient duration. However, we feel that when adequate data have been obtained, single case studies can give a sufficiently strong hint as to a possible cognitive effect of epilepsy, and that it is valid to present them as preliminary evidence, especially in the absence of better methods. This single case approach of course should be complemented, when possible, by the classical approach with larger groups using statistical methods and controls. Only this can give an idea of the range of the cognitive problems (if any) in populations of children with different epilepsy types and syndromes. However, decades of research using the latter method have not been able to identify the direct role of epilepsy among all possible factors in several situations, such as, for example, in benign partial epilepsy with rolandic spikes (see Chapter 8).

Studies with a single case, or only a few single cases, documented longitudinally in great detail, have shown, without any statistics, robust and clear data which have been amply confirmed later on in the domain of epilepsies with cognitive manifestations. Single case observations can generate new hypotheses which can be confirmed (or refuted) elsewhere and lead to further individual prospective studies using similar methods, which can be more focused and detailed.

The reader may be struck (and made suspicious) by the fact that that all the case illustrations in this book are pointing in the same direction, i.e. showing some kind of correlation (for the better or the worse) between epileptic activity and cognitive status – usually for the better when antiepileptic therapy is given. This could give the erroneous impression that therapy is always helpful and that it is easy to rely on it. This is far from being the case. One can only say that in the selected case illustrations (and the sample is obviously biased in favour of what we are trying to demonstrate) care has been taken to explore other possible variables and to produce sufficiently detailed data and follow-up to minimize errors of interpretation.

2
COGNITIVE EFFECTS OF EPILEPSY: EPILEPSY AS A NON-PAROXYSMAL DISORDER AND THE CONCEPT OF 'COGNITIVE EPILEPSIES'

It is important to examine the reasons for the relatively late recognition of the direct role of epileptic disorders on cognition and behaviour in children. It can give us interesting indications of our evolving thinking about epilepsies in general and hopefully prevent future exaggeration or confusion about this problem.

2.1 Historical perspective

In the classic textbook of child neurology of the first half of the twentieth century, Ford (1952) discussed the 'transient ' and 'persistent' effects of childhood epilepsies. Under the heading, 'Transient effects', he wrote: 'we may include the transient symptoms which often follow severe seizures as well as the cognitive and physical deterioration which eventually develops in so many epilepsies of long-standing. It is difficult to say whether these phenomena are the result of the convulsions per se or whether they are manifestations of the process which give rise to the convulsions.' Although Ford recognized ictal and postictal symptoms in other than the motor domain, there was no hint as to possible prolonged or even persistent direct effects of epileptic discharges on brain function. The view that cognitive deterioration was due either to the cause of the epilepsy or to acquired postepileptic brain damage, such as can occur after severe seizures or status epilepticus, remained for many years the prevalent one, as illustrated by the following historical examples.

2.1.1 Illingworth's Error or 'Mental Deterioration with Convulsions in Infancy'

In 1955, Illingworth, the famous British paediatrician, wrote a classic paper entitled 'Mental deterioration with convulsions in infancy' (Illingworth 1955). The paper carefully described the developmental arrest and regression in babies who probably had had infantile spasms (the EEG figures in the paper are very suggestive). He clearly noted the regression which sometimes preceded the onset of seizures but concluded that this was certainly the result of a progressive brain disease and not an effect of the seizures, which were brief and could not be responsible, because much more spectacular and severe seizures did not have this effect. He did not consider that a purely bioelectric disorder without severe clinical seizures could interfere with developing mental function.

2.1.2 Acquired Epileptic Aphasia or Landau–Kleffner Syndrome. From Landau to Morrell

The other example is the acquired epileptic aphasia or Landau–Kleffner syndrome. It took many years for it to be generally accepted that the language loss was due to a 'functional disconnection' of the language zones due to abnormal temporal epileptic discharges (as initially suspected by Landau and Kleffner). The idea that an unknown chronic insidious brain disease was responsible for both the aphasia and EEG abnormalities was for a long time a prevalent view.

The often slow onset of symptoms, their persistence for months or longer, and the apparent lack of correlation with other aspects of the epilepsy (EEG discharges, response to antiepileptic therapy) were thought to be incompatible with what was considered epilepsy. The gradual change of opinion towards recognition of the epileptic origin of the symptoms was illustrated in Menkes' classic textbook between the 1985 edition and the 1990 edition, in which Landau–Kleffner syndrome moved from a small paragraph under 'disorders of mental development' to a discussion in the chapter on non-convulsive status epilepticus, which is probably still not the right place for it! Morrell's electrocortical recordings of a cortical epileptic focus in the superior temporal gyrus, prior to multiple subpial transections carried out in severe cases, were a landmark in the recognition that Landau–Kleffner syndrome was an unusual form of focal refractory epilepsy (Morrell et al 1995).

2.1.3 Epilepsy is Not Only a Seizure Disorder

There are several very understandable reasons for the main resistance to, and late recognition and acceptance of, the idea that persistent cognitive and behavioural disturbances can be a direct manifestation of epilepsy. First is the deep-rooted belief that epilepsy is only a paroxysmal disorder with short-lived, rapidly reversible phenomena. Second, there are epilepsies with no cognitive or behavioural problems despite severe or frequent seizures, and there are also normal children with frequent epileptic abnormalities on the EEG who never have seizures. When the child with epilepsy has cognitive or behavioural problems, there is often an easily available explanation such as the underlying encephalopathy or side-effects of drugs. Finally, a rapid and clear improvement of cognitive or behavioural problems with antiepileptic drugs, which is for the clinician the most powerful argument for a direct link with epilepsy, is not as easily demonstrated as seizure control because it can take time to become manifest. In addition, in some particular situations, antiepileptic drugs can be unhelpful or even aggravate the behavioural disorder, so that it becomes very difficult to tease out what is due to epilepsy and what is due to a side-effect of medication.

Although it is acknowledged that epileptic manifestations can sometimes be more prolonged, such as in status epilepticus or in some postictal states, the very idea that epilepsy could manifest exclusively as a loss of cognitive function, a learning arrest or even as a developmental disorder without clinical evidence of seizures took a much longer time to emerge.

For example, although it has been known for a long time that a prolonged but fully reversible hemiplegia can be an epileptic manifestation (with only very brief and unrecognized motor seizures on that side prior to the deficit or true inhibitory seizures), it has taken time to realize that the same may occur with cognitive functions, for instance language.

A simple analogy can be drawn between the functional loss in the motor domain occurring after a focal motor seizure in a cortical motor area (postictal paralysis or Todd's paralysis) and the loss that happens with a focal seizure in a region devoted to a cognitive function, here oral language (ictal and postictal aphasia). It is important to note that the duration of the postictal motor deficit is not related to the duration of the seizure (a long postictal paralysis may follow a short seizure). This indicates that the postictal deficits are not due to neuronal exhaustion from the seizure but to (local) active inhibitory phenomena around the discharging focus (Efron 1961). This mechanism probably accounts for the so-called ictal hemiparesis (inhibitory seizure), which can be explained either by an immediate inhibition on the motor cortex following discharges in a closely neighbouring area or by discharges which directly activate an inhibitory circuit.

Prolonged epileptic dysfunctions in most instances are not true status epilepticus, but repeated focal seizures with a postictal state followed by a new seizure and a new postictal state without time for recovery in between. The term 'paraictal' is used to refer to a focal alteration in brain excitability with a strong functional inhibition and prolonged focal functional deficits (Shafrir and Prensky 1995, de Saint-Martin et al 2001), as occurs in the idiopathic partial epilepsies (rolandic epilepsy and related syndromes – see Chapter 8).

Each seizure, if it affects a region or network involved in a cognitive function, may not be recognized as such because the child must be involved in an activity in which this region

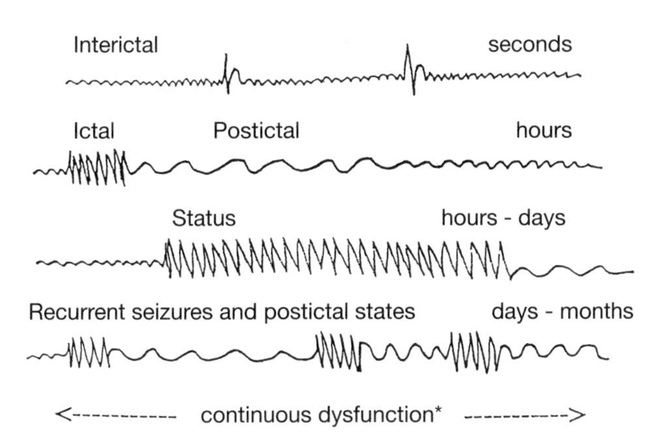

Fig. 2.1 Duration of cognitive-behavioural disturbances of epileptic origin and their EEG correlates. If seizures occur at frequent intervals with repeated ictal-postictal states, there may be no time for the child to recover and a continuous cognitive dysfunction ensues.

* In some idiopathic partial epilepsy syndromes, a continuous fluctuating dysfunction may occur which cannot be explained by such traditional ictal-postictal mechanisms and has been called paraictal (this is discussed further in Chapter 8).

or network is implicated at that precise moment, otherwise neither the child nor the people around the child will notice that anything is wrong. This idea is reinforced by the observations made during brain stimulation in conscious adults undergoing presurgical evaluation and mapping of the language areas (Ojeman 1983). If the patient is not listening to speech or talking at the time the stimulation occurs, they do not feel anything abnormal when stimulated in this zone, whereas they will be clearly aware of a temporary inability when they are engaged in these linguistic activities.

Importantly, the epilepsies with major cognitive impact often do not have severe, frequent or hard-to-treat typical seizures. This may also explain why they have been and are still unrecognized. One often cannot see the typical rapid, paroxysmal change and recovery of function, as is seen in usual epileptic manifestations, with clear-cut clinical–EEG correlations. The episodic nature of symptoms, considered characteristic of epilepsy, is often not immediately apparent. The clinical disturbances must sometimes be measured in days or weeks and, in special situations, possibly months or years. A gradual loss of cognitive functions, arrest or regression in development or a behavioural disorder may be the presenting problem with few or no hints of its epileptic origin. These special epileptic syndromes can rightly be called cognitive epilepsies.

2.1.4 A Definition of Cognitive Epilepsies

Epilepsies with 'cognitive' symptomatology, or 'cognitive epilepsies', can be defined as those epilepsies which manifest their effects mainly or exclusively in the cognitive sphere. In many forms of epilepsy, in fact, cognitive functions or behaviour are altered during the seizure itself, the postictal state and sometimes during what is thought to be the interictal period. However, the cognitive dysfunction is sometimes only one among other epileptic manifestations and is not recognized or considered the main symptom. It is thus somewhat arbitrary to draw a firm line in the definition of what constitutes a 'cognitive' epilepsy, and also to separate cognitive from behavioural epileptic manifestations (Deonna 2004). Indeed, behavioural disturbances can be the main or only epileptic symptom if the brain systems involved in social behaviour and control of emotions are primarily involved in the epileptic process. When cognitive disturbance or altered behaviour are the manifestations of an epileptic seizure, they may or may not be accompanied by other minor, visible, subtle signs of epilepsy, such as brief twitches, changes in posture or colour, pupillary dilatation, etc., but they are not the main element of the seizure.

2.1.5 The Notion of 'State-dependent' Cognitive Function in Epilepsy

Besag (1987) has used the term 'state-dependent', as opposed to permanent, cognitive dysfunction in epilepsy to point to the fact that many children with epilepsy do not have a regular and constant level of cognitive functioning but go through phases of transient cognitive decline or loss of mental efficiency, of variable duration. These are in direct relation to the activity of their epileptic condition but are not recognizable on the clinical level as overt seizures. The author does not refer, as we understand him, to a precise physiopathological state, but encompasses all potentially reversible abnormal bioelectrical events which may affect the child's cognitive functioning, and includes also side-effects of drugs. Although the term 'state', in this context, is potentially confusing because it suggests a specific condition or mental state, it is useful to draw attention to the fluctuating and variable level of cognitive functioning often seen in severe 'active' epilepsies. It implies that even a prolonged low level of mental efficiency or altered behaviour may not reflect the child's basic capacity and is potentially reversible.

3
EPILEPSY IN THE DEVELOPING BRAIN

3.1 Epileptogenesis in the immature brain

> In comparing the immature brain with the mature brain in regard to seizure susceptibility, one must remember that the immature brain is a dynamically changing structure, with the balance between excitation and inhibition varying as a function of age. The rate of development of inhibitory and excitatory pathways may vary from species to species and may reflect variations in synaptic organization or part of postnatal development. In addition, regional differences exist in developmental aspects of excitation and inhibition. Delays in the development of inhibitory input in one brain region may be balanced by precocious development of inhibitions in other brain regions.
>
> (Holmes 1997: 17)

The statement above shows the complexity of the innate developmental factors which will influence the onset, course, persistence or cessation of a tendency of a given infant's brain to develop epilepsy. This tendency can be either genetically determined (such as in neonatal familial convulsions) or the result of an early prenatally or perinatally acquired brain lesion or of a developmental structural brain anomaly. On the clinical level, this is reflected by the variety of paediatric epileptic situations, in which age at onset, semiology of seizures, circumstances of occurrence, and susceptibility to antiepileptic therapy can be very different and change over the course of time. This may explain puzzling situations such as the late onset of epilepsy in some congenital very epileptogenic brain pathology (such as focal dysplasias), or the apparently opposite responses to the same antiepileptic therapy at different ages.

3.2 Focal hyperexcitability, inhibition and spread of epileptic discharges

An epileptic seizure results from an abnormal excessive activity of a population of cerebral, usually cortical, neurons (Chang and Lowenstein 2003). This activity may propagate locally and implicate a larger number of neighbouring neurons (the so-called 'Jacksonian march' seizure), or at a distance along existing circuits such as the corpus callosum or the thalamus. In this latter case it leads to secondary generalization. In primary generalized epilepsy, there is a change in excitability within thalamocortical circuits. The local spread and inhibition and the distant consequences of an epileptic discharge will depend on the degree of functional development of the networks involved and on the balance between excitation and inhibition. For instance, a Jacksonian march of seizures is not seen in young infants. A focal epileptic discharge may spread to one or several of the pathways with which it is connected and be the trigger of a focal hyperexcitability at a distance. The immediate clinical and/or ictal/postictal manifestations may be misleading as to the main point of origin of the epileptic activity (Fig. 3.1).

It should be noted that epilepsy does exceptionally arise from neuronal structures other than the cerebral cortex. Abnormal epileptogenic tissue found in some malformations such as hypothalamic hamartoma or cerebellar gangliglioma can be the cause of an epileptic syndrome starting from these structures (Harvey et al 1996, Kuzniecky et al 1997).

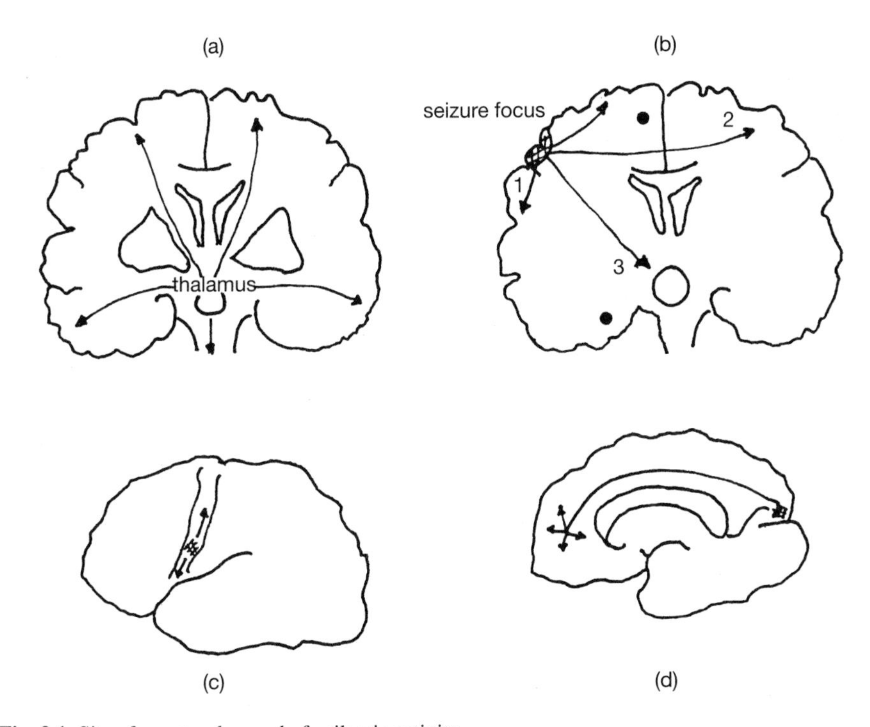

Fig. 3.1 Site of onset and spread of epileptic activity.

This figure shows the site of origin and possible spread of epileptic discharges in the brain of a child with epilepsy (see text). (a) Primary generalized seizures (e.g. typical generalized grand mal seizure): interconnections between thalamus and cortex (arrows). (b) Partial seizures: spread through (1) intra-hemispheric fibres (2) the corpus callosum (3) spread to thalamus with secondary generalization. Note that crucial areas for cognitive-behavioural functions, naturally very epileptogenic (black dot: medial-temporal and medial-basal frontal), are far from the brain surface. (c) Local propagation of epileptic activity from a primary cortical focus (e.g. 'Jacksonian march' along motor cortex). (d) Spread of epileptic activity from a cortical epileptic focus (here occipital) to a distantly connected area with trigger of a secondary focus. The recognizable clinical manifestations may be mainly or only related to the functional area in which this secondary focus arises. This spreading probably occurs through physiological pathways (e.g. commissural or intrahemispheric fasciculi) or through pathologically developed 'epileptic' networks. (Modified from Lothman 1993, in E. Kandel, editor. (2000) *Principles of Neurosciences*. New York: McGraw-Hill, p. 925.)

3.3 State of brain development (level of functional specialization) and onset of epilepsy

In the developing child, there is progressive lateralization of certain functions to one cerebral hemisphere and localization within that hemisphere to discrete cortical areas. This organization occurs gradually at different speeds and during preferential periods to form robust specialized networks. One can anticipate that the clinical consequences of focal epilepsy will be very different depending on its age at onset and localization. Fig. 3.2 shows this gradual process until the final adult stage is reached. The perisylvian region, which in normal ontogeny gradually becomes the seat of language functions in the left hemisphere in humans and also controls oromotor functions, is, for unknown reasons, the region where temporary disturbances of cortical excitability (the so-called focal sharp waves of genetic origin) most often arise. When this excitability manifests itself as clinical seizures, it is recognized as the 'partial epilepsy of childhood with rolandic spikes', and occurs at a preferential time period during early to mid-childhood (see Chapter 8, section 8.1).

The final state of organization is reached at different ages for different functions, so that the effects of focal epilepsy will be very different according to the network involved. Furthermore, the epileptic disturbance usually acts during prolonged periods and is often not strictly localized, spreading to the immediate surroundings of the focus or to distant areas, following functionally connected pathways. Therefore it is easy to conceive that a cortical area and the associated network which is in the course of specialization for a given cognitive function for which it has been programmed genetically will be particularly vulnerable to the effects of epileptic discharges. These discharges might prevent the network from recovering its previous state of organization and compromise the particular abilities and 'information' that were in the process of 'actualization'.

It is also obvious but not always fully realized by the clinician that the consequences of a focal epileptic activity experienced by the child or observed by the child's caregivers will depend on the functional role of the involved area. Epileptic discharges occurring in the primary motor, somatosensory, visual or auditory areas will have clinical consequences that can be recognized, or at least suspected, even in the nonverbal child. Those occurring in associative cortices involved in higher cortical functions, which occupy a much larger

Fig. 3.2 (*opposite*) Functional specialization (lateralization, specific localization) of brain functions.

(a) There is progressive lateralization to one hemisphere of some functions (usually left side for language and right side for visuospatial) and progressive localization of specific components in discrete areas within one hemisphere. The dotted area outlines the language areas in the perisylvian region (around the sylvian fissure) of the left hemisphere. (b) Major anatomic division of the brain into cerebral lobes and particular delineation of areas devoted to speech and language functions. The lower part of the motor cortex above the sylvian fissure is involved in movements of the articulators (lips, tongue, palate, pharynx). It is typically involved in benign partial epilepsy with rolandic spikes. Just in front of it is Broca's area involved in speech programming. The area below the sylvian fissure corresponds to the auditory area (involved in Landau–Kleffner syndrome). (c) and (d) These figures illustrate the small size of the primary sensory cortical areas (somatosensory, auditory, visual) shown in (c) contrasting with the much larger cortical areas shown in (d) involved in cognitive and behavioural functions: 'higher order cortex' (association cortex) and limbic and cingular cortices. (Modified from Bishop and Mogford 1988.)

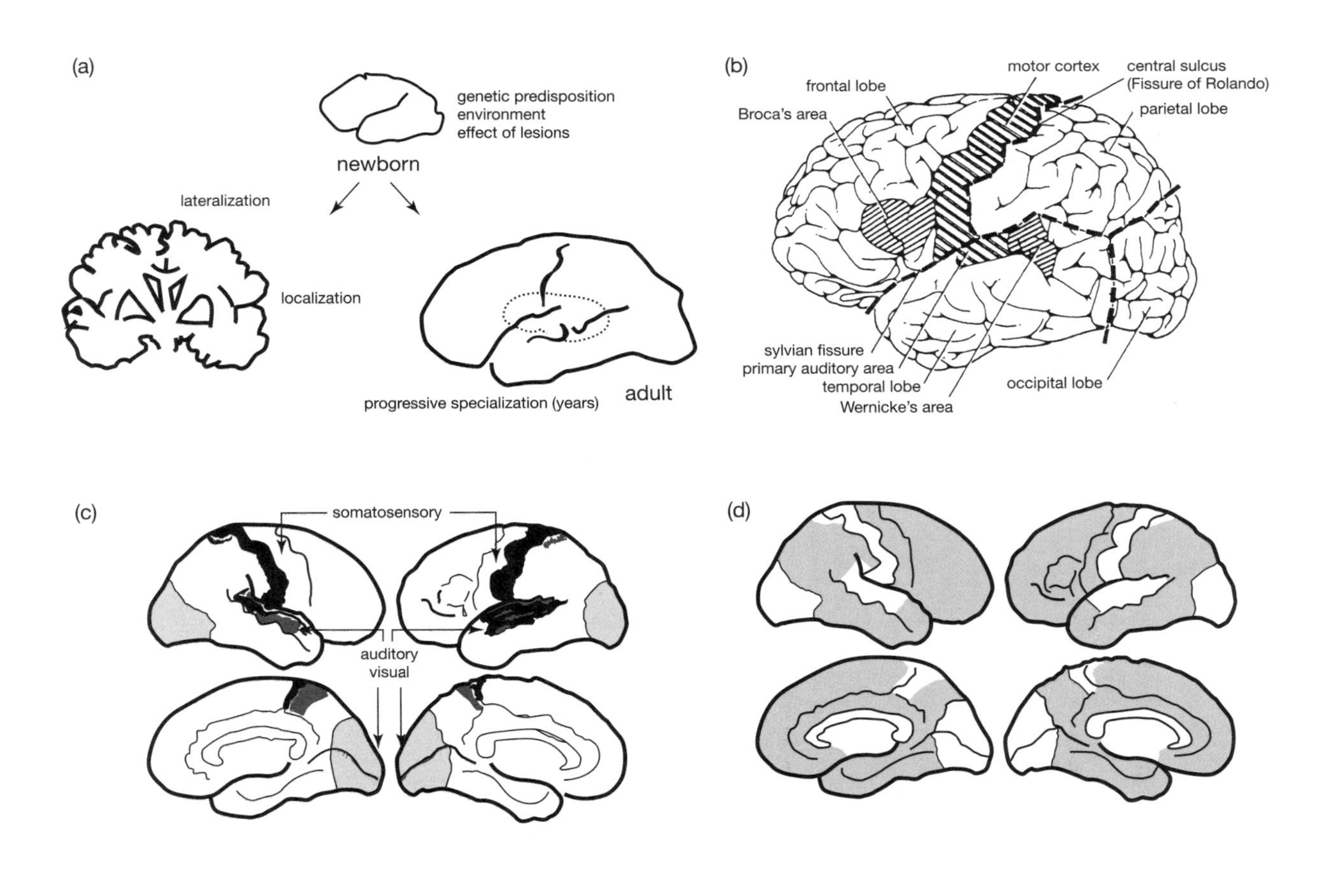
(a)
genetic predisposition
environment
effect of lesions
newborn
lateralization
localization
progressive specialization (years)
adult
(b)
motor cortex
central sulcus
(Fissure of Rolando)
frontal lobe
parietal lobe
Broca's area
sylvian fissure
primary auditory area
temporal lobe
Wernicke's area
occipital lobe
(c)
somatosensory
auditory
visual
(d)

part of the brain cortex (see Fig. 3.2d), will be either silent or manifest only when the function is operative at the time of seizure. In very young children, only unspecific behavioural changes or seizure manifestations due to propagation of the seizure may later on be observed (vegetative changes, secondary generalized motor seizures), with no hints as to the site of the initial discharge.

3.4 Structural pathology induced by epilepsy

There is a large experimental literature on the consequences of seizures on early brain development, brain structure and function, which will not be reviewed in detail here (Schwartzkroin et al 1995, Nehlig et al 1999). All of these data are of fundamental importance, but are still difficult to relate to the clinical reality of the various childhood epilepsies (Baram 2003). The first point to make is that seizures experimentally induced in animals are not the same as human epilepsy. The other is that the experimental work, done mainly on the hippocampal region, may not apply to other brain regions. Important variables such as age at onset, type of epileptic process, and circumstances of occurrence (fever, brain edema, etc.) will all influence the consequences of the seizure which may be either negligible or severe.

Experimentally, recurrent seizure activity may lead to disturbances of a wide range of developmental processes which depend on neurotransmitter and ion-channel-based activity. For example, slow waves of depolarization which are the basis of the development of synaptic activity in the young animal have been shown to be altered by epileptogenic activity. The formation of synapses, migration of neurons, arborization of dendrites, sequential expression of receptors and selection/removal of connections are all activity-dependent processes. These processes may be interrupted, slowed or accelerated and cause aberrant wiring or permanent damage to the involved circuitry. Alteration in normal connectivity may lead to disturbances of mental function, and to further epileptogenesis with sometimes direct seizure-induced injury (Baumbach and Chow 1981, Campbell et al 1984, Grigonis and Murphy 1994, Holmes and Ben-Ari 2001). All of these findings have not been clearly documented in pathological human tissue specimens. However, it is probable that in some focal childhood epilepsies affecting areas which are destined for, or in the process of, 'learning' a particular skill, the stabilization and organization of the networks involved might be delayed or permanently damaged. It is not known whether some original brain reorganization (different from that which occurs after destructive lesions) is still possible in these circumstances, and for how long recovery can take place (see Chapter 20).

3.4.1 Neuropathologic Correlates of Childhood Epilepsies

The effects of repeated seizures in the young human brain cannot be understood by examining autopsy or surgical material. These show various pathologies which can be either the cause of the epilepsy or unspecific changes due to general circulatory, metabolic or hypoxemic changes occurring during severe seizures. As was aptly noted by Caviness: 'The pathoanatomic correlates so far revealed in postmortem specimens of representative cases also represent abnormalities that have actually been observed, albeit within the relatively insensitive limits of routine pathologic analysis that are even further constrained by tissue sampling. This "visible world" of the clinician and the pathologist describes the workings of neural systems, on the one hand, and the histologic outcome of a complex and extended developmental history on the other. Neither this biology nor history is fully visible in the living human brain with epilepsy' (Caviness et al 1995: 114).

However, there are special situations in which damage from ongoing seizure activity (status epilepticus) can be documented with structural and functional imaging during the acute phase. This occurs in the so-called 'hemiconvulsions–hemiplegia–epilepsy syndrome' (HHE syndrome), in which unilateral hemispheric swelling develops during the acute seizure period followed by hemiatrophy. This is much rarer now, probably due to aggressive early treatment of status epilepticus, but its exact physiopathology and the possible role of a predisposing brain pathology are still poorly understood (Freeman et al 2002). The hippocampus is particularly sensitive to epileptic activity and this can now be visualized shortly after the acute epileptic state with cerebral MRI after prolonged febrile seizures in young children. A seizure starting from this area may lead to hippocampal swelling followed after a few months by atrophy. There might be a predisposing structural lesion (microdysgenesis) in this area (Mathern 1997, van Landingham et al 1998, Roulet-Perez et al 2000). If the damage is bilateral, severe developmental consequences may ensue. DeLong described a catastrophic 'clinical syndrome of early bilateral hippocampal sclerosis' which results from acquired bilateral hippocampal damage in one or successive episodes of status epilepticus. The children have a marked and permanent regression in language communication with autistic behaviour (DeLong and Heinz 1997). Fig. 3.3 shows such a course in a child we have followed from an early age.

3.5 Cerebral plasticity and epilepsy

Prolonged, recurrent epileptic discharges, with possible long normal intervals, may either disrupt or have no effect on the networks in which they take place. The age at onset and site of origin of the epileptic activity (i.e. its state of maturation when epilepsy becomes active), its duration, its spread to other regions, in addition to the etiology and age-specific disturbances of neurotransmission at the neuronal and synaptic level, will determine the presence (or absence) and severity of the structural brain consequences and the time course of their development (immediate, delayed, progressive). These are very difficult issues to study clinically and no generalizations can be made. Comparisons between humans and experimental animals and between children and adults have to be treated cautiously, at our current stage of knowledge. For instance, the possibility that recurrent focal seizures in a child can lead to chronic changes in excitability in the area concerned (or in the homologous area in the other hemisphere, the 'mirror focus') and be a source of later chronic epilepsy (secondary epileptogenesis) does not exist in functional partial epilepsies which always remit before adolescence, regardless of therapy. In addition to the changes in excitability that epileptic discharges themselves may engender, there might be other permanent structural changes that will influence cognitive functions. Focal epilepsy induced experimentally in a developing animal's brain at an early stage can interfere with the normal maturational programme of the affected neuronal networks, but the effects may be different if the epilepsy occurs later when the functional and structural organization of this region has been completed.

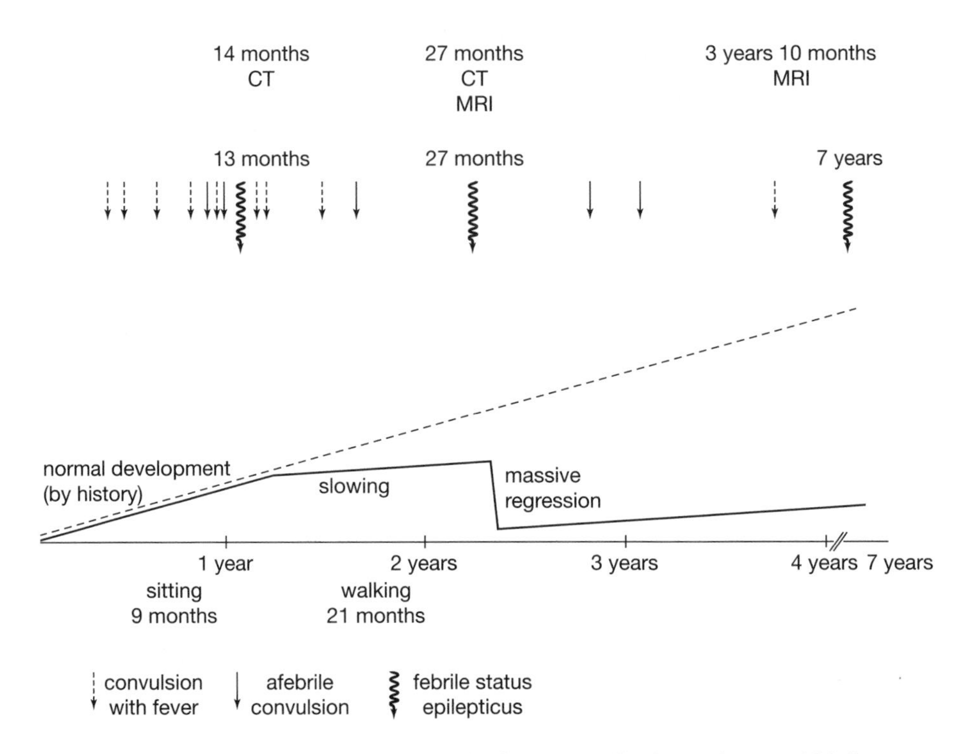

Fig. 3.3 Case P.G.: bilateral hippocampal sclerosis after status epilepticus and repeated febrile status epilepticus.

This figure shows the clinical course of a young girl who had an early onset of complex febrile and afebrile seizures. She had massive permanent regression in development after a second episode of status epilepticus at the age of 27 months which was at the time unexplained. MRI is shown in Fig. 3.4.

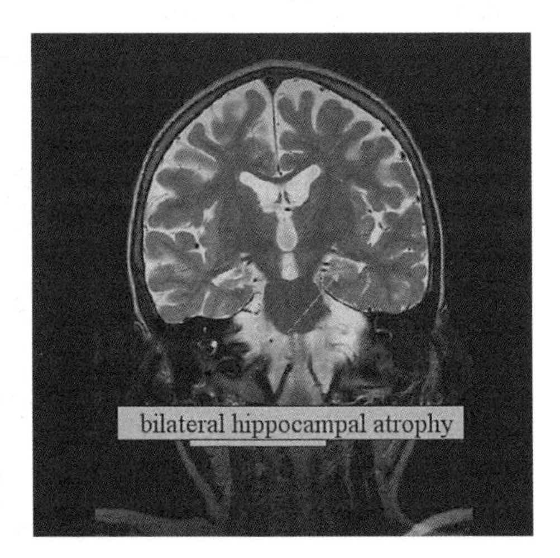

Fig. 3.4 Case P.G.: MRI at 3 years 10 months showing bilateral hippocampal atrophy.

Despite some general atrophy, both hippocampi, especially on the right side, appear small and hyperintense (T2 coronal slices).

It is known that plasticity and repair phenomena in the nervous system can be either beneficial or detrimental. For example, the motor function normally subserved by the damaged area may be taken up or reorganized elsewhere, with clear benefit, or it can create an additional disability, i.e. abnormal involuntary movements such as delayed onset dystonia and mirror movements. As far as brain excitability is concerned, the changes may be either protective against later epilepsy or, on the contrary, epileptogenic. One can also speculate that the epileptic activity does not always have negative effects. After all, the normal structural synaptic development which allows fixation in memory and learning is 'activity-dependent', i.e. repeated and regular paroxysmal electrical events are generated by the incoming sensory information (Luscher et al 2000). Epileptic activity in already developed or developing networks might contribute to their stabilization rather than always disturb their function.

3.6 Clinical consequences of epilepsy on developing cognitive-behavioural function

The abnormal electrical events and their consequences described above occur in developing brain regions in which function and structure may not be completely specified and stabilized. In younger children, one may be dealing with non-emergence or non-progression (stagnation) of a given function, or the disruption of a fragile just-acquired ability. In older children or adults one sees the loss of an already acquired cognitive skill or of a learned and mastered behaviour, which is a very different situation.

If the affected developing function is of fundamental importance for a particular emerging skill to appear and normally has to be present for subsequent capacities to unfold, one can envisage some important cognitive 'downstream' effects of the epileptic process. For example, a focal epileptic activity that affects a network involved in articulatory programming of speech will not have the same consequences on language functions as one affecting sound and verbal decoding (auditory and verbal agnosia), even though verbal production will appear strongly abnormal in both cases. In the first situation, communicative skills will be spared (see case H.J. in Chapter 3, section 3.7), and if speech recovers when

TABLE 3.1
Possible cognitive-behavioural consequences of epileptic dysfunction at different developmental ages (examples), contrasting very young children and older children in whom significant cognitive abilities had developed prior to the onset of epilepsy

Very young children (0–3 years)	Older children (>3 years)
Aberrant development	Slow learning**
Delayed development (non-emergence)	Cognitive arrest**
Developmental regression of one or more (global) function	Dementia Specific cognitive deficit (loss or non-acquisition) Psychiatric syndrome (psychosis, ADHD)

** global or specific

the epileptic activity stops, it will reveal intact linguistic skills. In the second situation, the absence of phonological decoding will have consequences on syntactic and semantic comprehension and expression of spoken words. The whole development of spoken language will then be severely disturbed, not because of an extended brain dysfunction affecting all language areas, but because of the 'knock-out' of a crucial initial step of language processing with downstream effects. This is well demonstrated when this step is bypassed by a visually coded language such as sign language, which reveals intact basic linguistic skills (see Roulet-Perez et al 2001).

3.6.1 Dynamics of Cognitive Development in Epilepsies with Onset in Early Infancy

We are concerned here with the evaluation of the direct effects of epilepsy on development, as a primary factor, or as an additional factor to the effects of an underlying brain pathology. It should be remembered that there are epileptic syndromes of infancy which do not affect cognitive development, so that no generalizations can be made as to the effects of epilepsy on brain function even at an early age (Deonna 1999).

The dynamics of development may be affected in different ways which are graphically illustrated in Fig. 3.5.

TABLE 3.2
Some epileptic syndromes of infancy and their influence on cognitive development

This table shows some epileptic syndromes with onset in infancy. Note that the consequences of epilepsy on development can be absent or severe, showing the variable effects of different types of epilepsy on brain development and function.

Seizures	Syndrome	Cognitive consequences
neonatal, multiform	BFNC	none
partial seizures (clusters)	BIFC	none
myoclonic	MEI	none
epileptic spasms	West syndrome	regression ± reversible
focal febrile, myoclonic status	SME	normal initial development (until 12–18 months); stagnation; marked mental retardation
partial seizures with 'spasms'*	not specified	variable; regression (± autistic-like?)

* Focal cryptogenic or symptomatic epilepsies of frontal or limbic origin. They are often associated with generalized spasms. In children over the age of 2 years, they are often called 'late infantile spasms'.

BFNC: benign familial neonatal convulsions
BIFC: benign infantile familial convulsions
MEI: myoclonic epilepsy of infancy (spontaneous or reflex)
SME: severe myoclonic epilepsy of infancy (also called severe polymorphic epilepsy of infancy or Dravet's syndome)

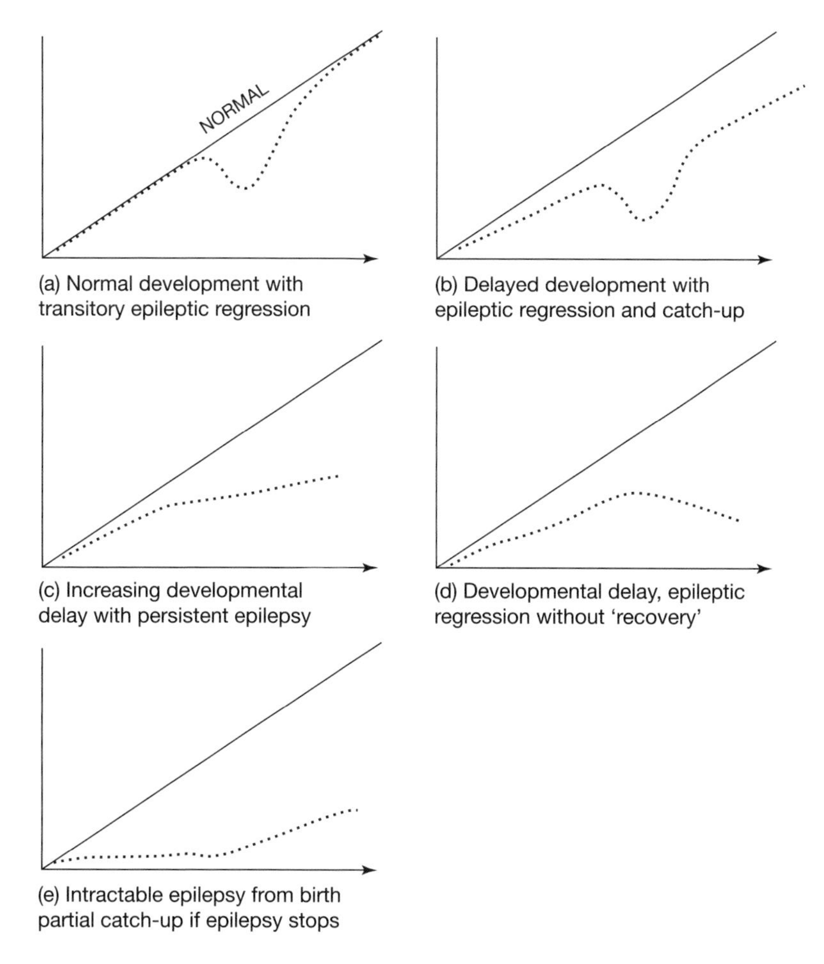

Fig. 3.5 Early onset epilepsies and dynamics of altered development.

This figure shows a graphic representation of altered developmental dynamics depending on age of onset, severity, duration of epilepsy alone or in addition to the consequences of the underlying brain disorder (see text).

(a) Normal development with transient epileptic regression: this is illustrated in babies with 'idiopathic' West syndrome, but also in some babies with symptomatic West syndrome associated with focal lesions such as cerebral infarcts or congenital tumours (see Chapter 8, section 8.5).
(b) Delayed development with epileptic regression and catch-up: in these cases, the child makes gains at various speeds if the epilepsy becomes controlled, but remains at a retarded level. This is the most frequent situation. The child develops to the level of his or her own basic potential.
(c) Increasing developmental delay with persistent epilepsy: in this situation, the direct or

indirect effects of the epilepsy contribute in a variable way to the delay, which is due to the basic cerebral pathology. The earlier and the more severe the epilepsy, the more difficult it is to separate these two components of the problem (Deonna 1999).

(d) Developmental delay, epileptic regression without 'recovery': in this situation, epilepsy once started is so severe that it not only precludes further development but does not even allow recovery of the developmental level that had been reached prior to the regression. Epilepsy-induced permanent brain lesions in crucial locations, such as bilateral hippocampal sclerosis, may be responsible (DeLong and Heinz 1997, Roulet-Perez et al 2000).

(e) Absent or minimal developmental progress due to early severe epilepsy, with partial later catch-up if epilepsy stops: this is probably exceptional but illustrates that some residual potential for development can exist despite months of uncontrolled epilepsy. Earlier surgical treatment of very epileptogenic focal dysplasias is likely to produce new data on this issue.

3.6.2 Dynamics of Cognitive Development in Epilepsies with Onset in Later Childhood

In school-aged children, who have mastered verbal language and the basic social skills, the possible chronic cognitive effects can manifest as:

1 Loss of an acquired skill. When there is loss of a previously acquired competence, and if this loss is rapid and major and out of proportion with other competences, there is not much of a diagnostic problem. When the loss is moderate, only a later further decline or recovery can indicate a significant problem in that domain. Note that a child may, because of epilepsy, fluctuate in abilities but still function within the normal range, especially if the child happened to be in a superior range initially.

2 Inability to learn a new skill. Learning is dependent on so many different factors that the possible role played by epilepsy, when it does not manifest with clear paroxysmal symptoms, is very difficult to demonstrate or may take a long time to become evident. The cognitive consequences will depend on the severity and duration of the epileptic process, its response to antiepileptic drugs, and whether the active epileptic period occurred in a critical learning period for the skill concerned. This will show mainly in the way the child is progressing in school. The result may be non-emergence, slow emergence or slowing of a new skill normally acquired or in the process of being acquired at that age, but it may take several months or even years to see or be convinced that the acquisition curve is far below the normally occurring variations. The child must of course have previously been normally exposed to the domain being evaluated at school and have had enough opportunity, help and motivation to learn. The speed, quality and amount of learning of new skills are typically not evaluated in formal neuropsychological tests and are often a subjective judgement on the part of teachers. Fig. 3.6 summarizes how epilepsy may interfere with cognitive development and school progress over time.

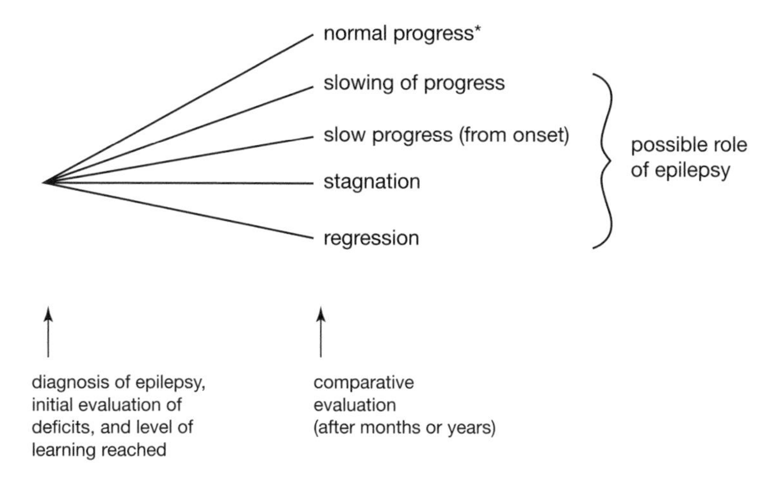

Fig. 3.6 Possible role of epilepsy in school-aged children.

This figure shows the possible role of epilepsy in learning in school-aged children and the different clinical situations observed. When the dynamics of progress is altered, epilepsy is one of many possible factors. The challenge is to identify the factors that determine these outcomes. Rapid recovery of abilities or a change in tempo of acquisitions when epilepsy is controlled can be strong indicators of a direct role of epilepsy.

* Note that a child can fluctuate in abilities but still remain in the normal range.

3.7 Effect of early focal epilepsy on specific developing skills

Focal epilepsy starting very early on in a baby with an otherwise normal potential, and affecting discrete brain areas in the process of specialization, could in theory interfere selectively and possibly transiently with a particular developing function. This appears difficult to demonstrate. The study briefly reported below (Mayor-Dubois et al 2004) in a child who displayed specific transient 'developmental' speech delay suggests that it can occur.

Case H.J.

This boy was first seen at the age of 26 months for evaluation of epileptic seizures which occurred mainly during sleep. At this time, he had a speech delay and the history suggested a probable stagnation after normal early development of babbling. A detailed quantitative study of videos that the family had made regularly from the age of 8 months indeed showed normal development of babbling up to the age of 12 months, followed by regression and a long stagnation in prelinguistic production. At the age of 26 months the diagnosis of an idiopathic partial rolandic epilepsy was made (in retrospect with an onset before 12 months). Under antiepileptic treatment, a rapid catch-up and normalization of speech was documented. Fig. 3.7 shows graphically the correlation between the evolution of the epilepsy and the language data, and the details of the linguistic study at successive ages.

The correlative data and the dynamics of the evolution with an early regression ruled out a transient, normally occurring speech delay ('slow starter') and led us to conclude that this epilepsy had interfered transiently with speech development. More specifically, it could be attributed to a selective deficit in speech programming (dyspraxia of speech) because the parallel studies of language comprehension, non-verbal communication and general cognitive development were entirely normal. Oromotor functions were affected, but not in a major way, as seen in the acquired epileptic 'opercular' syndrome, and could not account for the problem (Colamaria et al 1991).

This single case study is important in showing that early manifestations of epilepsy can be hidden, and present as specific developmental delay long before the epilepsy is recognized. It may seem at first surprising that such observations have not been made before. However, they had to wait for the development of video techniques, their routine use in various situations by families, new knowledge of normal prelinguistic development and

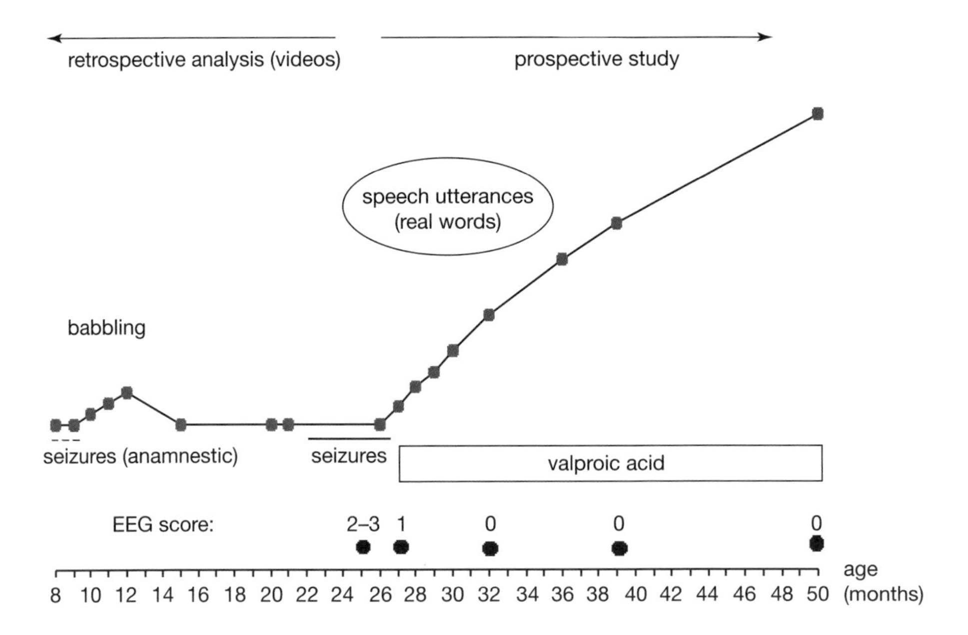

Fig. 3.7a Case H.J.: summary of clinical history.

Clinical summary (see case description) showing the dynamics of prelinguistic and early speech development, its prolonged stagnation due to interference of epilepsy and its recovery (EEG score: 0: no epileptic discharge, 1: rare, 2: frequent, 3: very frequent). (Modified from Damasio 1999.)

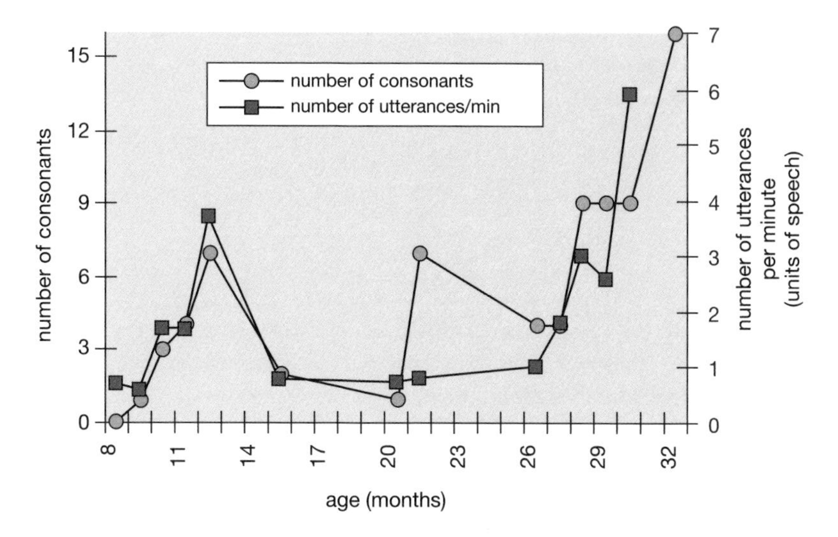

Fig. 3.7b Case H.J.: language production data.

Quantitative and qualitative evolution of babbling from 8 to 32 months as documented from family videos (8 to 25 months) and from personal clinical data (from 26 months). Note the normal early onset of babbling, the long stagnation and rapid increase after 26 months. (Modified from Damasio 1999.)

the creation of tools for its analysis. Finally, this had to be coupled with serial clinical and EEG follow-up over a prolonged period, which was possible only within a research project.

We do not know whether these situations are exceptional or simply not recognized, and we have no way at the present time to answer that question and to measure the practical implications of such privileged observations.

4
EPILEPSY AND COGNITIVE FUNCTIONS: IDENTIFYING THE DIRECT EFFECTS OF EPILEPSY

4.1 Overview of the main variables

Any clinician wishing to study one particular factor which can account for the cognitive, learning or behavioural problems of a child with epilepsy is confronted with an almost unsurmountable task. All of the potential factors are closely interrelated. Their specific importance at successive periods of the disease can be very different, sometimes insignificant, sometimes predominant. Each of the main categories of factors belongs to various domains of study and competence which are difficult to relate to the clinical epileptic situation at hand (see Fig. 4.1).

The epileptic variable, i.e. the direct effect of epilepsy itself, is a dynamic one. This characteristic allows us in some situations to isolate the effect of epilepsy 'proper' from other influences, and this is what we have chosen to emphasize throughout this book.

The underlying brain condition responsible for the epilepsy in the first place, the antiepileptic drug effects and the psychological consequences of the disease can almost always be proposed to explain a part or all of the child's problems. To make things more complicated, one must recognize that each of the broad categories of variables just listed can itself be subdivided into many different components. For example, an antiepileptic drug sometimes also has psychotropic effects independent of the antiepileptic action, which can be either positive or negative for the child. A minor decrease of cognitive efficiency due to epilepsy can lead a high functioning child to total frustration, discouragement and loss of self-esteem, with school failure out of proportion to any real learning difficulty.

These considerations could lead one to think that identifying the epileptic variables is a lost cause and that one should wait for universally efficient antiepileptic drugs or the availability of prolonged monitoring of electrical activity in all parts of the brain with non-invasive tools. Hopefully, the following discussion will help.

Table 4.1 shows the different factors involved for each of the broad causal categories which can account for cognitive and behavioural disturbances in a child with epilepsy. It should be noted that the presence of a brain lesion, the use of antiepileptic drugs, or psychological problems are not necessarily always a relevant aspect of the cognitive or developmental problems.

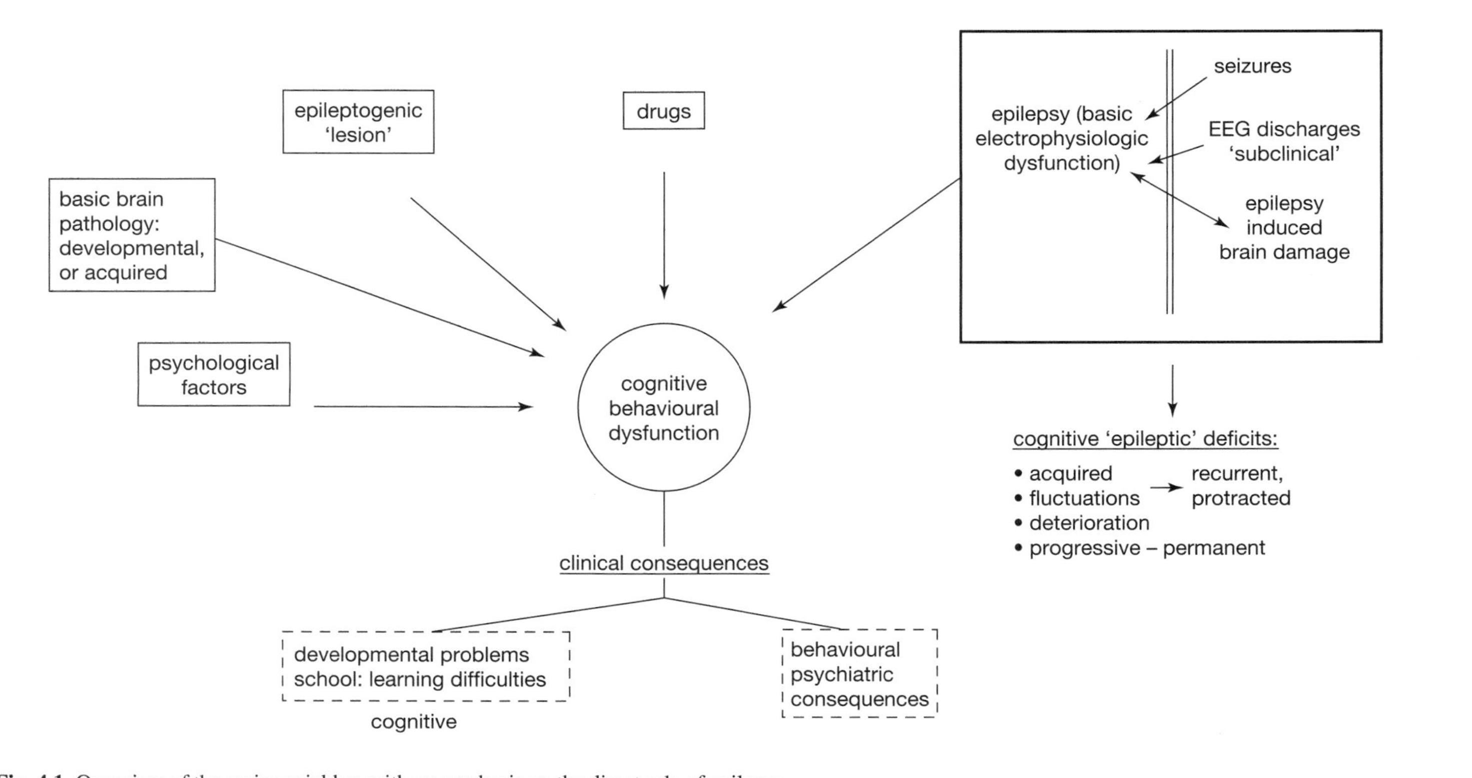

Fig. 4.1 Overview of the main variables, with an emphasis on the direct role of epilepsy.

This figure illustrates the different factors which can explain cognitive and behavioural problems in childhood epilepsy. The direct effect of the epileptic activity is given prominence because this is the emphasis of this book. The reader is encouraged to discover which other arrows could be drawn to show other indirect influences on cognition/behaviour. Note that the study of each variable is in itself a special field of expertise and research.

TABLE 4.1
Cognitive disorders and epilepsy in children: relationships

This table summarizes and contrasts the general causes of cognitive disorders in childhood epilepsies as opposed to those which are directly linked with epilepsy *per se*, and indicates in what particular situation a given factor is likely to be significant or not. (Modified from Wallace and Farrell 2004.)

General causes	Effects on brain function (cognition, behaviour)	Comments
brain lesion(s) causing epilepsy	variable effects, possibly none	may be asymptomatic until becomes epileptogenic – do not a priori blame pre-existing damage
antiepileptic drugs	specific antiepileptic effects, but also other possible effects (psychotropic) on cognition and mood	final positive or negative clinical effect on cognition and mood depends on many factors (cf. text)
psychological/emotional reactions (child, family)	non-specific (chronic disease) and specific to epilepsy (unpredictable, loss of control)	direct psychiatric manifestation of epilepsy and mental triggers of seizures (e.g. frontal, limbic) can be confounding factors
Epilepsy *per se**		
ictal – postictal	fluctuating deficit of variable duration (status epilepticus, postictal)	repeated ictal-postictal states with no recovery of function between episodes may lead to prolonged deficits
brief unavailability of specific subsystem for cognitive function	transient cognitive impairment related to EEG discharges	possibly reduced cognitive efficiency
prolonged cognitive epileptic deficits (paraictal**)	cognitive epilepsies: nature of deficit (selective or global) depends on cortical area(s) affected (e.g. language in Landau–Kleffner syndrome) and related networks	usually sustained focal/diffuse epileptic EEG discharges with/without CSWS may occur without associated 'typical' seizures
pathology induced by epilepsy	epileptic 'damage' to developing networks	may apply only to early or special epilepsies; limits of animal models of epilepsy

* age at onset, location and spread of epileptic process, duration and type of epilepsy can be important additional factors
** paraictal: this term has been used for prolonged deficits observed in some partial epileptic syndromes not clearly attributable to a typical ictal or postictal state, but considered of functional epileptic origin

4.2 Direct effect of epilepsy on cognition at a functional level

In this chapter, we are dealing only with the transient functional changes due to epilepsy and not the more permanent structural ones; we are aware, however, that these variables may be interacting in the same child at a given period or at successive periods of the epileptic disease.

The epileptic activity may or may not have a direct impact on the ongoing cognitive activity, depending, among other factors, on the site of origin, duration, extent and spread of the excitation and the importance and duration of the locally inhibited neuronal function.

Cognitive functions can thus be transiently (and repeatedly) interrupted or altered for prolonged periods as a direct effect of this abnormal electrical activity.

These functional, acute or more prolonged changes may occur in the following different ways:

1 Temporary disruption of the normal functioning of a given focal cortical area involved in a cognitive function (a focal 'cognitive' seizure) or a distributed network (such as in childhood absence epilepsy). It may or may not have a visible impact on ongoing cognitive activity, depending on whether or not this area was 'operative' at the time of the discharge. If not, it will be unnoticed by the subject and may or may not have a negative impact on learning.
2 Repeated or prolonged epileptic dysfunction (non-convulsive status epilepticus, recurrent postictal states) with durable periods (days, weeks, months) of disturbed cognitive function. Depending on the particular network involved in the epileptic dysfunction and the period at which it occurs in relation to the acquisition of a specific skill, more or less serious problems will ensue.
3 Focally (or diffusely) and intermittently disturbed brain excitability with EEG discharges but without observable seizures. This may be seen with diverse structural pathologies, but also in idiopathic/genetic epileptic syndromes. The local spread and associated inhibitory phenomena probably do not have the same neurochemical mechanisms in all epilepsies and even in the same syndromes different ones may be operative or they may change in the course of the epileptic disease. The term 'paraictal' has been used to refer to persistent but reversible neurological dysfunctions observed in some partial idiopathic epilepsies with focal sharp waves and which cannot be attributed to a classical ictal-postictal phenomenon (Shafrir and Prensky 1995, de Saint-Martin et al 1999).

The epileptic activity may occasionally be triggered or facilitated by a specific cognitive activity. This is probably rare but can occasionally be demonstrated with videoEEG (Matsuoka et al 2000).

4.3 Clinical situations in which a direct effect of epilepsy or epileptic EEG discharges on cognitive functions can be studied

There are several distinct clinical situations in which the direct role of epilepsy on cognition or behaviour in children can be studied. They are quite diverse but have all been very important in shaping our views on the subject and continue to be a source of new information in this domain. Every clinician is regularly confronted with one or the other.

1 Ictal (including status epilepticus) and postictal cognitive and behavioural deficits in partial or generalized epilepsies
2 Transient cognitive impairment (TCI) during EEG epileptic discharges
3 Epileptic syndromes presenting with cognitive and/or behavioural manifestations as the main symptomatology

4 Surgically treated epilepsies
5 Newly diagnosed epilepsy with behavioural/cognitive disturbances antedating first recognized seizures

4.3.1 Ictal (Including Status Epilepticus) and Postictal Cognitive and Behavioural Deficits in Partial or Generalized Epilepsies

Overview or general aspects

The transient cognitive and behavioural changes which can be precisely documented and correlated with other evidence of ongoing epileptic activity (paroxysmal epileptic EEG changes, clinical response to antiepileptic treatment, or both) offer the best available evidence of the direct effects of epilepsy. They are difficult to document outside the simple situations such as childhood absence epilepsy or non-convulsive status epilepticus in which a very rapid and important change in responsiveness, activity, or level of performance can be measured. When the cognitive or behavioural changes are more complex or subtle in their manifestation and last for a longer period than can be measured in a laboratory session or at the bedside, it is clearly more difficult to find definite proof of the epileptic origin of the symptoms.

The symptoms can be either positive or negative (Gloor 1991), that is, epilepsy can produce an excess of function (i.e. verbalization, hallucination) or a deficit (i.e. loss of language) (Rosenbaum et al 1986). The simple analogy is usually made with a partial motor seizure and postictal paralysis in which these two components occur in succession. However, epilepsy may activate areas or networks whose normal function can be principally inhibitory (e.g. premotor inhibitory area). It is possible that the same occurs with simple cognitive processes, but the final effect on more elaborate and integrated cognitive activities is not known. For example, epileptic discharges in temporal regions during reading aloud can sometimes improve rapidity of decoding while comprehension of the text is, on the contrary, decreased. This would indicate a differential effect of epileptic activity on two components of a task.

Unresponsiveness, 'absence' and the problem of ' loss of consciousness'

Temporary unresponsiveness may be the only or main clinical epileptic manifestation. Failure to respond to environmental clues or to people (unresponsiveness) may be accompanied by arrest of ongoing activity, inadequate continuation of this activity, or the sudden onset of a new and apparently purposeless but sometime elaborate behaviour. The child may have no conscious recollection whatsoever of what happened during this period or, on the contrary, remembers a very vivid sensory perception, complex feeling or a scene at the onset of the episode but has no 'conscious' memory of what happened thereafter. However, it can sometimes be shown by forced choice experiments or by the child's later behaviour that he/she had registered some information during the episode. These episodes may last for seconds, minutes or hours. To the ordinary onlooker, the expression 'absence' or 'he/she looked absent' will be the first that comes to mind and may continue to be used to describe what are obviously very different epileptic symptoms. All they have in common is the fact that the child has been temporarily unresponsive to or 'absent' from the physical world and the human community around him/her.

The intuitive and common-sense view is that presence in the world is what defines consciousness, although epilepsy is a very spectacular model showing that there are different levels of being 'conscious'. Damasio, in his book *The Feeling of What Happens* (1999), describes what he felt when he witnessed for the first time a complex partial seizure: 'I did not think then, but I think now, that I had witnessed the sharp-razored transition between a fully conscious mind and a mind deprived of the sense of self.' What he calls 'core consciousness' seems preserved during some epileptic seizures.

Gloor, in a series of remarkable papers about the meaning of consciousness in the context of epilepsy, summarized his observations during seizures in which 'loss of consciousness' was the main alleged symptom, as follows: 'The cause of the "unresponsiveness" may be due to aphasia, inability to perform voluntary movements, ictal or postictal amnesia (sometimes with preservation of memory during the ictus itself) or diversion of attention by a hallucinated experience' (Gloor 1986: S14).

From the clinical point of view, it is classical and still very useful to separate the typical absence epilepsy from other types of seizures (complex partial seizures) in which unresponsiveness is also the main or only symptom but which have a very different etiology and prognosis and response to antiepileptic medication. The latter are what used to be called temporal lobe seizures, now referred to as 'complex partial seizures' because their site of onset may be somewhere other than the temporal lobe, mainly frontal. Table 4.2 summarizes the major differences between typical absence epilepsy, complex partial seizures and

TABLE 4.2
Temporary unresponsiveness: epileptic or non-epileptic?

This table shows the main clinical characteristics of temporary unresponsiveness in typical petit mal absences and in complex partial seizures contrasting this with the behaviour of the 'dreamy', 'absent-minded' child.

	Typical absence epilepsy	**Complex partial seizures (temporal or frontal 'pseudoabsence')**	**Inattentive, 'absent-minded', 'dreamy' child (non-epileptic)**
Duration	few seconds	longer, minutes, hours	difficult to state
Frequency/situation	usually several per day	variable, often in clusters with long free intervals	depends on activity and emotional state
Unresponsiveness	abrupt onset, total	often partial	no, usually responds when addressed vigorously
Autonomic symptoms	none	pallor, cyanosis, mydriasis	none
Other associated symptoms	none, or rhythmic jerks of head or eyes	simple or complex motor automatisms	none
Postictal state	none	often fatigue or need to sleep	none
EEG	3 cycles/second SW	variable, temporal or frontal spikes	normal
Hyperventilation	provokes absences in 80–90% of cases	most often no effect	no effect

non-epileptic 'absent-mindedness'. It should be said, however, that this usually clear distinction is not always easy to make, for many different reasons. It may be that the relevant clinical observations cannot be made or are not adequately reported, or that additional circuits are involved during the epileptic discharge resulting in more complex behavioural manifestations (see also Chapter 8, section 8.6).

Nevertheless, it is useful to have the information in this table in mind when confronted with the parent's or teacher's frequent complaint that the child is 'dreamy', 'in the clouds' – a complaint which often raises the question of possible epilepsy.

Cognitive ictal manifestations

The cognitive epileptic deficit can be exquisitely specific and temporarily suppress any component of a perceptive (i.e. ictal blindness) or cognitive function (aphasia, amnesia, apraxia, spatial disorder, etc.). The epileptic zone (i.e. number and spatial extension of discharging neurons) may be too circumscribed or in a location too far from the brain surface to show a clear epileptic focus on the scalp EEG (Williamson et al 1993, Regard et al 1994). The different types of deficit which have been studied in children during the ictal phase are described in Chapter 7 on neuropsychology.

Case M.A.

An 11-year-old girl with known epilepsy characterized by rare episodes of non-convulsive status at the age of 4 years and 9 years, and under valproate therapy, was seen on an emergency basis because of fluctuating inability to speak for the past 12 hours. Detailed language testing was carried out immediately on arrival, prior to EEG and treatment. She had an isolated fluctuating word-finding difficulty, both in a naming task and in conversation, which was not improved by a phonological prompt, but she had no agramatism. Repetition was difficult and there were some phonological errors. Oromotor skills were normal. Comprehension, reading, memory and executive functions were normal. The EEG showed rare left frontal spikes. Buccal midazolam was given and she regained normal verbal expression (subjective and objective) within 20 minutes. This was interpreted as a specific transient impairment of phonological programming skills without other linguistic problems.

Primary emotions as ictal manifestations

Probably all primary emotions, with the same experiential qualities as those normally triggered by appropriate stimuli, can occur as ictal phenomena. For example, ictal fear, as reported in adults from direct stimulation or spontaneous seizures originating in the amygdala (Biraben et al 2001), is occasionally reported in children (Cendes et al 1994). Ictal

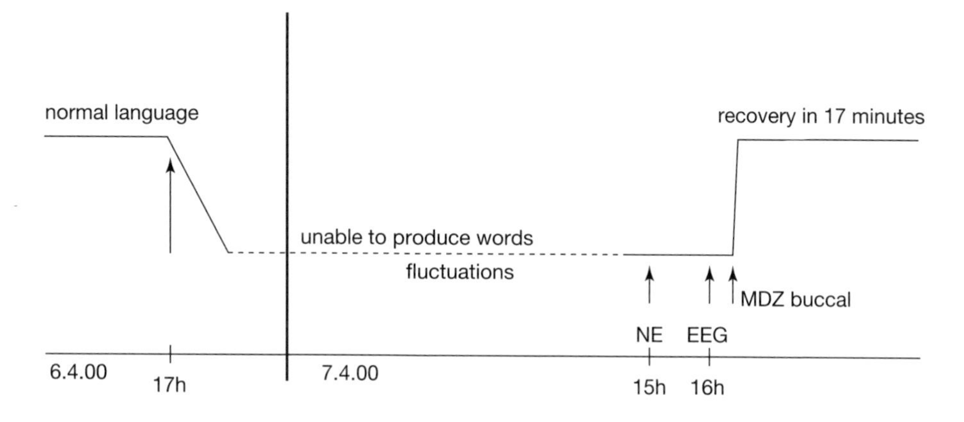

Fig. 4.2 Case M.A., girl, 11 years: aphasic status epilepticus.

This figure shows the clinical course and timing of investigations (see text). Note that the disability was fluctuating in severity from moment to moment during the symptomatic period.

fear may be diagnosed as a panic attack – a difficult differential diagnosis, because both have a very similar symptomatology and can even co-occur in the same patient (Mintzer and Lopez 2002). To complicate the issue, panic attacks in adolescents may be triggered by hallucinogenic drugs and cannabis some time after intake and without immediate triggering factors (Deas et al 2000). The final common pathway of the attack is likely to be the same in both instances (amygdala).

Laughing and crying are the earliest manifestations of pleasurable and unpleasurable physical and emotional life experiences which are gradually triggered by more elaborate or specific contents of consciousness or external events. They can be the sole or main manifestation of epilepsy (gelastic seizures and dacrystic seizures) (Lenard 1999). In children, they are typically seen in the syndrome of 'gelastic seizures, precocious puberty and hypothalamic hamartoma', but they can in fact occur in partial complex epilepsies of frontal and temporal origin of various causes (Arroyo et al 1993). Importantly, the 'non-natural', exaggerated quality of epileptic crying and laughing can, at least when it is frequent, be recognized by parents as different from the usual laughter or crying in their child, especially when these episodes are accompanied by abnormal vegetative, motor or other epileptic phenomena.

Complex perceptual-behavioural ictal manifestations

> As hallucinations produced by brain stimulation or epileptic discharges, dreams or the phenomenon of phantom limbs demonstrate, it is the brain that creates the reality we experience.
>
> (Gloor 1986: S16)

It is difficult to make a distinction between cognitive and emotional/behavioural manifestations because these different aspects are so tightly linked in normal mental function. However, when epilepsy involves brain systems (prefrontal, frontolimbic) subserving the experiencing of specific emotions or the regulation of mood, action and goal-directed behaviour, the main or only manifestations of epileptic discharges in these areas may consist of abnormal behaviours or emotional states.

Importantly, the involved frontal and limbic areas, which are intrinsically highly epileptogenic zones, are, for the most part, far from the brain surface. This means that epileptic discharges in these areas may not show on the surface EEG unless secondary generalization or spread to areas closer to the scalp occur.

These emotional symptoms and/or complex behavioural disturbances can sometimes be the only epileptic manifestation and must be distinguished from reactive phenomena to an unpleasant or frightening 'seizure' experience.

It is rare to have detailed descriptions of isolated ictal and/or postictal acquired and temporary behavioural abnormalities which can be attributed to the direct effects of epilepsy (Boone et al 1988, Jambaqué and Dulac 1989). A full-blown reversible frontal syndrome may be documented, but, more often, only non-specific, fluctuant and aberrant affective reactions or behaviours with attentional problems occur.

There may be no obvious associated cognitive impairment in these situations and only detailed neuropsychological testing can reveal specific signs of executive dysfunction. A remarkable case history recently reported by Manford et al illustrates the complexity of the interactions between organic (epileptic) and psychiatric factors in such situations (Manford et al 1998). The authors report in detail both the psychiatric and seizure history from early childhood and the investigations carried out from 10 years of age in a boy who eventually had successful left temporal epilepsy surgery at 17 years and was followed until the age of 21 years. This very intelligent boy (IQ 125) had increasingly severe behavioural problems and paroxysmal, initially only nocturnal, episodes (from the age of 8 years), then diurnal ones (from 11 years) consistent with complex partial seizures of temporal lobe onset, although his first EEGs were normal. His interictal behaviour was severely disruptive and intermittently bizarre with violent outbursts, which often appeared purposeful in a context of severe family problems. Several psychiatric diagnoses were considered, including borderline personality disorder, conduct disorder, organic personality disorder and malingering. He improved for a few months after inpatient psychiatric treatment. All these factors contributed to delayed diagnosis of epilepsy and prolonged psychosocial dysfunction. He improved markedly after epilepsy surgery at 17 years (resection of anterior temporal neocortex, body and head of hippocampus and amygdala). The author's analysis of ictal and interictal behaviours, and the description of the boy's relative insight into some of his problems, combined with aberrant behaviour, the family's violent reactions to his behaviour and the other psychological consequences of the disease are all impressively described and discussed from a joint psychiatric and neurological perspective.

The special case of paroxysmal rage or aggression as an epileptic manifestation
Child psychiatrists sometimes ask whether a child with repeated unexplained attacks of rage could have epilepsy. Among the so-called primary emotions, anger as an epileptic phenomenon has been much studied in adults, particularly because of its medico-legal implications of responsibility for violent behaviour. It is generally thought that unprompted paroxysmal rage directed against persons or the environment is practically never an isolated direct manifestation of epilepsy; in any case, it has never been directly proven (Ounsted 1969, Delgado Escueta et al 1981). An exception might be rage attacks described in hypothalamic hamartomas, a condition in which epilepsy arises directly within the malformation, but never as an isolated manifestation (see Chapter 9, section 9.1.3).

Abnormal behaviours, including aggressive reactions, may however be seen during seizures or in the postictal state when a confused patient misinterprets an onlooker's communicative intentions and resists restraint or any attempts to change his/her ongoing behaviour, leading to violence directed at the person concerned.

'Episodic dyscontrol' refers to attacks of paroxysmal rage or other emotional outbursts in children who display these behaviours in the absence of significant triggering factors. The child is usually completely exhausted at the end of the attack and has no apparent recollection of what happened, so that the question of an epileptic manifestation is sometimes raised. We do not recall ever having diagnosed epilepsy with confidence in such circumstances. This situation can occur in the context of adverse psychosocial conditions or as sequelae of brain trauma, encephalitis and sometimes epilepsy, which probably lowers the ability to exercise self-control, but the mechanism of the attack itself does not appear to be epileptic in the neurophysiological sense (Gordon 1999).

4.3.2 Transient Cognitive Impairment (TCI) during Epileptic Discharges on EEG

Since the EEG became a clinical tool, it has always been open to question whether the brief paroxysmal electrical activity seen in epileptic patients during the so-called interictal state could sometimes have clinical consequences which were either too brief or too subtle to be recognized by the patients themselves or an observer. Clinical observations have made it clear that there is no simple correlation between the amount of paroxysmal EEG activity as recorded on scalp electrodes and the clinical state of the patient, and, for a long time, the tendency was to dismiss the abnormalities as not significant if there were no recognizable clinical seizures (the view was 'treat the patient not the EEG').

Since the 1960s, several studies have shown that a drop in efficiency (i.e. simple reaction time) or increased error rate in some tasks (recognition tasks) can occur during some generalized spike-wave discharges on the EEG. Later on, with improved technology and more sophisticated cognitive paradigms, it became possible to demonstrate a laterality effect. Verbal and non-verbal tasks (short-term memory) were administered during continuous videoEEG monitoring, and error rates during the periods with and without focal EEG spike-waves were compared and correlated with the side of the EEG discharges. There were more errors on the verbal tasks with left-sided discharges and vice versa (Aarts et al 1984, Kasteleijn-Nolst Trenité et al 1990a).

Importantly this could be seen when no change in the patient's behaviour or cognitive ability could be recognized with the usual clinical observation. These EEG discharges could no longer be called, as previously, 'subclinical' EEG discharges.

These observations raised many hopes that one would soon be able to use this technology as a basic clinical tool to identify which children were actually symptomatic and needed antiepileptic therapy (Kasteleijn-Nolst Trenité et al 1990b). Twenty years later, we are still struggling with this difficult situation and not much progress has been made. There are several possible explanations for this:

1 Relevant tests can be done only in children old enough and intelligent enough to cooperate for a certain amount of time in usually rather dull and non-engaging tasks while under EEG monitoring, although more amusing and elaborate ones are being developed.
2 The EEG must contain enough periods *with* as well as *without* discharges to make a meaningful comparison (an EEG with too frequent discharges or with only rare occasional discharges cannot give useful information).
3 The interference with cognitive processing differs according to whether the stimulus to respond to or to remember occurs just before, during or just after the discharge. Furthermore, a given type of cognitive activity, its level of difficulty and the level of attention it requires may exacerbate or, more often, suppress the amount of discharges during the task at hand (Ounsted 1964, Binnie et al 1987, Boniface et al 1994, Kasteleijn-Nolst Trenité and de Saint-Martin 2004).
4 Finally, and probably the most important, is the fact that only simple cognitive tasks can be given for this type of correlation, so that a poor result is not necessarily predictive of the consequences for the learning process and for the various cognitive demands of ordinary life. The fact that some children with unrecognized frequent typical childhood absences continue to behave and learn normally indicates that a lot of cognitive activity can take place even if frequently interrupted. This is not to say that such absences are unimportant and should be ignored, but it leads one to think that there are different ways in which an electrical epileptic dysfunction can interfere with learning. One should take a differentiated view incorporating age, type of epilepsy, origin in the brain and spread, and amount of surrounding inhibition, in relation to the type of cognitive task to be solved.

Two important single case studies (Shewmon and Erwin 1988), one of which has passed largely unnoticed (Shewmon and Erwin 1989), illustrate the experimental difficulties in the detailed study of transient cognitive impairment. Shewmon et al tried to document the type of transient visual dysfunction during localized occipital discharges. Over a three-year survey of a large EEG laboratory in California, only three patients were found to be suitable for the protocol. Finally, only one patient was able to perform the visual recognition task as well as the reaction time task during and in between right occipital spikes on the EEG. The authors found increased misidentifications during spikes, but it could not be determined whether it was due to a transient impairment in visual acuity or to a transient visual agnosia. This is, to our knowledge, the only study – which has not been replicated – showing that a transient focal dysfunction could occur in direct correlation with single 'interictal spikes', and that 'The spike-related transient scotoma is not an all-or-none phenomenon, but fluctuates from spike-to-spike across a spectrum of degrees of visual impairment' (Shewmon and Erwin 1988: 687).

Recurrent transient cognitive impairment: leading to persistent cognitive impairment?
Having demonstrated that transient specific cognitive impairment during focal 'interictal' spikes can occur, the next question is whether an accumulation of these deficits innumerable times during many years could lead to a permanent deficit. The answer to this question is still not known, although it could be tested longitudinally, in theory, by a longitudinal study of subjects who have clearly shown transient impairment earlier on. In the behavioural domain, this is what has been postulated as the main cause of progressive behavioural changes in children with epilepsy before epilepsy is diagnosed and treated (Austin and Dunn 2002).

For the problem of treatment of transient cognitive impairment, see Chapter 14 on antiepileptic therapy.

4.3.3 Study of Epileptic Syndromes Presenting with Cognitive and/or Behavioural Manifestations as the Main Symptomatology

Landau–Kleffner syndrome and partial epilepsy with continuous spike-waves during sleep (CSWS) are the classic examples of these syndromes and will be discussed in more detail in Chapter 8. Their history illustrates in an exemplary fashion the debates and changes in concepts about how epilepsy, manifesting mainly as an age-related bioelectrical abnormality in discrete but crucial cortical areas for cognitive function, can give rise to prolonged cognitive or behavioural deficits, sometimes in the absence of recognized typical epileptic seizures. The various arguments given over the years for or against this viewpoint have been very fruitful in stimulating observations and studies which have shaped the way we now think about how epilepsy can cause delay, non-emergence, stagnation or loss of a given cognitive skill.

Landau–Kleffner syndrome and partial epilepsy with continuous spike-waves during sleep are often included by other authors under the 'epileptic encephalopathies' together with West syndrome and other epileptic situations in which acquired behavioural, cognitive and motor deterioration can occur as a direct result of the epileptic process, independently or in addition to the effects of the underlying cause of the epilepsy, of the visible seizures themselves (ictal or postictal) or side-effects of antiepileptic drugs. We do not favour grouping under this term what are in fact diverse epileptic disorders with probably very different mechanisms for the acquired dysfunction (see the discussion in Chapter 11 on mental retardation*).

Perusal of the literature and the successive positioning of Landau–Kleffner syndrome in child neurology textbooks, and in the International Classification of Epilepsies published in the last few decades since Landau and Kleffner's article in 1957, shows how it has moved from being considered a rare and obscure condition to being regarded now as the most

* Equivalent UK usage: learning disability.

severe end of a spectrum of cognitive abnormalities encountered in age-related, genetically determined partial epilepsy syndromes (see Chapter 8). Although how these particular focal epilepsies can cause such chronic and sometimes irreversible deficits is far from being completely understood, research is now focusing on how this paroxysmal bioelectrical disorder and the inhibitory mechanisms which prevent seizure spread can interfere with neuronal function in a developing brain both in the short term and in the long term.

4.4 Other special circumstances in which the direct role of epilepsy can be observed

4.4.1 Study of Surgically Treated Epilepsies

When a child with intractable epilepsy can be made seizure-free with surgical removal of the epileptic focus (or other techniques which prevent seizure spread), the cognitive and behavioural improvement that one can observe has many possible causes. The interruption of the damaging effects of continuous abnormal electrical neuronal activity in developing brain circuits is thought to be the main factor that will restore or improve development. This is, however, difficult to prove, because there are several other variables which can play a role, in addition to the direct suppression of the epileptic focus. The relief from antiepileptic drug side-effects, as a result of partial or total withdrawal, the restored independence and self-confidence and the emotional relief from constant threat of seizures, as well as the increased amount of time with adequate brain functioning (i.e. time not in a seizure or in a postictal state) and therefore increased capacity for learning, all contribute to the improvement.

The issue is very important because the tendency to propose earlier epilepsy surgery originates from the belief that cognitive development is mainly delayed or hampered by the seizures and that there is a potential for catch-up and even normalization when seizures are brought under control. There are no pre- and postoperative detailed longitudinal data of sufficiently long follow-up to answer these questions, which are both practically and theoretically important. When contemplating epilepsy surgery, one needs to distinguish clearly the objective of achieving seizure control (with many possible positive indirect, but uncertain, benefits in terms of psychological benefits and future social integration) from that of maintaining the intellectual potential and preventing cognitive deterioration which may or not be dependent on the epilepsy variable (see also Chapter 10 on epilepsy surgery).

4.4.2 Newly Diagnosed Epilepsy

Some neurologically and intellectually normal children with 'epilepsy only' present with school difficulties and/or behavioural problems which antedated their first recognized seizures (Austin et al 2001, Schouten et al 2001, Austin and Dunn 2002, Austin et al 2002). Clinical experience occasionally shows that these problems sometimes disappear or are much improved with antiepileptic treatment. Such cases constitute a convincing but completely neglected argument for the direct role of epilepsy on mental function (Deonna 1993). In these cases, despite the diagnosis of epilepsy with all its potential psychological consequences and the antiepileptic drug therapy, the child is much better. This indicates that the effect of epilepsy on behaviour was the determinant variable.

Detailed research in this area is surprisingly almost non-existent, but this is in some ways understandable. Physicians and parents are focused on the new diagnosis of epilepsy which is at the time the main preoccupation. Previous behavioural problems are sometimes not mentioned or are otherwise explained. For instance, the natural tendency to see the child's preceding difficulties as a psychological triggering factor of the epilepsy rather than another manifestation of the disease is very strong and has been in the past reinforced by psychodynamical theories on the genesis of epilepsy in children. The very striking and sometimes rapid improvement seen after the diagnosis and treatment makes this latter hypothesis quite unlikely. Several explanations for this improvement must be considered:

1 Seizures involving frontal or other areas important for cognition or behaviour and manifesting themselves only in these domains.
2 Brief and repeated intermittent losses of awareness or of cognitive efficiency due to brief generalized seizure discharges (so-called 'subclinical seizures') or disturbances in the quality of sleep due to unrecognized nocturnal seizures.

Only two studies, to our knowledge, have approached this problem (Austin et al 2001, Schouten et al 2002). Austin et al studied 224 children with 'epilepsy only' compared to control siblings. Epilepsy type and syndrome were defined and the possible occurrence of seizures prior to the time of firm diagnosis was looked for. A behavioural checklist was used as soon as the diagnosis was made (within three months) to document problems during the preceding six months. There was a statistically significant increased rate of problems in the group with epilepsy (31 per cent or 39 per cent respectively depending on whether or not prior suspect seizure events had been elicited in the history). Attention deficit was the most significant problem in the clinical group and was most marked in children with complex partial seizures. The associated cognitive problems and effects of antiepileptic therapy were not studied. None the less, this is a very important study, demonstrating for the first time what had long been suspected (Deonna 1996). It provides important evidence for direct cognitive/behavioural effects of epilepsy, independently of the presence of recognized typical seizures.

In Schouten at al's study, 69 recently diagnosed children with 'epilepsy only' were studied with a control group. Before the diagnosis, 22 per cent of those with epilepsy had repeated a grade (11 per cent in mainstream schools) and in 54 per cent remedial teaching had been requested (23 per cent in healthy classmates). Importantly, the group with epilepsy did not differ significantly from the control group in general intelligence. The authors concluded that 'the cause of poor school performance requires further study'. The documentation of changes in behaviour or cognition before and after the child is given treatment (the child being their own control) is the obvious next step. The following case study illustrates this.

Case R.A.

R.A., a boy with diabetes, was first seen at the age of 7 years for evaluation of two brief episodes of loss of awareness in the previous three weeks. He had never had similar episodes or developmental-cognitive problems, but his mother insisted that his behaviour had become very difficult in the last six months and he had almost stopped going to school. These episodes were wholly different from those due to hypoglycemia, which were already familiar to the mother.

EEG during drowsiness showed a 12-minute electrical seizure with a right frontal onset. MRI showed a small cortical arteriovenous malformation in the right prefrontal area. He had an allergic skin rash with carbamazepine and later phenytoin so that behavioural improvement with medical antiepileptic therapy could not be evaluated (clobazam was poorly tolerated). Surgical removal of the malformation was performed three months after diagnosis of epilepsy.

Subsequently, his behaviour dramatically improved and he had no further seizures. This was confirmed by semiquantitative questionnaires completed by parents, and interviews with teachers and the school psychologist. Neuropsychological evaluation showed mild signs of executive dysfunction which was also improving. This improvement could not be attributed to drug withdrawal since it occurred while still on clobazam postoperatively and was closely related to the surgical removal of the epileptic focus.

TABLE 4.3
Case R.A., boy, born 27.07.94. Evolution of frontal behavioural syndrome (questionnaire)

See text for clinical history. This table shows the results of the behavioural questionnaire (Q) before (Q1 to Q3) and after (Q4 and Q5) surgical therapy of epilepsy. Q1 was completed retrospectively. 0 no problems, + mild, ++ moderate, +++ severe. Note that in addition to possible non-specific problems in mood, attention and initiative, there were also new aberrant behaviours reported, such as 'our son is becoming crazy'.

	Q1 (11.01) retrospective	**Q2** (04.02)	**Q3** (07.02)	(08.02) surgery	**Q4** (11.02)	**Q5** (03.03)
mood problems	0	++	+++		0	0
inattention, hyperactivity	0	++	+++		+	0
loss of initiative, creativity	0	++	+++		+	0
learning problems	+	++	+++		+	0
aberrant behaviours (confusion, hallucinations, 'forced movements')	0	++	++		0	0

In summary, this boy had a six-month history of increasingly severe behavioural problems and school absenteeism without any hint of epilepsy. The precise documentation of his behaviour from several sources before successful therapy of epilepsy, and its nature (frontal syndrome) and the follow-up thereafter, with rapid spectacular improvement, suggested that his behavioural and learning problems could be directly attributed to the effect of a frontal epilepsy which lasted for many months before it was recognized and treated.

5 EPILEPSY AND COGNITIVE FUNCTIONS: THE OTHER VARIABLES

5.1 Brain damage (focal symptomatic epilepsies)

There have been many studies on the cognitive-developmental effects of early focal brain lesions in children (Vargha-Khadem et al 1994, Stiles 2000). These have looked at their general effects on cognition, the influence of the side of the lesion, and the consequences of a special localization within the cerebral cortex, mainly in school-age children. Only a few useful generalizations can be made in the context of this discussion. First, strictly unilateral, even large lesions can be compatible with normal cognitive development. This is especially true in lesions around the perisylvian region. Knowing this, one has to seriously consider an additional effect of epilepsy when children with such lesions present with cognitive or behavioural problems.

Each cortical region has its own developmental tempo, vulnerability and a variable capacity to compensate for the effects of lesions. Very little is known, for example, about the effect of isolated lesions of the frontal and occipital cortex occurring very early in development (Stiles 2000, Kiper et al 2002, Knyazeva et al 2002).

5.1.1 The Developmental Effect of Early Focal Brain Damage

The dynamics of early development in such situations has to be taken into consideration (and not only the later outcome), if one wants to distinguish between the cognitive effects of the lesion and of the epilepsy itself. Only rare attempts have been made to look for the course and possible catch-up of development of a given function (such as language or vision) and to document what reorganization of function can take place in the early years (Bates et al 1992, Stiles 2000, Kiper et al 2002, Knyazeva et al 2002). In the domain of language, at least, longitudinal studies from infancy have shown that transient delays in language development can occur which are later completely compensated for (Bates et al 1992). One can infer from these data that, depending on the function concerned, the age at which the child is examined and the age at onset of epilepsy, the temporal dimension of the 'lesion-reorganization' process can itself be an important variable.

5.1.2 Non-epileptogenic vs Epileptogenic Lesions

Any focal cortical lesion is potentially epileptogenic. Even when there is no clinical epilepsy, an epileptic focus can often be recorded around the site of the lesion and in homologous areas of the opposite hemisphere. In most studies on development of children with congenital focal cortical lesions, epilepsy is not studied as a possible variable (Dall'Oglio et al 1994).

Vargha-Khadem and co-workers' study (1992) of children with congenital hemiplegia is an important exception. They showed that side and size of a unilateral lesion did not significantly influence cognitive performance. The children with epilepsy (history of seizures or epileptic EEG) had a significantly lower score than those without. Although these findings are not proof, they are very suggestive of a direct role of epileptic discharges (Chilosi et al 2001).

In an individual child with a fixed focal brain lesion and partial epilepsy starting from that area, it is often very difficult, if not impossible, to know if an active interictal epileptic focus on the EEG plays a negative role on cognitive function. Fluctuating cognitive abilities or a gradual loss of function related to this area associated with increased discharges during sleep (CSWS) or documented transient cognitive impairment during EEG testing are very suggestive, but this latter information is almost impossible to obtain in practice.

Sometimes there is only a stagnation or slowing of progress in a given skill (Rosenblatt et al 1998). The following case illustrates the interaction between brain damage, epilepsy and genetic factors and how a longitudinal study can help to separate the different components of the problem.

Case A.Y.

A.Y., a 9-year-old boy, started with a right-sided motor seizure. He was left-handed with mild clumsiness of the right hand, which was smaller than the left; his EEG showed a left anterior epileptic focus and on MRI he had a prenatal focal ischemic lesion in the sylvian region (see MRI shown in Fig. 5.1).

His tested intelligence was normal but he had some difficulty learning to read and write. After seizures he had some language difficulties and his documented reading abilities fluctuated, suggesting that his epilepsy was interfering with his progress in this domain. There was a family history of dyslexia and, although he has much improved after seizure control, he remains weak in the area of written language.

5.1.3 Cognitive Consequences of Focal Symptomatic Epilepsies: Effect of Basic Lesion or Epilepsy?

Many studies on the cognitive consequences of focal epilepsies are based on the semiology of the seizures, the site of epileptic focus and, more rarely, on a documented focal brain lesion. Most cross-sectional studies on a given type of epilepsy (e.g. 'frontal epilepsy in children'), however, do not specifically address the role of epilepsy but are concerned with the effects of focal brain damage or focal brain dysfunction with many additional uncontrolled variables. It is usually assumed that the abnormalities found are the result of epilepsy rather than the result of the focal lesion from which the epilepsy has started. This can be

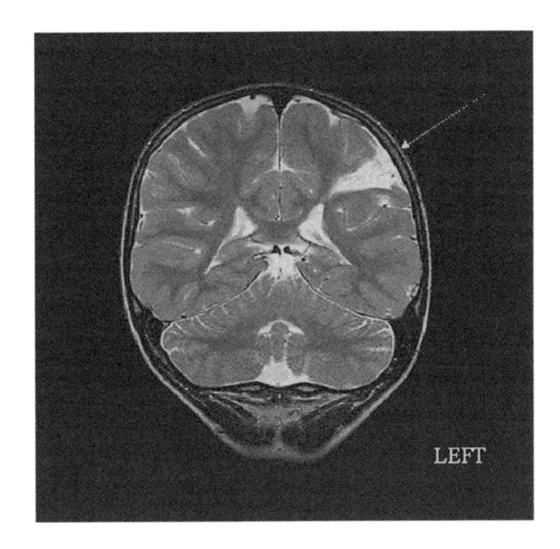

Fig. 5.1 Case A.Y.: MRI showing a prenatal focal loss of cortical substance in the left frontal area of probable prenatal origin (ischemic?).

accepted if the possible effects of the focal lesion have been completely compensated for, so that localized findings are the result of an acquired epileptic dysfunction in that area. As discussed above, one cannot make any generalizations here, because the potential for compensation is variable and is certainly different according to lesion site, age at onset, presence of associated lesions, genetic brain organization, etc.

Effect of early focal cortical pathology: non-epileptogenic and epileptogenic
Although direct evidence is difficult to obtain, the consequences that one can anticipate in face of an early fixed cortical lesion can be envisaged as follows. In the absence of an epileptic disturbance, an efficient organization (or relocation) of function will gradually take place, depending on timing, size and nature of the lesion. When the lesioned area becomes epileptogenic, this organization will not occur, or will occur less efficiently, because the area is constantly or intermittently disturbed by the abnormal electrical activity which spreads locally or at a distance, for instance towards the contralateral hemisphere. In the first case, there is a fixed, or often no, disability; whereas when the lesion is epileptogenic, the region is never in optimal conditions to allow the function to be consolidated locally, or, if a transfer of the function occurs, this process may be slower to develop or frequently interrupted.

5.2 Antiepileptic drugs

5.2.1 General Facts about Effects of Antiepileptic Drugs on Cognition/Behaviour

There are a few basic and generally accepted facts about the relationship between antiepileptic drugs and cognition, which one should keep in mind at all times.

Most antiepileptic drugs at a moderate dosage and used as monotherapy do not have significant cognitive consequences. Here is a quote from a review by Bourgeois (1998), showing the difficulty of evaluating this problem: 'Vermeulen et al reviewed over 90 investigations conducted over 25 years on the effects on cognition [Vermeulen and Aldenkamp 1995]. On the basis of their review, these authors concluded that they were not "in a position to provide a straightforward answer to the most pertinent question, i.e. whether antiepileptic drugs in therapeutic dose have any cognitive effects at all good or bad"' (Bourgeois 1998: 919).

Any antiepileptic drug can have marked side-effects in rare cases while being well tolerated by the vast majority, due to individual pharmacogenetic differences, or it can be the cause of worsening of seizures (Guerrini et al 1998, Perucca et al 1998).

Antiepileptic drugs may also have psychotropic effects independently of their antiepileptic effects. Anxiety and mood disorders frequently seen in children with epilepsy, either as a reaction to the disease or as a manifestation of the brain dysfunction, can sometimes be positively influenced by antiepileptic drugs. This may have an indirect positive impact on cognitive functioning. One must take this into account when evaluating improvement, particularly in learning and attention in cases where there is a complex mixed cognitive and affective component to the disorder. (See also Chapter 14.)

5.2.2 Balance Between Positive and Negative Effects

The consequences antiepileptic drugs can have on cognitive functions and behaviour depend greatly on the individual situation. Both direct and indirect positive and negative effects can occur.

In a high functioning child whose epilepsy has no cognitive impact, even minor side-effects will be noticeable. If the epilepsy has a major cognitive impact and if the treatment is effective, the benefits will far outweigh possible slight side-effects.

When the antiepileptic drug is inappropriate and exacerbates the cognitive problems (where these are direct manifestations of epilepsy), the pitfall is that this aggravation may be mistaken as an indication that the cognitive disorder is not epileptic in origin, whereas the opposite is true.

5.2.3 Positive Effects of Antiepileptic Drugs

On the one hand, antiepileptic drugs may directly improve cognitive function if the focal epileptic activity directly involving the relevant network (or spreading from it) is controlled by the drug. The discontinuity in cognitive functioning (from repeated absences or 'transient cognitive impairment') is no longer a problem, there is an increased amount of time for effective learning, and the unpleasant subjective experiences related to seizures disappear. On the other hand, the antiepileptic drug may have a positive psychotropic effect (antidepressant or anxiolytic).

Indirectly, the emotional reassurance of seizure freedom (or believing one is free), for the family even more than for the child, the increased desire and capacity for action, the 'discovery' of a 'new' cognitive state, and the gain in self-confidence in a child who previously was not functioning to their best potential, may all be mutually reinforcing, and there may be an additional placebo effect.

5.2.4 Negative Effects of Antiepileptic Drugs

The negative effects on cognitive functions are perhaps the most known and talked about, typically the effects on vigilance, memory and speed of processing. In addition, antiepileptic drugs may have negative psychotropic effects, for instance on mood, initiative, or quality of sleep. Monotherapy in moderate doses does not seem to affect the usually measured parameters of cognitive functions (see below; Aldenkamp et al 1993, Chen et al 2001). However, one must be very cautious about this aspect, especially with newer antiepileptic drugs. This is particularly important in young children and may not be taken into account by the general physician or adult neurologist.

In order to evaluate critically the possible negative role of antiepileptic drugs, one needs to have adequate indices of cognitive function to be compared before, on and off medication in similar types of epilepsies, without confounding basic cognitive problems and with comparable antiepileptic drug regimens and known serum drug levels. The comparison should be made after a sufficient time period. Finally, the magnitude and significance of any effect found, especially if minor, should be critically assessed.

Aldenkamp et al (1993) studied 83 children with epilepsy and matched controls with normal cognitive function; the children with epilepsy had had no seizures for one year and were on monotherapy with normal serum drug levels. A series of psychometric tests measuring speed, information processing and memory was administered before and after drug withdrawal (three months). The authors found no difference in 11/12 of the items tested and a moderate improvement in one item, psychomotor speed.

Williams (1998) studied children with newly diagnosed epilepsy before onset of therapy and after six months of monotherapy and compared the results with diabetic controls. There were no changes in neuropsychological tests and no differences from the controls.

It should be emphasized that the absence of measurable changes on standard intelligence tests before and after withdrawal of an antiepileptic drug does not necessarily mean an absence of cognitive side-effects, because important functions such as attention, speed of processing and fatigability, which are so important for learning, are usually not measured precisely in these types of evaluations. Future studies should focus on these aspects and also on finding new sensitive neurophysiological indices of dysfunction in selected cases in which it appears clinically significant. P300 (auditory event-related potentials) appears not sensitive enough (Chen et al 2001). Comparisons of large groups on standard neuropsychological or neurophysiological tests are unlikely to produce significant results. Also, much more attention should be paid to self-reported subjective benefits or side-effects, since this aspect is too often neglected in childhood pharmacotherapy.

On the psychological level, the fact of taking medication can put the child in a 'sick role' and this can have major consequences, regardless of the drug's effect. It can change the parents' view of their child, and sometimes the child's view of him/herself, from regarding the child as healthy to regarding the child as chronically ill. Sometimes, objective improvement in seizure control and cognitive capacities may have unexpected negative psychological consequences. The child may be better able to perceive the limitations imposed by their disease, they may have better insight into their disability, and realize what they were missing when they were unwell. They may have to face increased demands and constraints from caregivers, which, at least initially, may not be easy to live with.

Documentation of cognitive side-effects

Case A.V.: History (see Table 5.1)

This girl was first seen at 4 years 3 months for evaluation of paroxysmal intense pain in the right foot. Initial work-up was negative but partial seizures were suspected and she improved on carbamazepine. A definite diagnosis of epilepsy was finally made at 6 years 4 months with videoEEG during sleep showing numerous complex motor seizures suggesting a frontal onset or spread. MRI was normal. Seizures did not improve with add-on clobazam, valproate and phenytoine, but were much reduced with topiramate which was gradually increased over several months to a maximum of 200 mg/day (7 mg/kg). The blood level was within the accepted range.

Her development and behaviour since onset of epilepsy had been clinically normal, but a gradual stagnation in her school progress and decreased spontaneous speech had been noted by the parents since topiramate was introduced. This was very striking on neuropsychological examination and was confirmed by her school teachers. Despite the positive effects on her epilepsy, a side-effect of the drug was suspected. Topiramate was stopped and replaced by lamotrigine. Behaviour and language normalized and this was confirmed on comparative repeat neuropsychological examination.

The child is presently being worked-up for possible epilepsy surgery. The marked cognitive improvement clearly coincided with the drug withdrawal and could not be explained by decreased epilepsy severity or other drug changes. Particularly striking, before withdrawal of the drug, was the child's lack of initiative to speak, with almost complete mutism. Adults with epilepsy treated with topiramate often mention word-finding difficulties, a complaint not usually encountered with other antiepileptic drugs. This feature has not been systematically studied in adults and has not been specifically reported in children. Our observation does not allow us to draw the firm conclusion that the drug had a specific effect on speech because the child also exhibited a general slowness, although she was not demented and performed much better on visuospatial tasks. This issue of possible selective cognitive side-effects of different antiepileptic drugs needs further study.

5.3 Psychological factors

We will discuss here only the direct relationships between the cognitive and behavioural manifestations of epilepsy and the psychological-emotional state. Seizures with mainly a

TABLE 5.1
Case A.V., girl: neuropsychological evaluation on and off topiramate

This table shows the results of the neuropsychological evaluation on and off topiramate (see case history). Note that apart from the introduction of topiramate and its withdrawal, no changes in the other drugs or in the epilepsy frequency could account for this regression and its recovery.

	7 years 6 months	**8 years 2 months**
	topiramate 7 mg/kg carbamazepine	lamotrigine carbamazepine (off topiramate three months)
Frequency of seizures	marked decrease during therapy with topiramate (one year)	more seizures since withdrawal of topiramate
Behaviour	slow, lack of initiative	alert, rapid
Performance IQ (WISC-III)	69	84
Language	almost mute, latency of responses, two- to three-word sentences when intensely encouraged	initiates exchanges, spontaneous long sentences
Verbal fluency (MacCarthy)	3	16
Attention (Code WISC-III)	Standard score: 4	Standard score: 7

cognitive-perceptual or emotional content can have psychological consequences and, inversely, the psychological state of the child may be a triggering factor for this particular type of seizure. The general psychological consequences of epilepsy on the child and their family and the indirect effects of the disease on the child's personality and cognitive development are discussed later (see Chapter 15). (See also Chapter 14 on drug therapy.)

5.3.1 Mood Changes and Behaviour Problems in Relation to the Epilepsy Activity

Most children with epilepsy are better off from the behavioural and emotional point of view when their epilepsy is in remission and/or well controlled with antiepileptic medication. But there are striking exceptions to this, especially in severe epilepsies. Some children have a better mood and an easier behaviour during periods with frequent seizures than when epilepsy is well controlled. Worsening of behaviour may be a regular warning of a seizure in the hours or days to come, or, on the contrary, children may be better in the days or hours just before a recurrence of seizures. Parents of children in whom this pattern is regular consider it as the surest warning of a recurrence of seizures.

Such old and well-known observations reported by parents and people working with individuals with severe epilepsy probably have several different possible explanations, but to our knowledge they have not been systematically studied. These patterns are probably the best example of the complex interrelationship between epilepsy and behaviour (Fenwick 1992). The special problem of 'forced normalization' will be discussed in Chapter 14, section 14.2.

5.3.2 Psychological Consequences of Seizures with Direct Cognitive-Perceptual-Emotional Manifestations

Adults with epilepsy usually have enough life experiences to interpret what they subjectively feel and observe in different circumstances and what triggers 'normal' emotions. They can differentiate these from sudden 'forced' thoughts, emotions or distorted perceptions due to epilepsy. How young children deal with the same manifestations has not to our knowledge ever been studied in any detail (Soulayrol 1999). It is difficult to know, especially in a young child, whether the visible manifestations of emotion (fear, anger, surprise) in an epileptic seizure have the same experienced quality as those that occur in natural circumstances, and what significance this can have for the child. There is an abundant adult literature on these phenomena which is difficult to extrapolate to children. Does the child internalize the whole physical and mental experience of the seizure and incorporate it into his/her general understanding of him/herself as a feeling human being, and how can he/she further trust his/her emotions?

We are not aware of data on these questions, other than isolated retrospective accounts of childhood experiences in autobiographies of adults with epilepsy (Gloor et al 1982, Pineau-Valencienne 2000). Children certainly experience acute fear, loss or acceleration of sense of time, *déjà vu* (memory recollections) or *jamais vu* (complex new experiences) and memory loss, which could be a source of distortion of their own identity and also of chronic anxiety. Personal testimonies written in adulthood about such childhood experiences are suggestive, but it is difficult to know how far these have been distorted or reconstructed with the passage of time (Alajouanine 1963, Pineau-Valencienne 2000).

Young children may find it impossible to formulate these experiences verbally, or may be reluctant to do so because they are unsure of how they will be received, or they may not realize that it is not a shared universal experience. They also may be so scared of the experience that the emotional reaction to it overshadows all other possible rational self-observation. An interesting analogy can be made with the perceptual or emotional changes that happen during some migraine attacks. Although, in contrast to epilepsy, these attacks are long-lasting and usually quite well remembered, children with migraine often do not volunteer their complex experiences to the physician and do not mention them to their parents, who are sometimes surprised to hear about them for the first time in a consultation. So, it should not be surprising that what is known about such events in children with epilepsy is less than what they actually feel.

The child may experience situations where his/her inner reality, memory and ideas are distorted in an incomprehensible way, and the child may question what is a normal and what is an epileptic experience. Older children may be aware of this, sometimes speaking of their epileptic brain as alien or not belonging to them. Such experiences might come to the surface during psychotherapy, but we have not found evidence of this in recent books dealing with the psychological or psychiatric aspects of childhood epilepsy (Beauchesne 1980, Soulayrol 1999).

Sometimes, the physicians or families may refer to these episodes as the child's 'absences', whereas this is in fact very far from what the child actually experiences (e.g. complex partial seizure with vivid auras). This is beautifully expressed in the autobiography of Valérie Pineau-Valencienne: 'Absence is a term which is miles away from the sensations one experiences during a temporal seizure: fear, anxiety, violence, yes, absence: no.'

The following clinical situation illustrates the interaction between normal emotions and perceptions and those that are triggered by an epileptic phenomenon probably occurring in the same (limbic) networks.

Case V.S.

A very bright and insightful 11-year-old girl had suffered many temporal lobe seizures with auras in which she relived a personal event or experienced an unknown one, until a fully effective treatment was found. She and her family said her seizures were well controlled but she still complained that she had some moments of thinking or feeling something special, but was unsure if this was normal or a residue of her aura. It raised an acute fear of seizure recurrence and her physical emotional reaction to that fear ('my heart beats very fast') was most unpleasant.

It must be recognized that the complex networks which are determinant for our emotional and intellectual life also include the most epileptogenic of all cortical areas, i.e. the frontal and temporal lobes. It should be no surprise that an acute activation of these networks during intense emotional circumstances can trigger a seizure with emotional manifestations in the same emotional domain, or provoke a fear that this could happen. Also, cognitive situations which have a strong affective component activate these same brain systems and may trigger connected epileptic foci. In such situations, family or professionals can easily make erroneous interpretations, mistaking the triggering emotional factor for the primary cause of the disorder.

5.3.3 Special Situations

Reflex seizures to specific sensory or cognitive stimuli

In addition to the fear of spontaneous seizures, the child may 'learn' that some specific sensory experiences or cognitive activities (e.g. reading, arithmetic) can precipitate seizures, and the child may engage in more or less conscious avoidance behaviour (Matsuoka et al 2000).

Self-induced seizures

This is a variety of reflex epileptic seizures in which the child self-induces seizures which the child has probably initially and by chance found to be pleasurable and wants to be repeated. This is mainly seen in epilepsies with photic sensitivity in children with mental retardation (hand flapping in front of a light or in front of the TV), but also in hot-water epilepsy.

In a study of such patients, seizures started with an aura and feelings of pleasure (Bebek et al 2001). One can speculate whether pleasurable epileptic experiences can be deliberately triggered by stimuli such as music or 'intellectual' games, particularly in children whose usual epileptic manifestations are spontaneously cognitive or emotional in nature.

Pseudoseizures

The differential diagnosis between true epileptic seizures and pseudo-epileptic seizures may be difficult, especially in those who already have true epilepsy (the majority), who have an intimate experience and objective knowledge of its manifold manifestations. Several characteristics of the semiology or circumstances of occurrence may be helpful for differential diagnosis but will not be reviewed here. They have been enriched by the now frequently reported videoEEG recordings of pseudoseizures, which may sometimes be necessary, but rarely so, for a diagnosis. One should distinguish between symptoms which are intentionally reproduced by the child and those of a more unconscious nature, corresponding to a conversion disorder.

Pseudoseizures should also be distinguished from the psychological reaction to a genuinely perceived epileptic emotional manifestation (e.g. fear) or sensory experience (e.g. visual hallucination or blindness), as discussed above, or to the consciously realized loss of normal self-control and social appearance.

5.4 Sleep and epilepsy: contribution to cognitive dysfunction in some epilepsies

We will restrict ourselves here to comments about the role of sleep as a decisive contributing factor to cognitive dysfunction in special epileptic situations, without discussing the close relationship between sleep and epileptic activity in general, which is fundamental in clinical diagnosis and management of many different epilepsies.

The importance of good sleep for adequate cognitive function and learning is well known. The cyclic organization of sleep, with alternating phases of slow oscillations and brief episodes of rapid oscillations, appears to play a fundamental role in learning, with information acquired during waking recalled and consolidated during slow sleep (Sjenowski and Destexhe 2000). Recently, new exciting but still controversial theories on the respective roles of NREM and REM sleep in different memory processes have been proposed (see Hobson and Pace-Schott 2002 for a detailed review).

Epilepsy during sleep can affect cognitive functions in several ways, indirectly or directly (Stores 2001). First of all, seizures may delay sleep onset, lead to frequent arousals during the night, disrupt the quality of sleep by interfering with the regular sleep cycles, and decrease the total sleep time. As a consequence, the child can have postictal diurnal fatigue, slowness and decreased vigilance. In fact, many parents can judge whether their child has had seizures during the night from the child's ease and rapidity of awakening, their mood when they awaken and quality of daytime functioning.

More directly, seizure activity during sleep, especially when originating in specific networks (limbic or frontolimbic) involved in memory functions, can lead to a failure of normal consolidation or a loss of the most recently learned material, even without awakenings. It is not exceptional to hear from parents of children with epilepsy that material that had been carefully learned and rehearsed, and seemed well retained, the night before was completely forgotten the next morning. We are not aware, however, of specific studies in this area. For failure of consolidation to occur, epilepsy must affect specific networks involved in memory, because there are many examples of frequent nocturnal seizures during sleep (e.g. benign partial epilepsy of childhood, familial nocturnal frontal epilepsy) which have no such consequences.

When epileptic discharges are recorded on the waking EEG, these are usually even more frequent during the sleep EEG. However, epileptic discharges are sometimes present only during sleep (sleep is the most powerful activating physiological state for epilepsy), whether the child suffers from clinical seizures or not. The electrographic epileptic activity, if brief and infrequent, is usually not associated with daytime sleepiness or evident cognitive disturbances. In one special and dramatic situation, however, the so-called 'continuous spike-waves during slow sleep' (CSWS) pattern is clearly correlated with cognitive dysfunction (see Chapter 8, section 8.4).

CSWS represent secondary bilateral synchrony of focal discharges and are a marker of an active focal epilepsy. Many clinical studies have now shown that there is a temporal correlation between the presence of CSWS, their density (percentage of sleep with CSWS) and duration, and the occurrence of cognitive dysfunction (Rousselle and Revol 1995, Robinson et al 2001). The clinical deficit is related to the specific functional role of the focal epileptic area. In addition, during the CSWS activity, the normal thalamocortical activity during slow sleep (Steriade and Contreras 1998), which experimentally seems to have a role in memory processes, is probably disturbed. Consolidation of information during sleep may thus be hampered in clinical situations with CSWS, in addition to the direct consequences of the focal cortical disturbance (see Chapter 8, section 8.4).

Acquired sleep disturbances may be an early and severe problem in young children in the weeks or months before, or coinciding with, a language or behavioural 'epileptic' regression (Neville et al 2000). This is often mentioned in case histories, but we are not aware of any systematic study on this topic.

6
COGNITIVE AND BEHAVIOURAL PROBLEMS IN CHILDHOOD EPILEPSIES: A LITERATURE REVIEW – WHAT CAN IT TELL US ABOUT THE DIRECT ROLE OF EPILEPSY?

6.1 General data

There is an extensive literature on the cognitive and behavioural abnormalities in children with different forms of epilepsy. This is a clear indication that this is a frequent, if not the main, problem in many children with epilepsy, although it is rarely possible in most types of studies to sort out the relative importance of the different factors involved. In a general population of children with epilepsy, major school problems occur in about 15–30 per cent, even when their IQ is normal, and only a minority will obtain university degrees (Sillanpää 1992).

The extent of the problem must first be put in an epidemiological perspective. The epidemiology of epilepsy is by the very nature of the disorder a very difficult issue because there are no simple clinically observable characteristics or biological parameters which would include all cases and rule out other paroxysmal disorders. The causes and frequency of brain damage (which can give rise to both epilepsy and cognitive problems, the so-called symptomatic epilepsies) in a given childhood population vary in different parts of the world. For these reasons, quantitative figures have to be treated cautiously, and these come mainly from developed countries. The prevalence of active epilepsy in a given childhood population is about 4/1000 (Sidenvall et al 1996). About 40 to 50 per cent of these children have an obvious symptomatic epilepsy, that is an observable neurological deficit or lesion, and 25 per cent of these have associated mental retardation. The other 50 to 60 per cent have 'epilepsy only' (no neurological or cognitive impairment), which is either idiopathic (probably genetic) or cryptogenic (i.e. without a definable cause, but with a probable hidden non-genetic one). In a whole population of children with active epilepsy about 20 per cent have either 'benign rolandic epilepsy' (15 per cent) or petit mal (about 5 per cent). The main question for our purposes is whether some epilepsy syndromes or seizure types are particularly associated with learning or behavioural problems and others not; this would help in evaluating the importance of these problems in a population of children with epilepsy. To some extent, this is the case. However, the same epileptic syndrome may sometimes be associated with major cognitive or behavioural problems in one child, and mild or even no problems in another.

The term 'epileptic encephalopathy' is sometimes used to designate epilepsies in which epileptic activity is the main cause of the neurological or cognitive disturbances (with the exclusion of progressive diseases) and includes situations as diverse as West syndrome and acquired epileptic aphasia. While it is definitely true and important to recognize that some epilepsies have major cognitive consequences, we do not believe that grouping them together under the term 'epileptic encephalopathy' allows a differentiated appraisal of the factors which contribute to the underlying brain dysfunction.

Table 6.1 gives an overview of the occurrence and importance of cognitive and behavioural problems in the different childhood epilepsies. The significance of the data is

TABLE 6.1
Cognitive-behavioural problems in various childhood epilepsies

Primary generalized epilepsies (genetic) and epileptic syndromes	Etiology	Cognition–behaviour	Comment
Grand mal epilepsy	Genetic, often with febrile convulsions (GEFS+)	Normal cognition	Grand mal seizures in children are most often secondarily generalized seizures or misdiagnosed non-epileptic phenomena
Benign myoclonic epilepsy of infancy	Genetic	Normal development	No long-term follow-up studies
Petit mal absence epilepsy	A subgroup associated with febrile seizures: have a single gene mutation	Normal cognition	See discussion on petit mal epilepsy
Juvenile myoclonic epilepsy (JME, Janz)	Genetic, several genes?	Normal cognition	'Frontal' deficits reported in some adults with JME (Devinsky et al 1997)
Benign familial neonatal convulsions	Single gene mutation	Normal	No long-term studies on cognition
Rolandic epilepsy and variants	Genetic, multiple genes?	Children with rolandic epilepsies typically have normal intelligence	Transitory and/or sectorial deficits and behaviour problems often occur (see text)
Landau–Kleffner syndrome	Idiopathic, related to rolandic epilepsies	Aphasia, by definition often severe and persistent	Less severe or minor transient aphasias do occur (see text)
Partial epilepsy with CSWS	Idiopathic and symptomatic forms	Often prolonged and persistent cognitive deficit	Epileptic focus is more often frontal (see also text)
West syndrome (infantile spasms with hypsarhythmia in infancy)	Cryptogenic and symptomatic forms (80–90% with many etiologies)	Cryptogenic forms may have normal or near normal development; symptomatic forms often, but not always, retarded	Prognosis related to many factors in addition to epileptic activity. Normal development before onset of spasms is important predictor of good outcome

Lennox–Gastaut syndrome	Multiple etiologies (non-specific)	Most have mental retardation, exceptionally normal despite same seizure syndrome	Often follows West syndrome
Febrile convulsions	Genetic	Normal cognitive outcome in uncomplicated febrile seizures, even if numerous	A convulsion with fever may be the first manifestation of epilepsy. Prolonged febrile seizures may cause specific brain damage (hippocampal sclerosis)
Severe myoclonic epilepsy of infancy	Genetic (SGM)	Mental deterioration in all cases starts in 2nd year after a normal early development	Cases may occur in families with GEFS+ , reason for severe outcome unknown
Myoclonic-astatic epilepsy	Genetic factors (SGM possible)	60% normal, 20% mild retardation, 20% more severe	Prognosis correlates with seizure severity (see discussion in text)
Localization-related epilepsies			
Frontal	Any lesion, but also genetic: autosomal dominant nocturnal frontal epilepsy (SGM) and possibly some variants of rolandic epilepsy	Depends on dysfunction in prefrontal areas. Motor seizures alone compatible with normal cognition	Special case of partial epilepsy with CSWS (most often frontal) with severe cognitive sequelae
Temporal	Any lesion, most frequent is hippocampal sclerosis, also genetic forms: autosomal dominant partial epilepsy with auditory features (SGM)	Most often normal cognition but behavioural problems more frequent than in other types of epilepsies	No or minor deterioration despite severe often intractable epilepsy. Behavioural-autistic-type problems and mental retardation may occur in early onset forms
Parietal	Any lesion	? Visuospatial problems	No systematic studies
Occipital	Any lesion, also 'functional' form closely related to rolandic epilepsy	Central visual impairment rarely reported (Gülgonen et al 2000)	Symptoms may be related to propagation (temporal or parietal)

GEFS+: generalized epilepsy with febrile seizures plus. There is co-occurrence of febrile seizures and grand mal epilepsy (e.g. afebrile generalized tonic-clonic seizures)

SGM: single gene mutations. The epilepsies mentioned have been found to be due to single gene mutations in ion channels or neurotransmitter receptor genes

very much dependent on knowledge of the underlying etiology of the epileptic disorder or syndrome, and one should be aware that many of the existing studies were done prior to modern brain imaging and molecular genetics. The quantitative figures given must be taken only as a rough indication of the frequency and nature of the cognitive-behavioural problems encountered in a relatively large group of children with 'similar' epilepsies/syndromes. The figures give limited or no indications as to the direct role of the epileptic dysfunction itself. The diagnosis of a well-defined epileptic syndrome, based on similar clinical and EEG characteristics, has been a significant advance over the idiopathic/symptomatic division or the simple seizure-type (focal, generalized) or localization (frontal, temporal, etc.) level of classification, and is mainly used here.

Although some epileptic syndromes have been found to be related to single gene mutations, it is also clear that the same epileptic syndrome at the phenomenological level may be due to diverse etiologies with a very different prognosis, e.g. West syndrome. In addition to the syndromic classification, which is still the most helpful at this stage of knowledge for our purposes, we have also considered the so-called primary generalized epilepsies and have made some comments on epilepsies where only a localization-based classification can be made.

6.2 Methodological problems in published studies: how to evaluate the direct role of epilepsy on cognitive functions

6.2.1 General Aspects

Considering that any study comparing children with epilepsy with normal controls will find that children with epilepsy as a group fare on the whole less well, and this for a number of possible different reasons, the study design must meet several precise conditions in order to reach more than very general or obvious conclusions. Any study on cognitive function in a group of 'children with epilepsy' without further definition is meaningless. The characteristics of the population chosen, its homogeneity and the source of cases included in the study are crucial pieces of information. There are conditions which are especially difficult to meet, such as the duration of epilepsy prior to the study, the timing of the tests in relation to the activity of the epilepsy (clinical and EEG), and whether the child is on medication or not. The main important variables that are usually studied are the following:

1. Etiology (symptomatic vs idiopathic)
2. Specific epileptic syndromes (e.g. primary generalized epilepsy with classical petit mal absences)
3. Lateralization of focus (right vs left)
4. Location (frontal, temporal, occipital, etc.)
5. Seizure type (absences, partial complex seizures, etc.)
6. Untreated vs treated group (newly diagnosed, before/on/off treatment)
7. Children with learning disability and epilepsy vs children with similar learning disability without epilepsy
8. Children with epilepsy vs children with other chronic disease (emotional, personality variables)

When all this is known, the next question is what aspect of cognition/behaviour should be looked at in the particular group chosen for study.

6.2.2 Cross-sectional Group Studies with Controls and Choice of Controls

Controlled studies can be important if they show that there is no difference between subjects and controls, in which case a negative role of epilepsy can be ruled out. However, this is almost never the case, and the differences found can have several explanations. Often these are minimal and of questionable significance. These studies will not be further discussed because they cannot answer the specific question of the possible direct role of epilepsy. Good reviews can be found on the numerous studies which have focused on one specific variable of the epileptic disease which can be important for one aspect or another of cognitive functions.

Depending on the question being asked, controls should include not only normal children (classmates or siblings when psychosocial variables are crucial) but also children with similar clinical problems (i.e. learning disability, attention problems) or similar brain pathology but no epilepsy. This is especially important when looking for specific differences which may be attributed to epilepsy.

6.2.3 Longitudinal Group Studies

Longitudinal group studies are essential when one is dealing with such a dynamic variable as epilepsy, ideally with a control group. One problem is that it is very difficult logistically to have group studies with more than two or three comparative time periods and with detailed data in all cases. There is usually one comparison at two periods far apart, with possibly many intervening variables. Overall group results may obscure the most significant individual differences, which is precisely what one would expect in an unstable situation such as epilepsy. Group studies are also difficult to pursue over long periods or when flexible schedules are needed. Only a limited set of correlative data is obtained because of time and other constraints.

If a rapidly changing 'epileptic' parameter can be studied in a large number of children with controls, this is, of course, the most informative approach. For instance, children with newly diagnosed epilepsy studied just before and shortly after diagnosis and treatment could show cognitive/behavioural effects of epilepsy which were already manifest prior to the time of its recognition. This has not been done so far.

In general, longitudinal group studies (of which there are very few) have been important in determining whether the many different factors involved have any significant effects on learning, cognition and social adaptation over time. They have shown that most children with epilepsy do not regress, but keep their intellectual capacities (Bourgeois et al 1983, Austin et al 1999, Bailet 2000). Such studies have also helped to identify types of epilepsies, or other factors, which can lead to stagnation or deterioration (Bourgeois et al 1983). They have limited value in predicting individual outcome. The better the selection and description of the original sample, the more interesting the study.

We have reviewed all clinical studies in which quantifiable cognitive or behavioural variables were examined (and not reviews or clinical impressions) in a reasonably defined group of children with epilepsy published in the last 40 to 50 years (from 1956). Of 93 studies reviewed, only 27 were longitudinal. A change occurring between two or more

TABLE 6.2
Longitudinal group studies of cognition/behaviour in childhood epilepsy: special variables studied

This table lists some longitudinal studies in which systematic quantified comparative data were obtained in at least two successive periods, and the specific epilepsy variables that were looked for.

Special variables studied	Selected references
1 Comparison with other chronic disease	Austin et al 1994, Bailet and Turk 2000
2 Stability over time, risk factors	Bourgeois et al 1983, Ellenberg et al 1986, Mitchell et al 1994
3 Severity variables (age at onset, frequency, refractoriness)	Chaudhry and Pond 1961, Szabò et al 2001
4 Epileptic syndromes	Sato et al 1983, D'Alessandro et al 1995, Gaily et al 1999
5 Behaviour problems preceding first recognized seizures	Austin et al 2002
6 Effect of paroxysmal EEG activity	Baglietto et al 2001, Metz-Lutz et al 1999
7 Antiepileptic drug variable	Aldenkamp et al 1993, Chen et al 2001
8 Cerebral metabolism (CSWS)	Maquet et al 1995

points in time (for the better or worse) may or may not be related to the epilepsy itself, depending on how firmly other factors have been ruled out. One particular difficulty is knowing how close a correlation can be made between neuropsychological/behavioural observations and parameters of epileptic activity. Table 6.2 lists the main longitudinal studies on cognition and behaviour conducted in childhood epilepsies, which are indeed very few. The studies listed are concerned with the long-term effects (or not) of different important variables of the epileptic disease and its treatment, and not primarily with those of the epileptic activity *per se*. The reader can refer to the specific studies on these aspects. Studies dealing with the direct effects of epileptic EEG discharges (in benign rolandic epilepsy and more generally in 'transient cognitive impairments' of epileptic origin) are discussed in Chapter 8, section 8.1.3.

6.2.4 Single Case Studies

In these studies, the child is their own control, so that one can study the effect of a single or limited set of variables. The results may not be generalizable to all similar cases, but they offer the possibility of studying in depth cognitive changes which can occur as a direct result of epilepsy (or its treatment), which would be totally impossible to do in a group study. Several different acute epileptic situations where a rapid change is expected can be studied and compared from different angles, for example:

1 Comparison between ictal or postictal state and normal interictal state
2 Longitudinal studies of developmental disorders in which epilepsy may be suspected to be the cause
3 Effects of EEG discharges on cognitive functions (transient cognitive impairment)

4 Epilepsies with persistent but fluctuating and reversible acquired deficits
5 Acute treatment studies, medical or surgical, i.e. study of the cognitive changes which occur with suppression of clinical seizures or suppression of EEG discharges or repeated changes in therapy (on–off studies)

When clear results can be obtained repeatedly in the same child, this reinforces the importance of the epileptic variable being studied. Of course, if several comparable cases can be added, this amounts to a small group study. However, one should not wait for this to happen before publishing convincing well-studied single cases (which in themselves involve an enormous amount of work). These can constitute a resource for someone else who may have the opportunity to carry out a similar study and add new data.

7
CHILDHOOD NEUROPSYCHOLOGY (DEVELOPMENTAL COGNITIVE NEUROPSYCHOLOGY) IN THE CONTEXT OF EPILEPSY

(with Claire Mayor-Dubois)

7.1 Overview

The study of the different facets of normal cognitive development (language, memory, visuospatial functions, etc.) using increasingly sophisticated tools and study designs has for long been a major concern of childhood neuropsychology. The systematic and longitudinal study of populations of children with congenital or acquired disorders of cognition is much more recent. When one is attempting to understand the organization and development of 'normal' cognitive function in children with abnormal brains, one has to be wary of the following. Brains which have been damaged after a normal period of formation certainly differ in their organization from those with developmental, often genetic, defects which have a special original structure. Very special dissociated neuropsychological profiles are sometimes seen in these latter situations (e.g. in Williams syndrome) (see Karmiloff-Smith and Thomas 2003).

As far as epilepsy is concerned, a special approach has to be taken if one recognizes that epilepsy affects brain function and sometimes structure in a different way from any other static congenital or acquired brain disorder. In the latter case, cerebral organization and reorganization has to proceed with some given constraints, but development still evolves in a continuous way. In contrast, epileptic activity affects cognition and behaviour and the development of underlying brain mechanisms in a discontinuous, potentially reversible, fashion, either during brief periods or for more prolonged but limited periods of the child's life, or sometimes throughout the whole of childhood. The child has to adapt to an irregularly functioning and often unreliable brain.

The few textbooks on childhood neuropsychology, in which epilepsy is discussed at all, rarely acknowledge this unique situation. Epilepsy is either treated as any other childhood neurological disorder (e.g. brain trauma, meningitis) or along traditional lines, considering in turn localization-related epilepsies (frontal, temporal, etc.) or seizure-type epilepsies (absence, grand mal). This makes it difficult to separate the effect of the brain lesion giving rise to the epilepsy from a possible added or original influence of the epileptic dysfunction itself (Culhane-Shelburne et al 2002).

Taking into account the epileptic variable, specifically, is a demanding task that requires both the child's and the family's cooperation and also that the child neurologist and neuropsychologist work in close association, with flexible schedules.

7.2 The problem of normal variations, dynamics of normal development and the role of epilepsy

In order to conclude that epileptic activity interferes with a developing function, one must be sure that slow progress or unusual patterns observed are not part of a normal developmental variation. Development is not linear as is sometimes suggested by simple graphs. There is a huge variability in the age at which a given milestone is achieved and in the strategies a child uses preferentially before final competence is reached. There are periods of relative plateau for some weeks or months, followed by rapid progress, although, despite the common experience of these phenomena, the longitudinal data are limited.

A confusing concept of 'normal regression' in mental development (Bever 1982) has been used by some developmental cognitive psychologists. The idea is that mental growth is the result of dynamic structuring processes and not simply accumulation of skills. As development proceeds, new strategies are used which may lead at some point to a transiently less good performance. In the clinical context, regression, as used in this book, refers exclusively to the loss of an acquired function which is not part of normal development.

Some skills are acquired 'naturally', whereas others, such as written language, depend on explicit teaching. Motivation and training opportunities are therefore essential dimensions which need to be taken into account when measuring speed of acquisition in these domains. When a significant and rapid 'catch-up' in cognitive development following successful medical or surgical therapy is observed, this strongly suggests that epilepsy interfered directly with development, especially if absence of progress for a certain period of time was documented prior to the catch-up phase. There are, however, several different reasons for such rapid progress. The child may only be recovering what they had lost since the time epilepsy started, without genuinely new gain. If there had been no prior loss but only slow development, one must suppose that some brain development had proceeded during the active epilepsy phase but could not be 'actualized'. Another possibility is that the child was simply not 'available' for learning because epilepsy was constantly interfering with cognitive processes and depriving him/her of formative opportunities. Once epilepsy is under control, he/she may fully benefit from new information and experiences. An analogy can be made with the rapid progress seen in deprived children as soon as they are put in a stimulating environment.

Prospective observations at repeated and close intervals are needed to show the dynamics of change over time in these situations, and to see if the rapid functional change will continue, at what speed and to what extent, especially when the child still functions at a significantly retarded level. Data on this point are emerging (Roulet-Perez et al 2003).

7.3 Specific neuropsychological dysfunctions and their relationship to epilepsy (functional deficits of epileptic origin)

We will discuss here the broad categories of commonly studied cognitive or behavioural deficits which can be a direct consequence of the epileptic disorder. These can be acute and transient or more chronic, typically with significant fluctuations.

It should be pointed out again that some epilepsies, even when quite severe, do not necessarily affect learning and cognitive skills in a significant way, so that specific epileptic mechanisms and/or brain networks must be involved to account for problems in these domains. A very specific brain network and the function it supports (for instance, language or visuospatial abilities) may be affected but other cognitive abilities remain intact. The learning disability is thus limited to specific domains and those strongly dependent upon them.

In other instances, several different areas can be affected by the epileptic process, at the same time or at different periods, together or independently, with varying patterns of dysfunction. The study of each domain needs specific tools and expertise that cannot all be easily captured in a classical neuropsychological evaluation.

7.3.1 Attention

> Attentional systems represent the highest level of cognitive accomplishment.
> (Geschwind 1982: 185)

The different cognitive abilities, which are referred to under the global term of attention (alerting responses, sustained attention, divided attention, inhibition, etc.), are among the most complex and also the most vulnerable of the human brain functions (Posner 1994, Valenstein 1997). It is thus not surprising that inattention is a frequent complaint of parents or teachers of children with epilepsy, and is a frequently reported deficit in neuropsychological studies (Stores et al 1978, Piccirilli et al 1994, Gross-Tsur et al 1997). It may be due to a direct effect of the bioelectric dysfunction, a side-effect of drugs, or a basic feature of the brain dysfunction responsible for the epilepsy, to mention just a few possible factors (see Chapters 5 and 14). The important question is whether epilepsies have a predominant or exclusive impact on attentional mechanisms and whether this is the main reason for school or learning failure. Considering the many factors involved, it is very difficult to do a proper study in which attention deficits can be directly related to epilepsy and not to other problems such as antiepileptic drugs. Furthermore, an additional specific weakness in the domain (visual, auditory, etc.) in which attention is being tested may complicate the interpretation.

Two studies of children with idiopathic epilepsy (epilepsy only) compared to controls have approached this problem. One has been done in children with benign rolandic epilepsy (Chevalier et al 2000). The other involved children with newly onset idiopathic epilepsy (epilepsy not further defined) before formal diagnosis and without therapy (Schouten et al 2002). Children with epilepsy had more problems in some attention tasks in these two studies, but the differences compared to controls were minor and were not seen in all domains of attention tested.

The role of epilepsy as a direct and isolated cause of attentional problems could be clearly proven if a very inattentive child with epilepsy (or with paroxysmal epileptic EEG discharges without seizures) and no other problems improved rapidly and in a major way in this domain when the epilepsy became controlled with antiepileptic drugs. Clinical experience indicates that this occasionally occurs. More often, when epilepsy is controlled with an antiepileptic drug, attention is unchanged, suggesting that it was not the crucial 'epileptic' factor. Some children with focal epilepsies and a significant cognitive deficit (such as language) may have fully preserved attentional capacities, indicating that epilepsy in general does not necessarily impinge on attentional mechanisms. In partial epilepsies of frontal origin, attentional deficits are a major problem, sometimes initially the only one before other deficits become evident. In epilepsy with CSWS, which often has an origin in the frontal regions, inattention is also a prominent feature, but not as an isolated deficit (Deonna et al 2002). It can sometimes be a feature of the more common 'functional' partial epilepsies (rolandic epilepsies and variants) which occasionally show a focus of sharp waves in the prefrontal regions and cause temporary and isolated or predominant deficits in this domain, although this is not largely documented (de Saint-Martin et al 2001).

The frequency of attention deficits in childhood epilepsies, sometimes without, or with rare, seizures, raises the question of whether epilepsy can be a cause or important factor in children diagnosed as having an 'attention deficit disorder' (ADD), with or without hyperactivity. The data on this topic and the main clinical considerations concerning the complex interrelationships between disorders of attention and epilepsy are summarized in Table 7.1. It should be emphasized immediately that, with a few exceptions (Laporte et al 2002), children with attention deficit disorders do not have more seizures or paroxysmal EEG abnormalities than control children, so that 'hidden epilepsy' or 'subclinical seizures' are rarely if ever found in children presenting with a pure ADHD clinical phenotype.

Attentional problems, with or without hyperactivity, are frequent in children with epilepsy, as compared to a control population. These are directly or indirectly related to the effects of epileptic disease.

Severe deficits of attention are prominent in some forms of prefrontal epilepsy in children (e.g. partial epilepsy with CSWS) but they are associated with other cognitive and behavioural problems.

Children with a 'typical' attention deficit disorder (ADD) do not have more epilepsy than a control population, so that an EEG is not necessary in most cases. In a recent study, 27/483 children (5.6 per cent) with attention deficit disorder attending a tertiary child psychiatric centre were found to have rolandic spikes on the EEG, 'significantly higher than the rate of focal discharges of 2.4 per cent in normal children' (Holtmann et al 2003: 1242). The significance of these findings, possible biases and the link to epilepsy are open questions and are discussed by the authors.

A subgroup of children with ADD may present frontal lobe dysfunction in specific tests, but without epilepsy.

Epilepsy rarely presents with isolated attention problems in the absence of other behavioural or cognitive difficulties, but attention problems can occasionally be the first symptoms very early in its course, before clinical seizures are recognized.

TABLE 7.1
Deficits of attention and epilepsy: important considerations

This table summarizes the very different clinical situations in which a possible relationship between attentional problems and epilepsy is often raised and when it may (or may not) be significant.

Attentional problems, with or without hyperactivity, are frequent in children with epilepsy, as compared to a control population. These are directly or indirectly related to the effects of epileptic disease.

Severe deficits of attention are prominent in some forms of prefrontal epilepsy in children (e.g. partial epilepsy with CSWS) but they are associated with other cognitive and behavioural problems.

Children with a 'typical' attention deficit disorder (ADD) do not have a higher incidence of epilepsy than a control population, so that an EEG is not necessary in most cases.* A subgroup of these children may present frontal lobe dysfunction in specific tests, but without epilepsy.

Epilepsy rarely presents with isolated attention problems in the absence of other behavioural or cognitive difficulties. They can occasionally be the first symptoms very early in its course, before clinical seizures are recognized.

Attention deficit hyperactivity disorder and epilepsy often co-occur in the same child without a clear link. It may be the coincidence of two separate disorders or independent consequences of the same brain pathology. Symptomatic therapy of hyperactivity can be helpful and epilepsy is not a contra-indication (Gross-Tsur et al 1997).**

---

* In a recent study, 5.6% of 483 children with attention deficit disorder attending a tertiary child psychiatric centre were found to have rolandic spikes on the EEG, 'significantly higher than the rate of focal discharges of 2.4% in normal children' (Holtmann et al 2003: 1242). The significance of these findings, possible biases and the link to epilepsy are open questions and are discussed by the authors.

** The risk of precipitating seizures with methylphenidate in ADHD children with paroxysmal epileptic EEG abnormalities only is controversial (Hemmer et al 2001, Gucuyener et al 2003).

Attention deficit/hyperactivity disorder and epilepsy often co-occur in the same child without a clear link. It may be the coincidence of two separate disorders or independent consequences of the same brain pathology. Symptomatic therapy of hyperactivity can be helpful and treated epilepsy is not a contra-indication (Gross-Tsur et al 1997). However, the risk of precipitating seizures with methylphenidate in children with ADHD with paroxysmal epileptic EEG abnormalities, but no seizures, is controversial (Hemmer et al 2001, Gucuyener et al 2003).

7.3.2 Memory

> Epilepsy is a 'natural laboratory' for the study of memory.
>
> (Snyder 1997)

Ictal-postictal memory disorders

In adults, transient memory disturbances can be the only clinical manifestations of some complex partial seizures (so-called epileptic amnesic attacks (Palmini et al 1992, Zeman et al 1998)). In some cases, memory functions can be dissociated: for instance, access to old memories can be totally lost during a seizure while the patient can retain new information given during the event (Vuilleumier et al 1996), or a specific component of memory can be transiently altered, as illustrated by the following observation.

Case F.G.: Selective postictal spatial memory deficit

This 11-year-old boy with a learning disability and personality disorder had complex partial seizures from the age of 3 years with loss of contact, automatisms and postictal confusion. His EEG showed a left-sided frontotemporal spike focus and on MRI there was an unusual position of the left hippocampus (dysplasia?), but no hippocampal sclerosis. His mother insisted that he was amnesic for events preceding seizures and for some time after them. He was therefore evaluated in some detail on this aspect. At 8.30 a.m. one day, he was subjected to the Rivermead memory test and had normal results. At the end of the test (9 a.m.) he had one of his habitual seizures, although 'a short one' according to his mother. He was watched and rapidly recovered from his confusion. At 10.15 a.m., he was again given the same test to see if he remembered each item which he had succeeded in remembering before the seizure (locus of hidden objects, images and recognition of faces). Results were normal, indicating that he had not lost all recently learned material, except the item relating to spatial memory (learned route) which had been normal previously. This finding suggests a transient domain-specific epileptic memory disorder (spatial memory) in the postictal period. The role of the hippocampus in the recall of spatial orientation/location has been shown in experimental animals and in humans (Astur et al 2002).

Memory problems in children with epilepsy

The systematic study of memory functions in children with brain disorders and the availability of standardized tests are relatively recent. Memory is difficult to measure, especially in children in whom motivation and emotional context are so important. The aspects of memory typically tested in the laboratory may say little about how different types of information are consolidated in real and ordinary life beyond these short periods. In one interesting study, there was a poor correlation between everyday memory in children with epilepsy as measured by a questionnaire compared with traditional objective tests (Smith and Vriezen 1997).

TABLE 7.2
Possible alteration of memory during/after seizures

This table shows the severity and type of different memory disturbances which can be encountered in epileptic seizures.

Total amnesia of attack and of postictal period (primary generalized epilepsy)
Amnesia as the 'only' epileptic manifestation (so-called epileptic amnesic attack)
Partial memory dysfunction during attack, i.e. some encoding and retrieval possible
Failure of consolidation of material learned just before or shortly after attack

Complaints of parents of children with epilepsy do sometimes suggest a direct influence of epilepsy on memory. For instance, they mention that the child has forgotten school material that he/she had studied and known perfectly the evening before. This suggests that there is a rapid decay, typical of weak memories, or that the normal consolidation which occurs during sleep not only had not taken place, but that the material had been erased, possibly because of a nocturnal seizure. Also, some parents insist that their child needs more rehearsing to remember a new fact, but that once it is learned, it is very solidly acquired. It may be that the mechanisms that allow natural consolidation to occur after initial exposure and minimal re-exposure are intermittently fragile and inoperative because of the epileptic activity; but other explanations are also possible (attentional, encoding, strategy problems).

Jambaqué et al (1993a), using a specific memory battery investigating verbal and visuospatial memory (Signoret 1991), studied 60 children (aged 7.5–14.5 years) with primary generalized epilepsies and partial epilepsies, and 60 normal controls. They found that children with partial epilepsies had significantly lower memory scores than those with idiopathic generalized epilepsy. In the group with partial epilepsies, those with temporal lobe epilepsies had lower scores than those with extratemporal epilepsies, and (as in adults) the type of deficit was related to hemispheric specialization (visuospatial memory was more affected with right-sided lesions and verbal memory with left-sided lesions). These data of course do not reveal the direct contribution of epilepsy as opposed to the underlying causal disorder.

There should be plenty of opportunities to study what happens during seizures and during postictal and interictal periods in children with temporal lobe epilepsies. These very epileptogenic mesiotemporal regions are often the site of early developmental anomalies (dysplasias, developmental tumours) and acquired pathology (hippocampal sclerosis), from which epilepsy arises. The seizures are often frequent and refractory to antiepileptic drugs, and are surgically treatable. There is now a large literature on adults but there is much less on children in these situations (Jambaqué et al 1993a, Lendt et al 2000, Szabò et al 2001, Mabbott and Smith 2003). When and how seizures which start in or spread to areas closely involved with memory systems affect the organization of memory, learning, and more generally the cognitive and psychological development of the child remains a complex problem (Mabbott and Smith 2003).

Specific memory problems in adults with temporal lobe epilepsy

In adults with temporal lobe epilepsy, there is usually no memory loss of material learned during the interictal periods and in close proximity to the next seizure, except sometimes in the period just before a seizure and in the immediate postictal period (Bergin et al 1995). This is not surprising if one considers the fact that such patients generally maintain quite normal cognitive and learning capacities despite uncontrolled epilepsy over many years.

When memory problems are present, verbal memory is usually more affected with left temporal epilepsy and visual spatial memory with right temporal epilepsy, and this can be accentuated during the postictal period. The specific issue of memory consolidation in epilepsy has only recently begun to be studied systematically, but so far only in adults.

Memory consolidation is a particularly crucial issue during childhood, the most important learning phase in life.

Blake et al (2000) have compared adults with left and right temporal lobe epilepsy on verbal memory tasks repeated after an eight-week interval. There was a clear difference in memory consolidation of verbal material in those with left temporal lobe epilepsy after that period. This could not be attributed to other confounding factors that could have occurred in the interval. It was concluded that a failure of memory consolidation did account for these differences, because these patients had had normal results when tested in the laboratory (after 30 minutes) and these were comparable to the results of the individuals with right temporal epilepsy and controls.

There are good reasons to believe that the same can occur in children who constantly have to learn and consolidate new material, indispensable to building academic knowledge. These children would not be recognized in the laboratory as having poor memory unless tested repeatedly. This problem with memory consolidation may not be apparent for ordinary life events or facts, where there are plenty of natural opportunities to 'rehearse' and to tie them to other experiences.

7.3.3 Long-term Memory Deficits in Children with Temporal Lobe Epilepsy? Comparison with Adults

There are very few 'modern' studies specifically dealing with memory disorders and epilepsy in children (Hershey et al 1998, Williams 1998, Lendt et al 2000, Szabò et al 2001, Gleissner et al 2002) and they concern mainly children with refractory temporal lobe epilepsy before and after surgery.

When a postoperative memory improvement can be documented after successful surgery (and if other confounding factors can be ruled out, such as alleviation of drug therapy), this suggests that there was a direct negative effect of epilepsy on memory systems, presumably in the healthy contralateral mesial temporal lobe (hippocampus). Studies in adults have shown that memory is either unchanged postoperatively or temporarily decreased, but rarely improved. This would seem to depend also on the quality of memory preoperatively, those with previously better memory having a measurable decline and feeling subjectively more disadvantaged.

Long-term follow-up data on adults with surgically treated temporal lobe epilepsy are starting to emerge. Helmstaedter et al (2003) have followed memory and non-memory functions in 147 surgically and 102 medically treated patients with temporal epilepsy at baseline (T1) and after 2 (T2) to 10 years (T3). Fifty per cent of the medical and 60 per cent of the surgical patients showed significant memory decline at 10 years, with little change in non-memory functions. Seizure-free surgical patients showed recovery of memory and non-memory functions at T3. The authors concluded that chronic temporal lobe epilepsy is associated with progressive memory impairment, but that memory decline may be stopped and even reversed if seizures are fully controlled. Overall outcome measured by work and educational status mirrored clinical and school results.

This study showed that many years of uncontrolled temporal lobe epilepsy could lead to memory decline, but these data, of course, cannot simply be extrapolated to children. The mean age at onset of epilepsy in the medically and surgically treated groups was respectively 17 and 12 years (and the duration of epilepsy prior to surgery was 19 years). A younger age at onset of the epilepsy may allow a reorganization of memory which is not possible, or less so, at a later age.

Mabbott and Smith (2003) have assessed memory in 44 children and adolescents who underwent right temporal, left temporal or extratemporal excisions. A striking finding was that there was no significant decline of memory after surgery in any of the groups, but follow-up only ranged from a few months to a maximum of less than two years. The authors found 'a substantial variability in performance' and that 'lesions typically associated with memory impairments in adults do not show the same effects in children' (Mabbott and Smith 2003: 1004).

Research on outcome after temporal lobectomy in children and the representation of memory functions in the young brain is just beginning. Beyond some general statements about the lack of memory decline in the short term in successfully treated children, more precise predictions for future cognitive achievements in adulthood are lacking. Age at onset of epilepsy, characteristics (severity, spread or not beyond the epileptogenic lesion), and duration of epilepsy prior to surgery are crucial variables. Future studies with a large number of comparable patients will be necessary but hard to obtain.

Plasticity for memory functions and the future of children who have had temporal lobectomy for intractable epilepsy

Epilepsy of temporal origin is frequent in children and often refractory to medical therapy. Nowadays, epilepsy surgery in resistant childhood temporal lobe epilepsy is proposed increasingly earlier if seizures persist for more than two years and where there is a definite lesion on MRI (mainly hippocampal sclerosis). This is justified because of the social and psychological consequences of this severe epilepsy and the excellent results of surgery.

The remarkable benefits for a child's quality of life are now indisputable, but one must also think of the evolution of cognitive functions over an increasingly longer life trajectory. Temporal lobectomy has been performed for more than 40 years and long-term follow-up into early adulthood of the children treated in the 1960s to 1970s has shown definite durable benefits in social life and behaviour (Lindsay et al 1979, 1980). No cognitive decline or memory problems seem to develop, at least in early adulthood, and episodic memory can be maintained with a single hippocampal system, although this has not been formally tested in these early series (S. Oxbury, personal communication). A single case of the original series operated on by Falconer (Lindsay et al 1979) had status epilepticus in adulthood, with a severe residual amnesic syndrome, and at autopsy bilateral hippocampal damage (Oxbury et al 1997). This suggests that he was fully dependent for memory on the contralateral 'healthy' side and that no reorganization elsewhere in the affected hemisphere had taken place before surgery. We are not aware of other cases with temporal lobectomy in childhood who sustained late contralateral hippocampal damage and permanent amnesia, and this case may be exceptional. The reorganization of functions may be different depending on the etiology, duration of epilepsy, and age at time of surgery, but it appears that hippocampal functions cannot be taken up by other structures, regardless of age.

In the clinical syndrome of bilateral hippocampal sclerosis after status epilepticus (with devastating clinical sequelae) sustained in infancy (described by DeLong and Heinz (1997) and discussed in Chapter 3), the clinical context and the age at which the hippocampal pathology occurs are very diffferent from the surgical temporal lobe epilepsy cases.

It is not known if memory capacities will be maintained in individuals who had temporal lobectomy for epilepsy in childhood, when they reach late adulthood, or whether the physiological memory decay will put them at an extra disadvantage from that point of view. This worrying question could now be approached by restudying patients with similar pathologies operated on at different ages and after a long period of follow-up. This of course has to be balanced with the memory decline which could have occurred if the epilepsy had remained active for many years.

In conclusion, the systematic study of memory in children with early focal brain pathology, particularly that affecting structures known to be crucial for memory in adults, is only beginning. Unexpected dissociations between different aspects of memory in children with early acquired hippocampal damage have been reported (Vargha-Khadem et al 1997a). Epilepsy is adding another dimension to the problem and new data should be expected, especially since many of these cases can be cured by surgery, allowing pre- and postoperative comparisons and special aspects of memory to be studied. This is illustrated by the following case.

Case E.J.:
Deficient autobiographic memory in temporal lobe epilepsy

E.J., a dizygotic twin, started to have complex partial seizures with olfactory hallucinations due to focal dysplasia of the left uncus, at the age of 8 years. He had normal intelligence (WISC PIQ 93, VIQ 92), and standard verbal and visuospatial memory tests (Signoret and Rey) were near normal. His mother insisted that he had problems remembering facts of his own life (autobiographic memory) and needed more rehearsal than his twin brother when learning new material, although he was not failing in school and had no recognized episodes of acute amnesia. A questionnaire about family life events over the preceding three years (22 questions/events) was constructed using the mother's diary and was given separately to E.J. and his twin, with the following results: number of events spontaneously recalled (8/22 versus 16/22 in his twin), number of different souvenirs per event (14 versus 32); number of prompts necessary for recall (25 versus 10). E.J. had surgical removal of his dysplasia, with cessation of seizures. Autobiographic memory was much improved thereafter.

Memory may also be disturbed in epilepsies of frontal origin, but the nature of this impairment is very different from that found in temporal lobe epilepsies. This has only recently begun to be studied in children (Hernandez et al 2003).

7.3.4 Language

Oral language disorder and epilepsy

Language development is remarkably resistant to adverse external circumstances and can occur despite significant congenital and early acquired brain damage (Bishop and Mogford 1988). At the same time, it can be selectively affected in its quality and speed of acquisition and can regress or even be totally lost at any stage of development, in its oral or written forms, in some types of epilepsy. This paradoxical combination of high resistance and marked vulnerability is probably related to the role that different brain systems play in subserving language acquisition at successive developmental periods (Neville et al 1991).

Prospective studies of language development from a very early age in children with known focal brain damage, and functional imaging studies in normal very young children (Chiron et al 1997) have shown that the brain regions predominantly involved in early language are located in the right hemisphere with a progressive specification and shift to the perisylvian region of the dominant left hemisphere in the majority of subjects. This may explain why language development may be delayed with pathology outside the classical language areas in some early focal pathologies (Bates et al 1992).

Among the cognitive dysfunctions which can be a direct consequence of epilepsy in children, language has been by far the most studied dimension, whether it is transient impairment of acquired language or delayed acquisition. The availability of normative developmental data and the possibility of obtaining a corpus of language repeatedly for longitudinal follow-up make systematic studies of language easier than those of other functions. Another reason for this particular interest in language in epilepsy is probably the fact that an acquired disturbance of verbal language, especially distortion or loss of verbal expression, is immediately recognized as a dramatic change, even in a very young child.

Language disorder and epilepsy in children: possible relationships

Both language disorders and epilepsy are frequent in children (Robinson 1991), so they can co-occur in the same child for different reasons. For instance, a child with a familial developmental language impairment can also have an unrelated lesional or genetic epilepsy. On the other hand, a language disorder and epilepsy may be separate consequences of the same brain pathology, for instance encephalitis in infancy.

There are several situations in which a proven or possible direct causal link between epilepsy and language disorder exists:

1. Loss of language during seizures (ictal and postictal aphasias). This can occur at quite an early stage of language acquisition and depends more on the developmental level reached at the time epilepsy manifests than on actual chronological age (Deonna et al 1982). It is remarkable that a very discrete component within the language system,

including prosody, can be affected during epileptic seizures (or the postictal period) originating in the language areas (Deonna et al 1982). Aphasia or dysphasia may be an isolated epileptic manifestation or only one among other epileptic symptoms. It may be acute in its onset and resolution. Sometimes, it is more protracted and even persistent, as in (2).

2 Acquired epileptic aphasia (Landau–Kleffner syndrome) is probably the most severe end of a spectrum of cognitive disturbances which can be seen in these frequent genetic syndromes (see Chapter 8). It is an important model for the possible role of prolonged focal epileptic discharges in the developing brain, and will be discussed in detail in Chapter 8 on specific epileptic syndromes, and Chapter 12 on developmental language problems (section 12.3.1).

3 Focal epilepsy and developmental language disorder. The question of whether a developmental language delay can be the only manifestation of a focal epilepsy (or focal paroxysmal EEG abnormalities) in relevant brain areas has attracted a lot of attention since acquired epileptic aphasia was recognized as an unusual epileptic syndrome. Several EEG studies (including sleep recordings) of children with developmental dysphasia, now usually named specific language impairment, and some therapeutic trials have not produced any convincing evidence that epilepsy is, even rarely, the cause of typical developmental dysphasia. In special situations, however, this possibility should be taken into consideration and warrants an EEG (see case H.J., Chapter 3, section 3.7 and Chapter 12 on developmental disorders and epilepsy).

Le Normand and Cohen (1997) carried out a series of very detailed longitudinal developmental linguistic studies in a few children with simple partial epilepsy of early onset (frontal focus not further specified and onset of epilepsy before 1 year) but no longer active at the time of the study. The most striking feature was the variability in type of linguistic aspect involved, severity and rapidity of progress (sometimes to full normalization) between the different children and the age at which the improvement occurred compared to normal controls. Unfortunately there were no details about the type, exact location (except an initial frontal EEG focus), duration and cause of epilepsy, so that the possible role of epilepsy itself cannot be separated from all other factors.

Although there is a high incidence of language disorders in children with focal epilepsy (Parkinson 2002), the possible direct role of epilepsy often remains uncertain.

Atypical language representation has been found in earlier studies done in adult patients with severe epilepsy before undergoing epilepsy surgery (Ojeman 1983). These findings may be the consequence either of the basic epileptogenic pathology itself or of the direct and persistent effects of epilepsy during the period of language organization, or even both. More recently, Devinsky et al (2000) have also performed language studies during cortical stimulation in adult patients with refractory epilepsy before epilepsy surgery. The epilepsy had a childhood onset in all patients. They found that 'language cortex had a wider distribution in those with lower IQ, poorer education and worse verbal and memory skills' (Devinsky et al 2000: 400). These patients with atypical language organization and a wider distribution of language cortex may be more vulnerable to a focal epilepsy originating outside the perisylvian zone and thus present with unusual patterns of development or acquired deficits.

Written language disorder and epilepsy

Epilepsy arising in language areas subserving written language can give rise to reading and spelling problems, e.g. an acquired epileptic dyslexia. This has very rarely been documented as an isolated temporary cognitive deficit in children. It appears very likely in the following case.

Case P.L.:
Intermittent deterioration of reading of epileptic origin

P.L., a boy, was seen at 6 years 5 months after a first nocturnal seizure. His development was normal, but he had been evaluated by a child psychiatrist because of behavioural problems. An EEG showed a left temporal electrical seizure and independent bilateral frontotemporal focal sharp waves. MRI of the brain was normal. A diagnosis of idiopathic partial epilepsy was made.

In the following months, mother and teacher noted periods of agitation, intermittent deterioration of ability to read, and occasional nocturnal urinary incontinence. Neuropsychological testing showed normal oral language and cognitive abilities but a specific delay in reading acquisition. Videotapes of P.L. reading aloud the same text, recorded at two different periods (one recorded at school by the teacher during the reported difficult phase, and the other by the mother at home in a 'normal' period), showed a marked difference on several parameters of reading competence (Table 7.3).

Antiepileptic treatment with sulthiame was given. Behavioural problems, urinary incontinence and fluctuations in reading disappeared and the EEG normalized.

Importantly, there was no problem with oral language and behaviour coincident with the intermittent reading problems, so that this would have passed unnoticed if exercises in reading aloud had not taken place regularly in school and at home.

A very difficult and debated question is whether a partial epilepsy starting early during the course of written language learning in cortical networks relevant for this function could be responsible for a developmental reading delay. There have been many EEG studies in children with specific developmental reading problems (developmental dyslexia), some showing an increased frequency of epileptiform discharges. These studies cannot tell whether these discharges represent a fortuitous association or a marker of an underlying disturbed brain organization, or (even) whether they play a causal role in the abnormal written language acquisition.

TABLE 7.3
Case P.L., 8-year-old boy. Epileptic dyslexia: analysis of videotaped recording of reading at two different periods before commencement of sulthiame*

This table shows an analysis of reading accuracy and fluency using video-recordings of the child reading the same text two weeks apart (one at school by the teacher and the other at home), during a period of 'difficult reading' compared to a 'normal' period.

	At school (15.11.01)	**At home** (02.12.01)
Fluctuations	yes ++	no
Accuracy	many mistakes	mostly accurate
Speed	slow ++	faster
Words far from target	yes	no
Simple grammatical words	omitted	present

* Sulthiame is an old drug which had not been used for many years until recently, when its efficacy in rolandic epilepsy and its good tolerance in monotherapy were established in several studies, mainly in Germany. Sulthiame (Ospolot R) is produced in Germany by Desitin and is currently used in Germany and several other European countries (but not in the UK, and not in the USA), including Switzerland where it has recently been officially licensed.

Case R.C.

We have studied a 7.5-year-old girl with left-sided onset complex partial seizures and postictal conduction aphasia who had unexpected difficulty learning to read and write and in whom fluctuating problems in this domain, correlating with the activity of the epilepsy, could be demonstrated (Deonna et al 1993c). At the time of publication, etiology was not known, but on the first MRI at the age of 23 years she had a large area of left temporal dysplasia (Fig. 7.1).

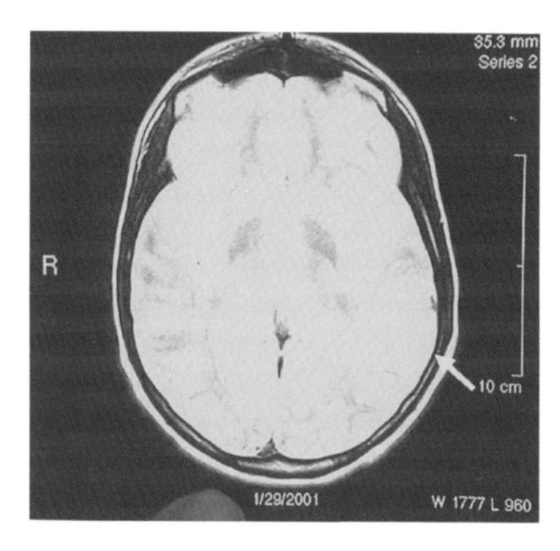

Fig. 7.1 Case R.C.: MRI showing large left 'transmantle' temporal dysplasia.

We have also documented an isolated stagnation and later a regression of written language acquisition in a child with benign rolandic epilepsy.

Case R.G.:
Specific reading disability as a direct consequence of epilepsy in BPERS (Fig. 7.2)

This right-handed boy happened to be included in our study on BPERS (Deonna et al 2000, participant 8) at the age of 6 years when he was just starting to learn to read. He had a normal IQ, no history of delayed language acquisition, no history of familial learning disability, normal measured oral language skills and metaphonological abilities, and no attention problems. With these data, there were no reasons to expect any difficulty with reading. After normal learning of the alphabet and first decoding of simple words we documented a complete plateau in his reading progress for more than two years, followed by a regression, whereas learning of mathematics,

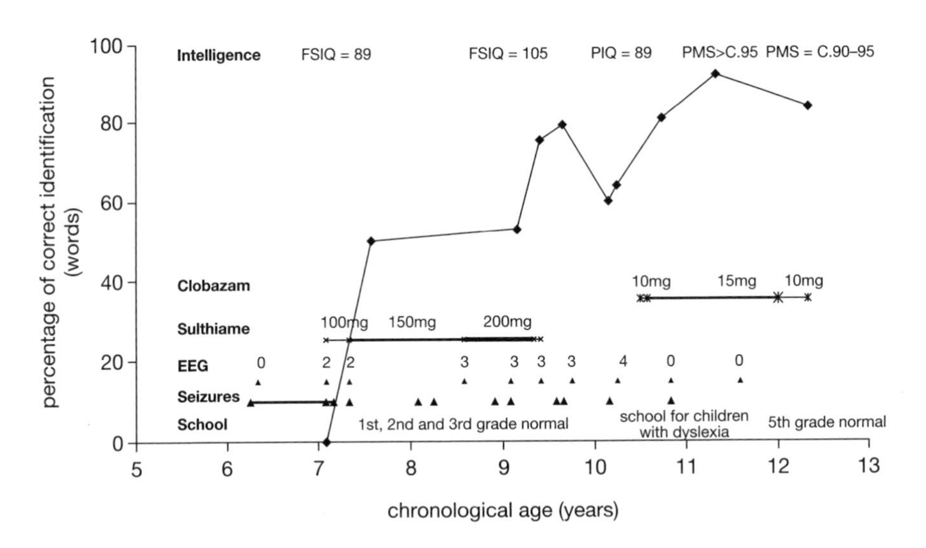

Fig. 7.2 Case R.G., boy: evolution of reading acquisition in rolandic epilepsy.

See case description. This figure shows the evolution of measured reading ability and course of epilepsy (clinical and EEG) from 7 to 12 years. Note the long stagnation, subsequent fluctuations with lowering of performance and regression when EEG epileptic activity was the most intense, followed by rapid progress in relation to change of therapy and disappearance of discharges. The improvement in reading was specific to this domain, because general cognitive abilities and other learning capacities tested in parallel remained unaffected (Mayor Dubois et al 2004). The numbers (0 to 4) under 'EEG' mean: O: no epileptic discharges, 1: rare, 2: frequent, 3: very frequent, 4: subcontinuous. FSIQ: full-scale IQ, PIQ: performance IQ, PMS: Raven's progressive matrices, C: centile.

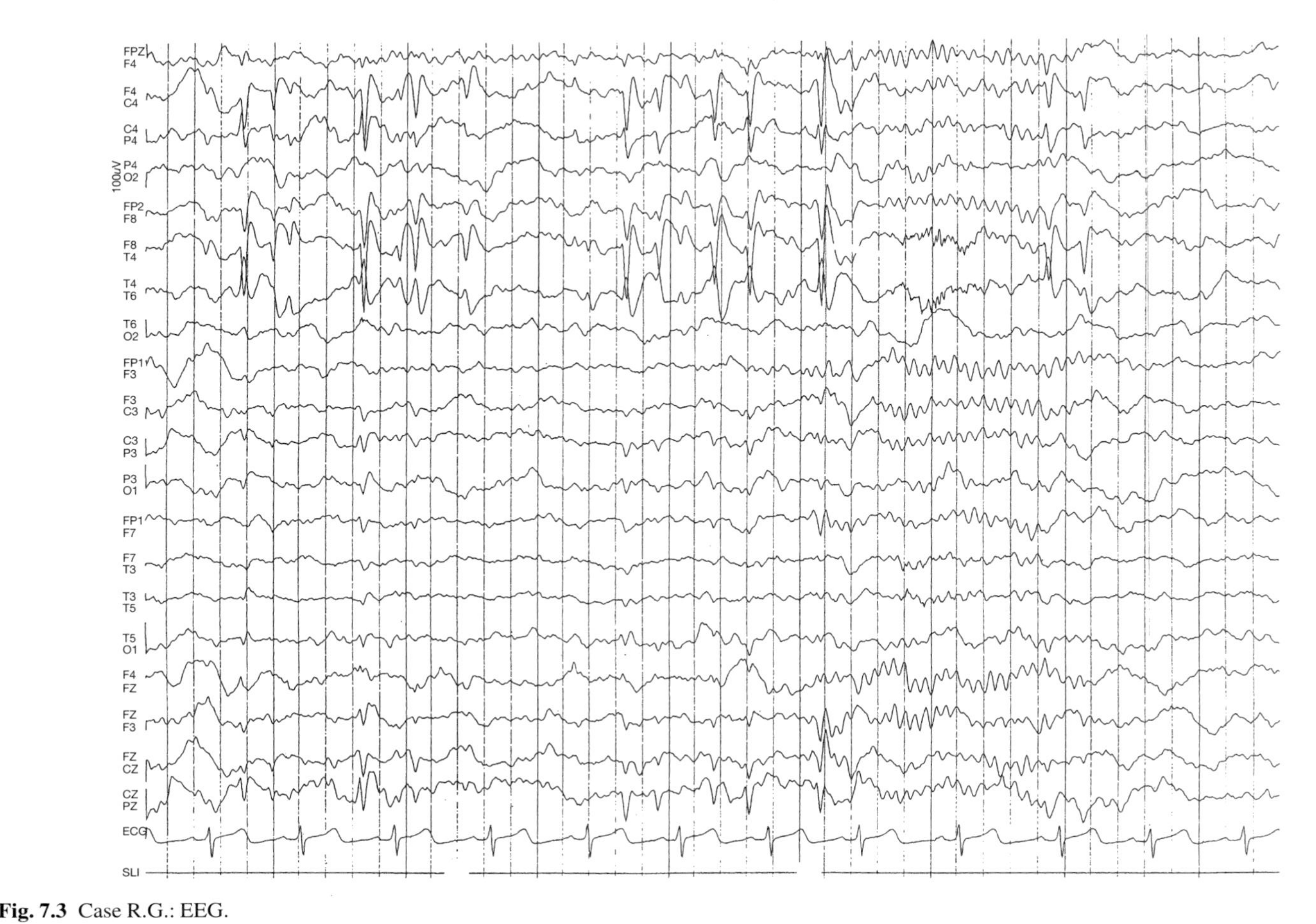

Fig. 7.3 Case R.G.: EEG.

EEG at 10 years at the time of regression in this boy's reading abilities (see case description). Note right-sided centrotemporal frequent focal sharp waves (F4–C4). These occasionally spread to the contralateral side. There were also, though very rarely, independent spikes on the left side.

and other cognitive skills that were monitored, remained normal, including attention skills. During this period, he had a very active sharp-wave EEG focus in the right frontotemporal region, which was not influenced by antiepileptic therapy with sulthiame (Fig. 7.3). After this long stagnation, there was some slow progress despite persistence of the EEG discharges. At 10 years, a regression in his written language skills (without clinical seizures) was documented, coinciding with worsening of the EEG. Clobazam was then given. The paroxysmal EEG activity was for the first time suppressed and this coincided with rapid and continuous progress in reading (although not completely normal) during the next three years, with repeated normal EEGs.

In summary, this course could not be attributed to a global cognitive regression, attentional difficulties, general learning failure or a reactive depression, as all these aspects were regularly evaluated along with reading skills at successive periods throughout the six years. It appeared to be the direct result of the epileptic activity in cortical areas important for the learning and consolidation of written language forms (Mayor Dubois et al 2004).

Effects of epileptic discharges on reading and reflex reading epilepsy

Spontaneous epileptic EEG discharges are often suppressed or attenuated by the act of reading – as they are during other cognitive activities. During focal EEG discharges, one study has shown that the speed of reading was not slower, but on the contrary more rapid, while reading comprehension was decreased (Kasteleijn-Nolst Trenité and de Saint-Martin 2004). It is probable that many different components of a reading task may be preserved or compromised depending on which part of the involved network is implicated. Brief generalized EEG discharges in typical absence epilepsy may alter the reading efficiency or quality of reading (bradylexia, dysprosodic reading, reading loudness reduction) without visible interruption of activity (Poblano et al 2001).

A very rare situation, reading epilepsy, is a variety of cognitive reflex epilepsy in which the act of reading can trigger seizures. Cases in which only reading provokes seizures can be distinguished from those in which seizures may also occur spontaneously or in other circumstances. Seizures usually start rather late in childhood or in adulthood so that they are very unlikely to be a cause of reading problems in childhood.

7.3.5 Other Specific Cognitive Dysfunctions

If focal epileptic activity anywhere in the brain can interfere selectively with the function of a limited group of neurons within a given network, or spread locally, or at a distance in the same hemisphere or contralaterally, an infinite number of possible epileptic cognitive dysfunctions can be expected. Many different types have occasionally been reported in children (e.g. apraxia, visuospatial disorientation, visual agnosia) and could be expected to occur, but they are either infrequent or difficult to capture in existing laboratory tests (Matsuoka et al 1986). They can sometimes be suspected from a parent's description of a transient very unusual or new behaviour or the loss of an apparently common and simple ability. It is difficult for a child to observe rationally and express verbally changes in his/her perception of the outside world (or of his/her inner world, such as body perception), and this must be taken into account.

7.3.6 Lateralized 'Modular' Epileptic Deficits vs Supramodal Cognitive Dysfunction, and the Notion of Executive Dysfunction

The question often arises whether the cognitive deficits are related to disturbances of modular functions related to the side and localization of the epileptic focus or to supramodal 'executive' functions or even to less specific more widely distributed functions such as attention, reaction time or speed of processing. Deficits in executive functions such as planning, problem solving, shifting focus of attention or inhibition of non-significant stimuli may arise when the epileptic process involves the relevant frontal lobe circuits, by the focus itself, local spread or generalized discharges. These types of deficits, in addition to slowness and inattention, may therefore occur alone or in association with lateralized, modality-specific deficits in the case of multiple independent foci or secondary generalization. Alternatively, one or the other deficit may predominate at one period of the evolution of the epileptic disease. Any longitudinal study on this problem needs to acknowledge these facts and seek neuropsychological and EEG evaluation in order to obtain the best possible 'image' of the 'epileptic' problem.

7.3.7 Psychological–Psychiatric Symptoms

Emotional symptoms and/or complex behavioural disturbances of acute or more chronic expression can be the direct consequence of epilepsy in relevant brain systems (prefrontal, frontolimbic). Behavioural disturbances can be the first and, for some time, the only epileptic manifestation. The occurrence of behavioural problems preceding the first recognized seizures (Austin et al 2001), which sometimes disappear as soon as the epilepsy is diagnosed and treated, is a potential example of a purely behavioural manifestation of epilepsy, but this has not been studied systematically (see Chapters 4, 5 and 16 on newly diagnosed epilepsy).

7.3.8 Autistic Type Behaviour as an Epileptic Manifestation

This complex and controversial issue is dealt with in Chapter 12.

7.4 Global problems in cognitive function and learning

7.4.1 Learning Failure and the Notion of Underachievement

Significant cognitive stagnation or inability to learn may be a direct effect of epilepsy. Failure to learn in school and/or documented decrease of IQ (due to the non-acquisition of new skills) can be found in a minority of children with epilepsy and can have many different causes or a combination of causes (Besag 1987). A normal IQ and unchanged scores on repeated testing does not necessarily mean normal performances in school.

The notion of 'underachievement', typically observed in many children with epilepsy, refers to the discrepancy between normal cognitive capacities as measured by IQ and insufficient school progress. It often cannot be explained by purely emotional or motivational factors (Seidenberg et al 1986, Trimble and Cull 1988, Mitchell et al 1991, Seidenberg and Berent 1992). Some abilities which are crucial for good school achievement are not addressed by ordinary IQ tests: for instance, sustained attention, dual task performance, ability to consolidate new memories and to perform under speed constraints. These abilities can easily be disturbed by the epileptic activity, even without overt seizures, and a deficit in any of these, alone or in combination, may be the main reason for a learning failure. Studies looking for a global explanation, in terms of attention, memory, or a 'problem with sequential information', to account for school problems in children with epilepsy, as often occur in the literature, have to take this into account. The capacity to plan and organize one's own activities, to imagine alternative strategies, to inhibit irrelevant information, to shift from one topic to another – abilities referred to as executive functions – is of course crucial and can now be studied to some extent with formal tests in children (Chevalier et al 2000).

7.4.2 Cognitive Deterioration (Cognitive Arrest) and Dementia

In a young child who is normally making constant and rapid progress, any stagnation in cognitive skills should raise a strong suspicion that epilepsy may be playing a direct role, having excluded of course a progressive brain disorder with symptomatic epilepsy. The term 'dementia' refers to a true global loss of skills and not only stagnation. The same epileptic process, however, depending on its severity, can interfere with the 'normal' developmental progress at a variable rate, and may lead first to stagnation for a long time, but later to true dementia.

The most dramatic examples of this can be seen in partial epilepsies of frontal origin with a tendency to spread and which are often accompanied by continuous spike-waves during sleep (CSWS). In the rare cases where the epilepsy is rapidly controlled, the restoration of cognitive functions is the best demonstration of how epilepsy can dramatically and reversibly alter cognitive functions, sometimes in the absence of major seizures or even any visible seizures (see Chapter 8, section 8.4).

8
EPILEPTIC COGNITIVE DYSFUNCTION IN SPECIFIC EPILEPTIC SYNDROMES OR EPILEPTIC CONDITIONS

We will discuss here specific epilepsy syndromes which are potentially important for their consequences on development and cognitive function. These syndromes are also quite frequent. It should be emphasized that the many different childhood epilepsies and epileptic syndromes are very unequal in their consequences for cognition, ranging from none to severe. Furthermore, those with the most severe impact in this domain may not be severe epilepsies in the traditional sense, that is, with frequent or difficult to treat seizures. Sometimes no 'visible' seizures occur at all.

No special attempt has been made here to discuss the different epilepsies based on seizure classification. For instance, discussing children with 'complex partial seizures' would include seizures of frontal or temporal origin and of various underlying causes such as hippocampal sclerosis, focal dysplasias, ischemic lesions, and some focal epilepsies of genetic origin, which would make it difficult to identify the direct contribution of the epilepsy.

8.1 Benign partial epilepsy with rolandic spikes (BPERS) and variants

8.1.1 BPERS as Part of a Spectrum of Idiopathic Partial Epilepsies with Focal Sharp Waves

The syndrome of 'benign partial epilepsy with rolandic spikes' (BPERS) is a model for the debate on the cognitive manifestations of focal epileptic discharges in a developing brain, and therefore must be dealt with in some detail. The syndrome is frequent, representing 8–23 per cent of all epilepsies in children aged 0–15 years. There is no obvious brain lesion, the focal EEG abnormalities are usually numerous, and the epilepsy most often starts at a relatively advanced stage of brain maturation. Most of the children are intellectually and behaviourally normal and thus can easily cooperate in neuropsychological tests. The study of this syndrome may also help us to understand what can happen with other focal epilepsies in which presence of a lesion and other confounding factors complicate the issue.

BPERS is a genetically determined syndrome in which certain cortical brain regions (mainly the perisylvian areas) present abnormal focal electrical activity with partial seizures of variable frequency. This bioelectrical disturbance may last for a brief or a more extended period of childhood, but it normalizes at or before puberty. It manifests on the EEG as focal sharp waves mainly in the centrotemporal areas. These focal sharp waves have been extensively studied and show special characteristics (increase during sleep, modification by sensory stimuli, etc.) (Pan and Luders 2000). Seizures, as expected from the localization of the EEG abnormalities, are simple partial motor and sensory seizures involving the lower face – the so-called sylvian seizures – and tend to occur during sleep (after falling asleep or before arousal in the morning), sometimes with extension to the hemibody or with generalization to the whole body.

The seizures are usually rare and disappear before puberty, and the children have no cognitive or neurological disability. Ten to 20 per cent of the children experience only a single seizure. This typical picture of 'benign partial epilepsy with rolandic spikes' is the most frequent type of idiopathic epilepsy in children. It was long considered the prototype of a specific epileptic syndrome with sharp boundaries. Children with cognitive problems or with EEG abnormalities in locations other than the centrotemporal (rolandic) region were excluded from initial clinical studies.

Over the years, it became apparent that some children with the typical syndrome had epileptic foci in other locations, either at the time of initial diagnosis (as an additional focus or as the only focus) or later. These could occur in the same or the contralateral hemisphere, sometimes with a changing preponderance of left- or right-sided discharges. Some children were found to have learning and/or behavioural problems which could not be explained as psychological consequences of the disease or side-effects of drugs (Doose et al 1996). Finally, some children developed atypical features such as frequent or difficult-to-treat seizures, other types of seizures (Aicardi and Chevrie 1982, Hahn et al 2001), or acquired neurological or cognitive deficits. In addition, several studies, including family studies, also showed that not all children with these EEG abnormalities have clinical seizures.

All these data have led to the conclusion that BPERS is only the most typical and most frequent manifestation of a spectrum of genetically determined partial epilepsies of childhood with focal sharp waves on the EEG in different locations (Panayotopoulos 1999; see Table 8.1).

8.1.2 Cognitive Disorders in BPERS

> Although patients with gross motor deficits or mental retardation were excluded, some patients did nonetheless have behaviour problems or scholastic difficulties. Slight mental retardation was found in a proportion to be expected in a total population. As to personality disorders, it is nearly impossible to establish their relation to the convulsive disorder, and a number of children with epilepsy have such difficulties because of the psycho-affective effects of the seizures (difficulties the patient has adjusting to his condition and his relation with the family).
>
> (Beaussart 1972: 806)

Recognition that children with BPERS often have cognitive and behavioural problems has been a slow process over the last 30 to 40 years, despite the fact that such problems

TABLE 8.1
The spectrum of idiopathic (genetic) partial childhood epilepsies with focal sharp waves

This table shows the clinical epileptic syndromes with their major clinical features, which are considered as belonging to a continuum or spectrum of different epileptic manifestations within the 'idiopathic partial epilepsies with focal sharp waves'. The most frequent and best known is 'benign partial epilepsy with rolandic spikes'. Note that in partial epilepsy with CSWS, focal lesions are now increasingly found, so that its place in this table is debatable.

Clinical epileptic syndrome	Major features	Comment
Benign partial epilepsy with rolandic spikes*	'Sylvian' seizures	For link see discussion (BPERS–LKS connection)
Acquired epileptic aphasia (Landau–Kleffner)	Acquired auditory agnosia	
Benign partial epilepsy with other neurologic/'cognitive' disorders	Gait disturbances; oromotor deficit (ant. operculum syndrome)	Transient deficit related to upper and lower rolandic (sylvian) area
Atypical partial epilepsy of childhood ('pseudo-Lennox syndrome')	Myoclonic-astatic seizures in addition to partial seizures with FSW	Severe epilepsy with variable cognitive deterioration, sometimes none
Benign occipital epilepsy (early and late onset forms)	Early form: nocturnal eye-deviation, vomiting, often status Late form: seizures with visual symptoms (elementary), migraine-like headaches	(a) Overlap with rolandic epilepsy in some cases (rare) (b) Cognitive outcome normal (no systematic studies) (early form) (c) Late forms: cognitive outcome not largely studied, cases with cognitive delay or regression
Partial epilepsy with CSWS**	Cognitive arrest – dementia, psychiatric disturbances	Link with above syndromes less clear. Some are clearly lesional epilepsies. Role of thalamic damage?

* There can be variability in the location of spikes in the course of the disorder. Frontal foci may be associated with transient behavioural regression

** Sometimes defined as EEG syndrome, 'epilepsy with CSWS'

were clearly mentioned in early descriptions of the syndrome, as illustrated by the above quotation. Table 8.2 summarizes the historical evolution of the thinking of child neurologists and epileptologists and the data which led to the gradual awareness of the possible direct effects of epilepsy on cognition.

Beaussart had indeed recognized that many children had cognitive/behavioural problems, but he attributed them to psychological factors – a view which has changed over the years. The commonly held view was that children with BPERS did not have cognitive or behavioural problems because of their epilepsy. Indeed, the first long-term follow-up study, by Loiseau et al (1983), showed that, on average, such children had higher professional qualifications as adults than a control group, suggesting some inherent cognitive superiority. This was subsequently questioned, as the patients in the study came from a private practice with a social selection bias (Aicardi, personal communication).

TABLE 8.2
Cognitive-behavioural disorders in benign partial epilepsy with rolandic spikes: historical perspective 1967–2004

This table summarizes the change in perception of the importance of cognitive-behavioural problems in many children with BPERS, and the data that are gradually accumulating showing a direct link with the epileptic activity itself. Note that the latest question, which is still being investigated (not mentioned in the table), is whether BPERS can give rise to a specific learning disability as a direct consequence of epileptic activity starting in the relevant circuitry at a crucial learning period.

• Behavioural/school problems mentioned in initial descriptions of the syndrome	**1967**
• Rolandic epilepsy: benign epilepsy syndrome, normal children; other problems dismissed	
• Close relationship between BPERS and acquired epileptic aphasia (Landau–Kleffner syndrome) recognized	
• Prolonged reversible oromotor deficits during active epilepsy phase reported in some children with otherwise typical BPERS	
• (Transient cognitive impairment during EEG discharges suspected, but not largely confirmed)	
• Neuropsychological studies confirm normal intelligence but show variable attentional or selective (language, others) deficits in a proportion of children as compared to normal controls	↓
• Longitudinal EEG–neuropsychological studies have shown that acquired temporary cognitive-behavioural problems can be the direct consequence of the epileptic activity (EEG)	**2004**

An influential view on the cause of the associated cognitive and behavioural problems in children with BPERS was proposed by Doose (Doose et al 1988, 1996). After extensive clinical and EEG studies of affected children and their siblings, Doose proposed that children with focal sharp waves had a 'hereditary impairment of brain maturation (HIBM)' which was manifested either by seizures or intellectual impairment or both. However, most children with this syndrome, even those with many seizures and/or frequent EEG discharges for prolonged periods, do not generally show any intellectual decline, or learning or behavioural problems. That is to say, the hereditary impairment can manifest either as an epilepsy or as a developmental problem in a totally unconnected way, which would be surprising if both were manifestations of the same basic disorder. Doose (Doose et al 1996) did not consider that the paroxysmal EEG abnormalities could by themselves interfere directly with cognitive function, a possibility which, as will be seen below, has proved difficult to demonstrate and accept. The major systematic quantified neuropsychological studies performed on this topic in the last 20 to 30 years in children with BPERS are shown in Table 8.3.

These studies have dealt with a range of widely different questions, and only a few use a longitudinal methodology to show or exclude a direct role of epilepsy or epileptic discharges on cognitive functions (D'Alessandro et al 1995, Deonna et al 2000, Baglietto et al 2001, Massa et al 2001). Surprisingly, the possibility of transient cognitive impairment during EEG discharges in this syndrome has rarely been studied (Binnie and Marston 1992, Pressler and Brandl 1995, Pressler 1997), and this will be discussed separately below.

Most studies have looked for either a global or specific cognitive deficit (general intelligence, or visuospatial, language or executive functions), for a relationship between side of the focus and cognitive dysfunction (D'Alessandro et al 1990), for the presence of behaviour problems, or for a special pattern of language lateralization (Piccirilli et al 1988).

The first quantitative assessment of cognitive function in these children was made by Heijbel in 1975, who found no difference in IQ between the probands and their normal siblings. The probands had only slightly lower results in visuospatial tests (Heijbel and Bohman 1975). As a whole, these results tended to confirm the preponderant impression that these children had no cognitive problems.

Piccirilli et al (1994) were the first to conduct detailed neuropsychological assessments including attention tests. They were very restrictive in their selection of children: they included children aged 9 to 14 years, but excluded those with an IQ of less than 80, and those who had presented with seizures in the last six months or who were taking medication. This is important to underline, because this selection of the most benign cases studied in an inactive phase of the disease made it unlikely that a significant deficit would be found. In their first paper, Piccirilli et al questioned whether the epileptic focus had an influence on the brain organization for language, comparing right- and left-sided cases on a paradigm of concurrent verbomanual tasks (Piccirilli et al 1988). They also looked for attention problems in relation to the side of the focus (Piccirilli et al 1994). They found problems when the focus was right-sided or bilateral but not in those with left-sided foci. In a follow-up study of these same children four years later, the original minor differences between cases and controls were not found any more. This was the first longitudinal study which documented transient minor cognitive dysfunctions in BPERS (D'Alessandro et al 1995).

Several subsequent cross-sectional studies all found that, despite normal average intelligence, about half of the children with BPERS had some sectorial weaknesses and school problems as compared to controls, but these appeared to be quite variable (Weglage et al 1997, Staden et al 1998, Croona et al 1999). Staden et al studied 20 children with typical BPERS and found that 13 out of the 20 had 'difficulties with 2 or more of the 12 standardized language tests' (Staden et al 1998: 242). In 8 out of these 13, IQ was within the normal range, indicating a specific language deficit. Weglage did not find any difference in language abilities in children with BPERS compared to controls, but did find differences in visuospatial abilities. In our series we found all types of profile without any specific pattern (Deonna et al 2000).

Why do so many children with BPERS have scholastic difficulties despite normal intelligence and, in general, no or only minor and transient deficiencies in one domain? This raises the further question of whether an 'executive dysfunction', which is not easily captured in standard tests, can be a feature of BPERS. Chevalier et al (2000) studied 13 children with BPERS (7/13 on medication), and controls, on a range of tasks measuring impulsivity and control of inhibition, and found that children with BPERS scored significantly less well than controls on these tasks, but not on 'nonexecutive function measures' (selective attention and memory span, no other cognitive measures reported). Croona et al (1999) also found differences between children with BPERS and controls in some executive functions. One should be careful not to attribute low performances in some computerized attention tests or positive responses in questionnaires to a specific isolated attentional deficit in order to explain the learning problems encountered in some of these children. However,

TABLE 8.3

Types of published neuropsychological studies and areas studied in BPERS

This table shows the neuropsychological studies conducted in typical benign partial epilepsy with rolandic spikes, the most frequent form of idiopathic childhood epilepsy. It shows the variety of neuropsychological questions explored and the fact that very few studies have been set up to investigate a possible direct role of epilepsy.

Author (year)	Domains studied	No. of children (age)	Control data	Longitudinal study	Tests used	Conclusions
Heijbel Bohman (1975)	Intelligence, behaviour, school adjustment	16 (7–12 years)	yes	no	IQ, Bender & behaviour scale	Patients worse than controls for visuomotor coordination
Piccirilli et al (1988)	Language lateralization	22 (9–13 years)	Comparison of left- and right-side EEG focus	no	Verbomanual concurrence task	Atypical cerebral organization
D'Alessandro et al (1990)	Neuropsychological abilities in relation to side/bilaterality of EEG focus	44 (9–13 years)	yes	partial (11/44)	IQ, attentional tasks, language, visuomotor	No IQ difference from controls, slight problems in some subtests, no specific deficits, no difference from controls four years later (11/44)
Piccirilli et al (1994)	Attention problems in relation to focus side	43 (9–13 years)	yes	no	Figure cancellation task only	Patients with right and bilateral EEG foci worse on visual attention , left focus was same as controls
Weglage et al (1997)	Neuropsychological and behaviour characteristics in children with and without seizures (EEG with focus only)	40 (6–12 years)	yes	no	IQ, psycholinguistic tests, motor performance behaviour checklist	Children impaired in visuomotor skills, short-term memory, positive correlation with frequency of spikes, not with side or presence of seizures
Staden et al (1998)	Search for specific language dysfunction	20 (6–13 years)	no	no	IQ, 12 standardized language tests (oral)	13/20 children with two or more low performances
Croona et al (1999)	Cognitive abilities, behaviour compared to controls	17 (7–14 years)	yes	no	Standard tests, questionnaire to parents	Lower scores than controls, more behaviour problems

Chevalier et al (2000)	Action regulation and inhibition	13 (6–12 years)	yes	no	Tasks measuring impulsivity and control of inhibition	Deficits on some measures of impulsivity and inhibition
Deonna et al (2000)	Types of cognitive problems/evolution in relation to EEG activity	22 (4–11 years)	no	yes	Standard tests	Transient dysfunction related to EEG activity/various profiles
Baglietto et al (2001)	Role of sleep activation of discharges (CSWS) in cognitive evolution	9 (6–11 years)	yes	yes	Standard tests	Improvement in IQ score with remission of CSWS
Massa et al (2001)	Search for clinical and EEG markers of cognitive, behavioural problems	35 (6–7 years)	no	yes	Standard tests	Certain interictal EEG patterns are predictive of cognitive problems

inattention can occasionally be a predominant, if not the major, factor. When we analysed the reasons for the low performances observed during a transient period in 8 of our 22 children, attentional deficits did clearly account for the low performances in two of the children. In none of the children of the whole series did we ever evoke the clinical diagnosis of an isolated attention deficit disorder with hyperactivity (Deonna et al 2000).

It remains a challenge to find out whether a deficit in executive functions could account for some of the school and learning problems in children with BPERS independently from the modality in which the tests are carried out.

8.1.3 Evidence for a Direct Link Between Epilepsy and Cognitive-Behavioural Problems in BPERS

Acquired prolonged reversible deficits in BPERS

Some children with BPERS develop prolonged but fully reversible focal neurological deficits topographically related to the perisylvian region. These deficits can be either mild, such as drooling or oromotor apraxia (Fejerman 1987, Roulet et al 1989, Kramer et al 2001), or more severe, with facial, lingual and pharyngeal motor dysfunction, resulting, in extreme cases, in an opercular syndrome (Boulloche et al 1990, Colamaria et al 1991, Shafrir and Prensky 1995, de Saint-Martin et al 1999, Gayatri et al 2002). Some of these children have additional phononological impairments or word-finding difficulties, indicating that neuronal circuits specific to speech and language can also be involved (Deonna et al 1993a).

During this very active epilepsy phase, the EEG usually shows abundant bilateral focal rolandic spike discharges with marked increase and sometimes generalization during sleep, but rarely reaching the usual and somewhat arbitrary definition of continuous spike-waves during sleep (CSWS), which is more than 85 per cent of slow sleep occupied by spike-waves. These cases offer a very striking demonstration that the intense focal epileptic activity occurring in this epilepsy syndrome can interfere in a prolonged and sometimes insidious way with a very specific aspect of a cortical function. The dynamics of these deficits, which typically fluctuate significantly and can last for prolonged periods, are illustrated in Fig. 8.1.

In some cases the neurological deficit happens without recognized seizures so that the diagnosis of epilepsy is delayed. Importantly, these children have clinical and EEG findings otherwise similar to the other cases of BPERS, with the same final benign course of the epilepsy, and no evidence of an underlying focal pathology on MRI. These findings suggest that they still belong to the spectrum of rolandic epilepsies and are not symptomatic epilepsies involving the rolandic area with a severe refractory course, as has also been reported (Otsubo et al 2001).

Do these frequent epileptic discharges in the lower rolandic areas have any impact on the maturation and further development of oromotor functions, especially in severe cases or those with an early onset? In the longitudinal study described below, this question was addressed using quantified evaluation of oromotor functions at two successive periods.

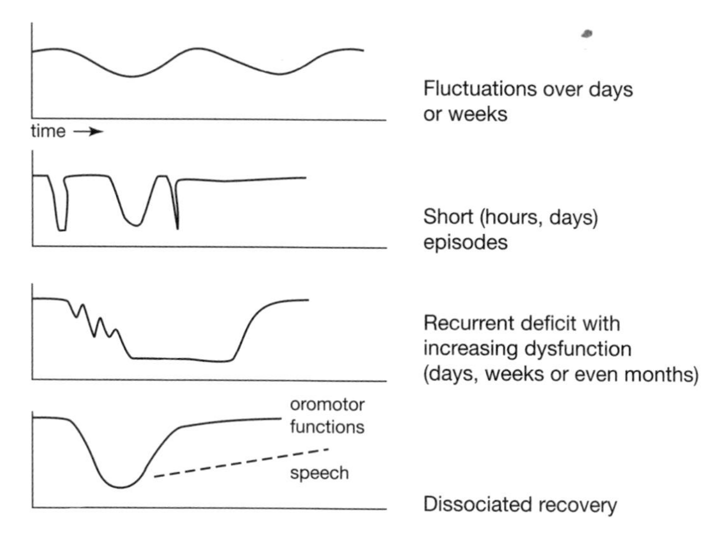

Fig. 8.1 Benign partial epilepsy with rolandic spikes: prolonged fluctuating speech and oromotor deficits. This figure shows the variable time course and dynamics of the observed deficits. The recovery of oromotor functions may precede that of speech (or vice versa), i.e. a recovery dissociated in time may be observed. (Modified from Deonna et al 1993a.)

Case F.M.

This boy had a typical early onset (at 3 years) of frequent hemifacial motor seizures (electroclinical seizure recorded) with final benign outcome (remission at 6 years) and diagnosis of rolandic epilepsy. He never had dysarthria, swallowing or drooling problems. The maturity of voluntary buccolinguofacial movements (56 items) was tested at 6 and 9 years and compared with norms established in normal children (Henin 1980: 'Evaluation of orofacial praxis', unpublished). At 6 years, he was well below the norms for movements – 'cheeks, jaws' (C, 7 items) and 'lips' (D, 14 items) – which were normal at repeated testing at 9 years. This was interpreted as possible delayed maturation of these functions due to epilepsy (see Fig. 8.2).

The predominant location of the epileptic activity (focus or foci), its extension and intensity and the specific role that this area plays at the time the disorder becomes active are what will determine the nature and severity of the deficit and the occurrence (or not) of cognitive or behavioural consequences.

Massa et al (2001), in a prospective study of children with BPERS, found six interictal EEG patterns predictive of neuropsychological impairments: five were qualitative –

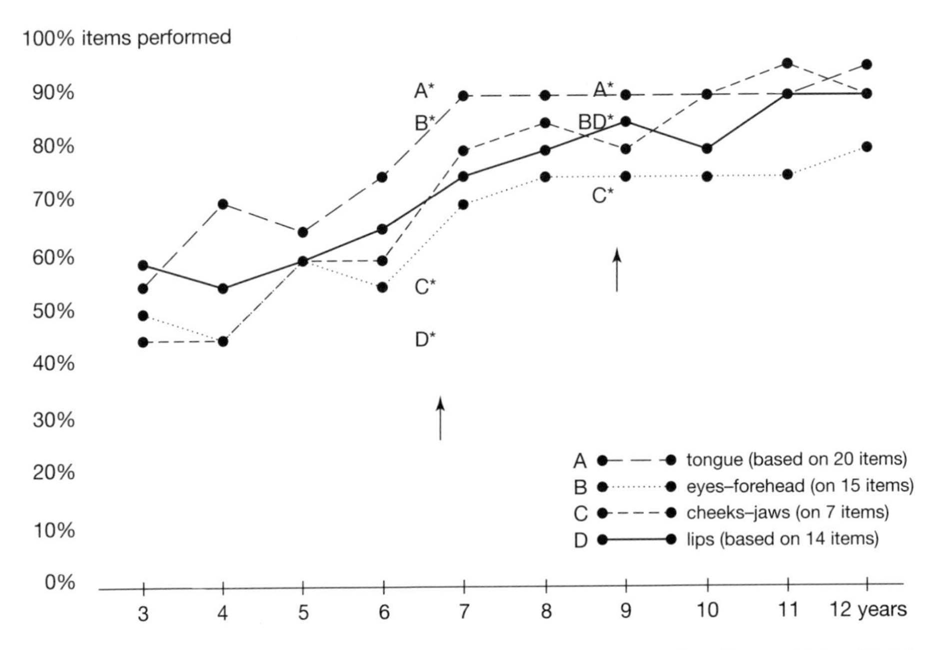

Fig. 8.2 Case F.M., boy: development of oromotor functions in early rolandic epilepsy with hemifacial seizures.

See text. Orofaciolingual movements were tested at 6 and 9 years (arrows) and the performances compared with those of normal children. Each line represents the results obtained by normal children according to age in one of four categories of movement (A to D). Capital letters with * represent F.M.'s results, each letter corresponding to one of the categories of movement. Note that between 6 and 7 years the child performed well below the normal level for cheeks–jaws (C) and lips (D) and that this normalized at 9 years. The performance of F.M. was videotaped and his cooperation was optimal at each session when tested at 6 and 9 years (Mayor-Dubois, unpublished).

intermittent slow wave focus, multiple asynchronous spike-wave foci, long spike-wave clusters, generalized 3 c/s 'absence-like' spike-wave discharge, conjunction of interictal paroxysms with negative or positive myoclonia; and one quantitative – abundance of interictal abnormalities during wakefulness and sleep. The 10 children with these EEG findings had neuropsychological impairments, whereas the others remained normal throughout the course of the study. These children clearly had a more severe disorder with a longer duration of epilepsy and EEG abnormalities and more seizures (although these were few in number in both groups). It remains to be confirmed whether any individual finding or a combination of these EEG findings has a special predictive value for cognitive problems early on in the course.

If the main epileptic activity is situated in a location other than the lower rolandic region, such as the superior temporal area (Heschel's gyrus), or spreads to it, it will impact on the decoding of sounds, that is, produce an auditory agnosia (Landau–Kleffner syndrome). In this frame of thinking, one can expect a variety of possible cognitive/behavioural problems in BPERS and variants, knowing that there is a great variability in the age at onset and localization of these focal sharp waves (Pan and Luders 2000). One must realize that when the epileptic activity is very intense, the surface EEG epileptic discharges may appear diffuse, whereas the point of departure is a highly localized cortical focus. This was well documented by Morrell with electrocorticographic studies of children with Landau–Kleffner syndrome who were treated with subpial transection (Morrell et al 1995).

Another example of this situation is illustrated by the following case, where the function involved and dynamics of recovery over a prolonged period and the relationship with the epileptic activity could be precisely documented because it occurred in a very specific, limited and quantifiable domain, the graphomotor function.

Case C.S.:
Rapid and protracted recovery of graphomotor deficit in a case of BPERS – a longitudinal study

This 11-year-old boy with typical BPERS from the age of 7 years was seen because of progressive deterioration of writing that could not be explained by a motor, praxic or sensory deficit. This could be documented by computerized analysis of the graphic act and compared to the results in normal age-matched children. His initial very low score improved spectacularly and very rapidly (within one to two weeks) in correlation with the reduction of the epileptic activity, probably due to withdrawal of carbamazepine, but it was still very far from normal. We thought that he had reached his best level, arguing that his focal epilepsy, which involved cortical areas concerned with fine motor control, had been active for a long time and had caused a permanent 'weakness' of this particular function.

Surprisingly, follow-up during the next two years showed a continuous regular improvement until normalization of almost all writing parameters. We could thus document a prolonged recovery period. Interestingly, his epilepsy had started at the age of 7 years and, from the history, writing had become difficult from that time on. We concluded that the acute reversible deterioration of his handwriting at 11 years was due to a sudden worsening of his epilepsy, but that the learning and automatization of this skill had been interfered with for a long time previously and needed a prolonged period to reach an almost normal function. Whatever the mechanisms for this, it has important implications for other dysfunctions of a more direct cognitive nature which can occur in the course of these epilepsies (Mayor et al 2003). (See Figs 8.3 and 8.4.)

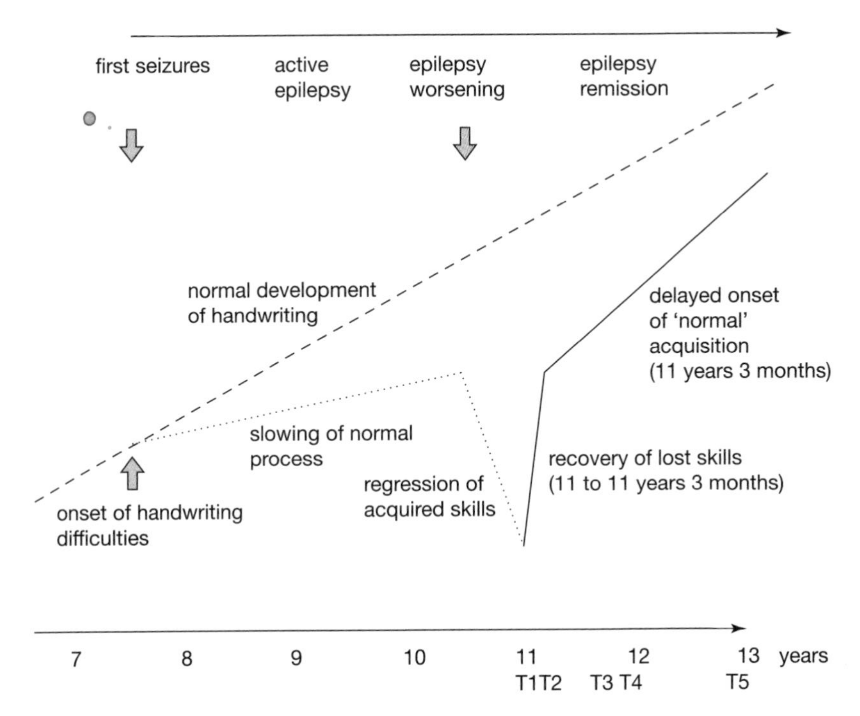

Fig. 8.3 Case C.S.: evolution of epilepsy and handwriting skills.

Evolution of handwriting skills in a child with typical rolandic epilepsy (see description in text). Note the different speed of recovery – fast (days) then gradual (years) – of this function in relation to the activity of the epilepsy. T1 to T5 refer to the points at which the computerized analyses of the graphic act were obtained (five times between 11 and 13 years). (Modified from Mayor et al 2003.)

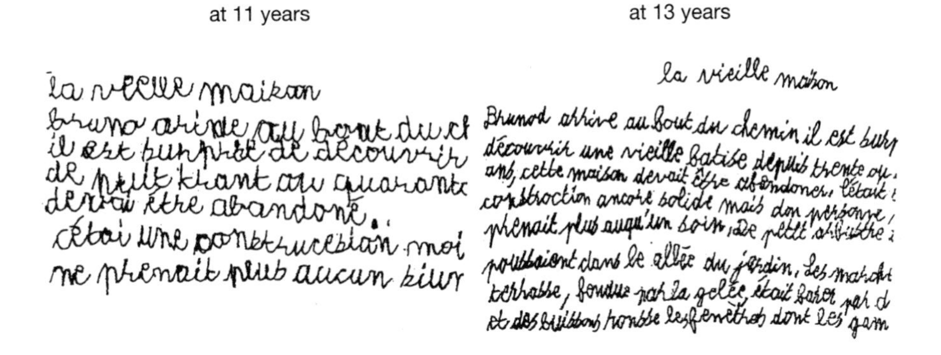

Fig. 8.4 Case C.S.: comparative samples of handwriting.

Comparative samples at 11 years (when at his worst) and at 13 years (after recovery). (Mayor et al 2003.)

Cognitive deficits during the active epilepsy phase

Despite the fact that there are many children with BPERS, who can fully collaborate in psychological testing and usually have frequent discharges on EEG (Deonna 2000a), it has proved very difficult to document a direct chronological relationship between the activity of the epileptic disease (measured by the intensity of epileptic discharges on the EEG and sometimes also clinical seizures) and cognitive functioning. Most children with BPERS and a moderately active epilepsy do not show evident measurable cognitive changes and possibly not at the time the study is done. A few prospective studies have suggested a relationship between the general activity of the epileptic disease at successive periods and the quality of cognitive functioning (Metz-Lutz et al 1999, Massa et al 2001). We have performed a neuropsychological and EEG follow-up study of children with typical BPERS from the time of diagnosis. Out of 22 children, 8 showed sectorial weaknesses in visuospatial or verbal short-term memory or in attention, which disappeared on follow-up, concomitant with improvement or normalization of the EEG (Deonna et al 2000). These transient difficulties were interpreted as a subclinical effect of epileptic EEG activity on cognitive functions, which was also reflected in school results. We felt that our data had to be treated with caution, as the differences measured between the active EEG activity and the remission were minor and could have had other explanations.

In an originally designed longitudinal controlled study of nine children with BPERS, Baglietto et al (2001) performed a sleep EEG every three months until remission of the discharges, and administered detailed neuropsychological testing at the peak of the disorder (T0) and at remission (T1), determined by the disappearance or the marked decrease of the discharges during sleep, 6 to 24 months later. They showed a significantly lower IQ and weaknesses in other test results (although still in the normal range) at T0 in the patients as compared to the controls. Marked improvement was found at T1 in the patients, who performed this time as well as the controls. Note that these children were probably a selected group of the more severe cases of this syndrome, because they had an intense EEG activity during sleep which could be quantified at different time periods of the disease and coupled with cognitive evaluations. These findings, however, strikingly support the view that cognitive dysfunctions can occur during the period of most active epileptic activity (the marker here being the EEG activity during sleep), but recover without evidence of a persistent dysfunction after remission of the discharges.

Transient cognitive impairment during EEG discharges

Studies looking for transient cognitive impairment during the focal EEG discharges in BPERS have been very rare, which is surprising given the importance of the problem and the availability of cases. Since the initial, often quoted study of Binnie (Binnie 1991, Binnie and Marston 1992, Binnie et al 1992), who found evidence of transient cognitive impairment in typical cases of BPERS, very few clear confirmatory studies have been published (Pressler and Brandl 1995, Pressler 1997). It is not clear whether this is due to the difficulty of demonstrating minor changes during these brief discharges (see Chapter 4, section 4.3.2 on transient cognitive impairment), or whether there are in fact no cognitive correlates of this particular type of EEG epileptic anomaly.

In a detailed longitudinal case study, de Saint-Martin et al (1999) described a child with BPERS who had a prolonged oromotor deficit and facial myoclonia. Long-lasting drooling, dysarthria and dysphagia occurred in the periods when interictal abnormalities were abundant and bilateral, but not during severe or repeated seizure episodes. The authors suggested that the deficits therefore did not represent true ictal or postictal manifestations but powerful enhanced inhibition around these 'interictal' spike foci.

In summary, it is still not completely clear and understood whether subtle 'on-line' brief epileptic dysfunction during the interictal EEG discharges is one possible cause of the cognitive or behavioural dysfunctions frequently observed in this syndrome (de Saint-Martin et al 2001).

BPERS as a cause of specific learning disability?

If BPERS can be the cause of stagnation or regression of an acquired cognitive skill such as reading and writing, could it also be responsible for a specific learning disability if the onset of the epilepsy coincides with the period when the skill in question is just starting to be acquired and affects the relevant neuronal networks? If such a situation is encountered and can be followed prospectively, it is also necessary to prove that epilepsy interferes with that skill directly and that predisposing or other general cognitive, psychological or medical factors (drugs) which could all prevent progress in that skill have been ruled out. This exceptional opportunity occurred in a case initially seen in our prospective study of 22 cases with BPERS (case 8, Deonna et al 2000). The patient had an isolated specific difficulty in learning to read and was regularly followed after publication for a further four years. The decisive data came only after this long period. (This case, R.G., was described in Chapter 7 – see p. 76.) In the other 21 cases, the time relationship between the learning of a specific skill and the epilepsy onset and activity did not allow this aspect to be studied so precisely.

Behavioural and emotional problems in BPERS

Although behavioural and emotional problems had already been noted by Loiseau et al (1967) and Beaussart (1972) during the active phase of the syndrome or even in the months preceding diagnosis, these problems have not been given much attention for a long time, although clinical experience shows that they are not at all uncommon. Such problems have been documented in recent studies using questionnaires (Weglage et al 1997). As in other epilepsies, they could easily be explained as a reaction to the diagnosis, with all its psychological and social implications, or as a possible side-effect of medication. However, when such problems occur even before the diagnosis is made, or in children with only one or a few nocturnal seizures, who are untreated and where all attempts have been made to convince parents of the benign nature of the condition, one can suspect that the problems may have a physiological origin more directly related to the epileptic process, possibly when the focus is more anteriorly situated in the frontal area.

Case L.S.

An 8-year-old boy was seen in an emergency outpatient consultation a few days after he suddenly started to have three to five seizures a day. An electroclinical partial motor seizure of frontal type was recorded on the EEG on the same day, with a right-sided frontal onset. Interictal bursts of high voltage spike and slow waves were seen in both frontal regions, with more on the right side. Neurological examination and MRI of the brain were normal. Carbamazepine was started, with immediate cessation of seizures.

On follow-up six months later, we learned that the child's behaviour had markedly deteriorated in the three months preceding the diagnosis of epilepsy, and was so disruptive to the family that the mother had to be treated for depression. All symptoms disappeared as soon as he was treated. The acute onset of frequent seizures that required immediate therapy and the omission by the family of the important information on his recent change in behaviour (and the failure of the physician to ask for it) precluded a detailed study of that dimension before therapy. Control EEGs one and two years after seizure onset were normal and therapy was stopped.

In retrospect, the diagnosis of idiopathic 'benign' partial epilepsy with 'frontal focus' was made, and the behavioural changes prior to the diagnosis were most likely due to a frontal epileptic dysfunction (de Saint-Martin et al 2001).

8.1.4 Cognitive Epileptic Deficits in BPERS and the Dynamics of Evolution: Summary and Questions

There are many clinical arguments for the theory that the prolonged cognitive deficits described in BPERS are linked to the epileptic activity. However, some facts remain difficult to explain in terms of classical ictal (including status epilepticus), postictal and interictal states. A very striking and puzzling aspect of the acquired 'epileptic' disturbances encountered in these partial epilepsy syndromes is how they develop and recover. The onset may be acute or insidious, and fluctuant, and the deficit may worsen or recover very gradually or in a stepwise fashion. The dynamics of evolution may vary in the course of the disease in the same child. This suggests that different epileptic mechanisms are responsible or that the resulting dysfunction depends on other factors.

The sometimes rapid recovery within a short time, followed by further progress at a much slower pace over an extended period, is worth noting. The rapid improvement phase is easier to explain – as due to the regained normal availability of neuronal circuits which were disturbed 'on-line' by the epileptic process. For the slower and often incomplete phase, one can speculate about whether there may be new learning and formation of an entirely different circuitry, or progressive repair of circuitry which had been 'damaged' early on in the course of the disorder.

At the moment, we do not have good answers to these questions, which will possibly be answered in the future by longitudinal clinical–EEG studies along with functional imaging. The type and level of ability attained at the time function was lost, how fully mastered, exercised and automatized the function was, and, in the case of an emergent capacity, at what age and in what main location the epilepsy started, are probably very important variables, which are rarely if ever similar in two children, even if they have the same epileptic syndrome.

Clinical importance of cognitive problems in BPERS

After many years during which cognitive problems in BPERS were either ignored or denied, one should not overstate their importance. After all, the majority of children with this syndrome seem to have no significant long-term consequences of their epilepsy. When cognitive disturbances occur in children with BPERS, they are usually neither spectacular nor severe, they may often pass unrecognized, and in most cases they are not the cause of major scholastic disabilities. One may therefore wonder why so much importance should be given to them. One reason is that a child whose cognitive competences fluctuate or are not in keeping with his/her potential, or who develops behavioural problems during important and prolonged periods of his/her childhood, may suffer, and his/her family too, more than one can imagine, especially when these problems are misunderstood. In these situations, to be able to recognize and discuss these problems is much more reassuring than to attribute them to other – for example, educational or motivational – causes. Finally, this syndrome

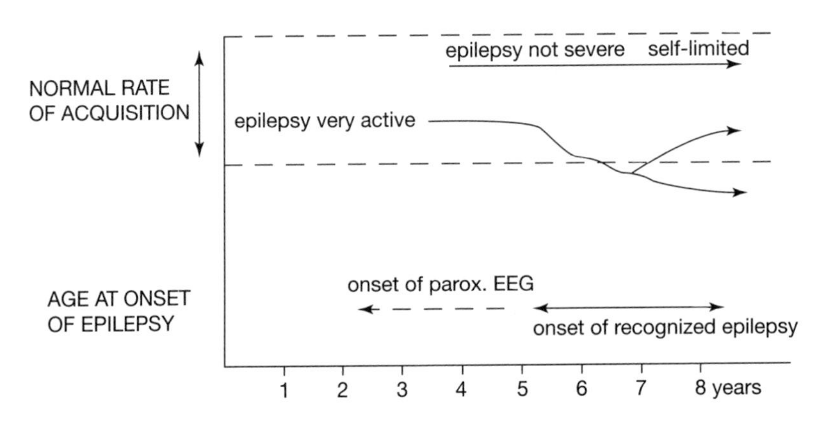

Fig. 8.5 Rolandic epilepsy: schematic representation of possible clinical courses of cognitive development.

Note that the epileptic disease may have started long before it is actually diagnosed and that spontaneous recovery may occur. In most children cognitive functions will remain within the normal range during the active course of the epilepsy, but in a few (especially those with multiple EEG foci, high density of EEG discharges and marked activation during sleep (see Massa et al 2001)), there can be an acquired reversible dysfunction, which, depending on the initial level of the child, may still be in the normal range, or clearly below for a period. Longitudinal studies may fail to document possibly significant changes if the comparative evaluations are made too far apart.

and its more severe variants, despite the great difficulties of evaluating the possible developmental effects of subtle, prolonged and fluctuating problems of epileptic origin, offer the best opportunities to study a great variety of cognitive and behavioural effects of focal epilepsy in childhood.

8.2 Acquired epileptic aphasia (see Table 8.5)

As already discussed, acquired epileptic aphasia has been of major importance in shaping our view about how some childhood epilepsies can present with persistent cognitive problems, sometimes without evidence of epilepsy other than a focal paroxysmal EEG (Deonna 2000b).

The nature and cause of acquired epileptic aphasia differ fundamentally from other types of acquired aphasias during childhood. These are summarized in Table 8.4.

We do not consider acquired epileptic aphasia (or Landau–Kleffner syndrome) as a rare, exotic and physiopathologically obscure condition, but as only one of the severe manifestations that can be encountered in idiopathic partial epilepsies of childhood, which involve mainly the perisylvian region and whose prototype is benign epilepsy of childhood with rolandic spikes (Dulac et al 1983). This view, which is now generally accepted on this side of the Atlantic and has been for some years (Dulac et al 1983, Deonna 1991, Deonna and Roulet 1995, Doose et al 1996), is still under discussion in the USA and Australia (Berroya et al 2004).

Interestingly, the clinical facts that speak for a close connection have gradually emerged from clinical considerations and follow-up observations in both syndromes, although the history of each of them followed its own path with little overlap between the two for several years. Clinicians studying children with Landau–Kleffner syndrome initially noted that the

TABLE 8.4
Characteristics of 'typical' acquired aphasias of childhood and of acquired epileptic aphasia (Landau–Kleffner syndrome)

This table shows the clinical language characteristics and the evolution seen in typical acquired aphasias of childhood after focal brain lesions, compared with those seen in the syndrome of 'acquired epileptic aphasia' (Landau–Kleffner syndrome).

	Typical (classical) acquired aphasia	Acquired epileptic aphasia (Landau–Kleffner syndrome)
Onset	Depends on type of lesion	Gradual with fluctuations, rarely acute
Type of aphasia	Mainly expressive (brief receptive phase)	Mainly receptive (auditory agnosia). Purely expressive speech can occur (cf. anterior opercular epileptic syndrome)
Recovery	Total and rapid (days or months)	Progressive, variable with remissions and exacerbations over years, often with sequelae
EEG	Slow waves on side of lesion, rarely epileptic focus	Focal sharp waves, often bilateral with temporal predominance, marked increase of discharges during sleep (± CSWS)

TABLE 8.5
Acquired epileptic aphasia (Landau–Kleffner syndrome): typical features

Note that we consider the etiology of this syndrome to be the same as that of the partial childhood epilepsies with focal sharp waves, and not 'unknown', as stated in most textbooks. Most children lose language because of epileptic auditory agnosia, but expressive language may be the main or only language problem.

- Previously normal child or pre-existing language delay
- Acute or insidious onset of aphasia* (3 to 7 years), but onset at younger or older age possible
- Clinical seizures not always present
- Etiology: probable severe end of spectrum of idiopathic partial epilepsies of childhood, e.g. rolandic epilepsies. Normal brain imaging
- EEG: paroxysmal bitemporal asynchronous focal sharp waves, often markedly increased during sleep (CSWS)
- Close relationship (not always) between severity, duration of aphasia and paroxysmal EEG abnormality
- Poor response (possible aggravation) to most conventional antiepileptic drugs except diazepines. Good response to corticosteroids
- Variable partial or total recovery with remissions and exacerbations (fluctuations), sometimes prolonged

* In fact, mainly auditory agnosia. Cases with predominant expressive language problems do exist.

benign course of the seizure disorder, its remission before puberty and the EEG features (focal sharp waves on EEG, increase of discharges during sleep) were quite similar to what was seen in idiopathic partial epilepsies, suggesting a functional disorder (Dulac et al 1983). Later on, what appeared initially unthinkable (that a severe aphasia could be a symptom of a partial epilepsy syndrome with the most benign prognosis) was gradually accepted. The idea of a spectrum or a continuum was also reinforced by family studies, especially those in which both syndromes occurred in siblings (Doose et al 1996).

On the other side, it was increasingly noted that some children diagnosed initially as having typical BPERS could develop oromotor or speech problems or auditory agnosia, together with the sleep EEG pattern of CSWS and the same variable dynamics of onset of and recovery from symptoms as in Landau–Kleffner syndrome (Deonna et al 1993a, Fejerman et al 2000, Yung et al 2000). Sometimes this evolution is a consequence of an aggravation of the epilepsy by drugs such as carbamazepine (Prats et al 1998). In one personal case, hemifacial seizures on awakening, typical of BPERS, were recognized only when the child, who had recovered language, told us and his parents that he had had them for quite a while but had not mentioned them. In addition, we have also encountered, and heard of from other colleagues, children who presented transient and brief periods of poor speech comprehension, difficult verbal expression or even written language problems during the course of an otherwise typical BPERS, which we believe are mild language manifestations of their epilepsy. These cases unfortunately have not been studied, let alone published.

Acquired aphasia with epilepsy has been reported in some children with a documented lesion in the language areas at the time of diagnosis (tumour, inflammatory disease) (Solomon et al 1993). In our opinion, it is inappropriate to use the term Landau–Kleffner syndrome for any focal epilepsy involving cortical language areas with aphasic manifestations, even if these are prolonged or persistent. One should limit the term to those cases without a demonstrable pathology and accompanied by the typical focal sharp waves on the EEG in the temporal areas, often with marked activation of discharges during sleep. There may be exceptional cases which have a closely resembling syndrome but in which a focal dysplasia can be found, sometimes later in the course of the disease (Roulet et al 1991, Roulet-Perez et al 1998). In such cases, it is possible that both the epileptogenic lesion and the focal epileptic syndrome do play a role.

Typical acquired epileptic aphasia is unique and devastating only because the epileptic dysfunction is specifically located in the primary auditory cortex (Rapin et al 1977, Paetau 1994, Morrell et al 1995, Boyd et al 1996, Korkman et al 1998, Seri et al 1998) and leads to a loss of ability to decode sounds (auditory agnosia). This in turn leads to a loss of language comprehension followed by deterioration of oral speech. Oral speech depends strongly on auditory feedback for its maintenance and proper output, and can be completely lost. Table 8.6 shows a unique recorded testimony of a 6-year-old child who shortly after a rapid recovery from auditory agnosia of two months' duration and return of fluent speech could describe the fluctuating symptoms and auditory hallucinations in his own way.

In the years following the recognition of this syndrome by Landau and Kleffner in 1957, only the most severe, persistent and sometimes permanently aphasic cases were studied and reported (Deonna et al 1977, 1989). We now know that a mild transient disruption of language, at times affecting only speech production, can occur in active phases of an otherwise benign partial epilepsy with rolandic spikes (Deonna et al 1993a).

Acquired epileptic aphasia can start in children who have had perfectly normal language development, but some children already have language problems before onset of the syndrome. In such children, and in those with a very early onset, evidence of language loss may not be obtained, so that the diagnosis is difficult. This issue is discussed further in Chapter 12 on developmental disorders and epilepsy (section 12.3.1).

The clinical presentation, evolution, associated problems and especially educational management of acquired epileptic aphasia are beyond the scope of this chapter and the

TABLE 8.6
Case A.G., boy, 6 years 6 months, with Landau–Kleffner syndrome: interview after recovery

This boy had a two-month history of auditory agnosia (Landau–Kleffner syndrome). This is taken from a transcript of his answers in an interview shortly after he had recovered comprehension of language and could express clearly what he had experienced during the acute symptomatic phase.

Comprehension during aphasic (auditory agnosia) phase:
'I hear but I do not understand'
'Noises within my head, that was scary'
'Even if I closed my ears I would still hear them, but there was nothing, I was looking outside'
'Sometimes I hear, sometimes I don't'
'I had the impression that there was a little man . . . two, and sometimes they close the ear with a key'

reader is referred to other sources (Hirsch et al 1990, Deonna 2000b, Metz-Lutz et al 2001, Vance 2001). The crucial issue of antiepileptic therapy is discussed in Chapter 14.

One of the many remarkable features of this syndrome is how some children can adapt and learn another communication system, namely sign language (Roulet-Perez et al 2001). Sign language, if it can be implemented, not only maintains crucial communication within the family but allows the child to acquire academic knowledge during the aphasic period. As soon as the child recovers oral language, sign language is no longer used, or only as a support (Vance 1991).

Case L.C.

A 4-year-old boy gradually lost all comprehension of language and ability to speak over a three- to six-month period. He soon started to use natural signs, and formal sign language was introduced about one year after onset of the disease. His mother, his 9-year-old sister and the speech therapist learned sign language as well, with surprising enthusiasm. He was able to attend the regular elementary school. He rapidly became very proficient in sign language, and his sister even more so. With steroid treatment, significant verbal language recovery occurred about six months after introduction of sign language, with spontaneous decrease of signing, but without loss of interest in that language.

8.2.1 Prognosis, Long-term Outcome of Acquired Epileptic Aphasia and Physiopathological Aspects

The initial severity, duration of the active phase of the syndrome and degree of recovery can be quite different. It is certain that the prognosis of children today, who are diagnosed rapidly and treated aggressively in order to suppress epileptic discharges, will be different from that of children 30 or 40 years ago.

Initially, only the most severe forms were recognized, and there is also a natural bias to report the more severe cases (Mantovani and Landau 1980, Deonna et al 1989, Zardini et al 1995, Baynes et al 1998, Rossi et al 1999). Adult follow-up studies of children are understandably rare, and residual language problems of variable severity have been reported. Even in those who seem to have recovered completely, short-term phonological memory deficits have been demonstrated clinically (Deonna 2000b, Metz-Lutz et al 2001). Electrophysiological studies and functional imaging (PET and fMRI) done many years after remission of the syndrome have shown persistent abnormalities in the auditory cortex. This suggests a permanent epilepsy-induced dysfunction in this system rather than simply the direct 'on-line' effects of the epileptic discharges, since these were no longer present at the time of these studies (Maquet et al 1995, Majerus et al 2003). It has been postulated that focal epileptic activity in a maturing neuronal network could disrupt its organization

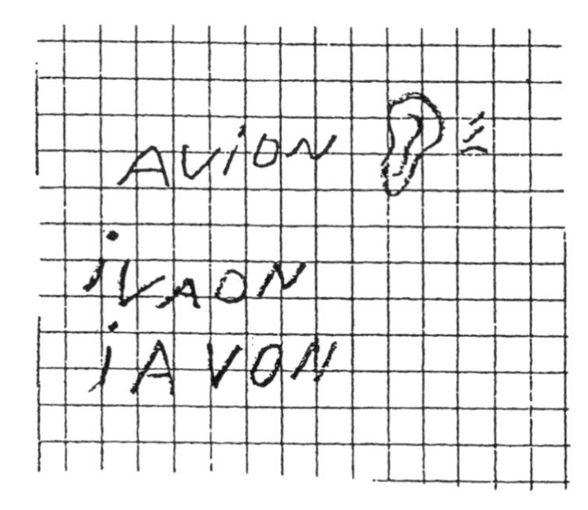

Fig. 8.6 Case A.G.'s drawing of his residual difficulties.

Spontaneous drawing done by A.G. at the age of 9 years of his residual difficulties with complex sound recognition. He explained that he sometimes hears 'avion' (plane) as 'ivaon' or 'iavon'.

permanently, for instance by maintaining active synapses which should normally have been eliminated (Morrell et al 1995).

A basic question, however, remains unanswered. How do we explain this prolonged, age-limited firing of local neuronal populations in preferential areas such as the perisylvian area (without underlying developmental pathology in the classic sense) in acquired epileptic aphasia and related disorders? A constitutional (genetic) imbalance between excitatory and inhibitory intracortical neurons in these areas has been postulated, but this is at the present time still a hypothesis (Metz-Lutz et al 2001).

Mild auditory processing residual problems

Fig. 8.6 illustrates the rather subtle auditory processing difficulties drawn for us by a child (A.G.) who has apparently completely recovered and has no difficulties in standard laboratory language tests. In this very bright child, this led to some errors in comprehension of oral texts which was mistaken at school as inattention.

8.3 Acquired epileptic aphasia 'plus': associated impairments and overlap with other acquired cognitive/behavioural epileptic disorders

If one accepts the notion that there is a variability in the exact location, extension and degree of the maximal focal epileptic activity at different ages and in different children, it is not surprising to observe this variability at the clinical level. Not all cases of acquired epileptic aphasia have the pure, isolated acquired auditory agnosia described above, and some have additional cognitive, general communicative and behavioural impairments which can dominate the clinical picture, either at onset of the disorder or later in its course (Deonna et al 1977, Robinson et al 2001). A child with global cognitive regression (dementia) initially may become mainly aphasic later on. In such severe cases, language may be affected not only at its structural level (phonology, syntax, semantics) but also in its communicative use (pragmatics) (Chival and Thibault de Beauregard 2000).

The catastrophic loss of communicative abilities resulting from auditory agnosia can be an evident cause of behavioural problems and hyperactivity in these children. It is remarkable sometimes to see the marked improvement that can be observed when the diagnosis is made, and substitutive language is given.

However, severe behavioural impairments can be a part of the epileptic disorder itself and not primarily the result of the loss of communicative abilities. Major behavioural improvements can be seen before and even in the absence of language recovery, due to a natural decrease of the activity of the disease or as an immediate result of therapy, either medical or surgical (Neville et al 2000, Robinson et al 2001). In these cases, the epileptic activity is located not only in the perisylvian region but also in the frontal regions (multiple foci or spread).

8.4 Partial epilepsies with CSWS

Continuous spike-waves during slow wave sleep (CSWS) is essentially an EEG finding. However, largely for historical reasons, it has received the erroneous status of a specific epileptic syndrome after the description of a group of children, not otherwise suffering from severe epilepsy, who had prolonged and usually permanent cognitive decline in conjunction with this striking EEG abnormality (Patry et al 1971, Roulet-Perez 1995, Veggiotti et al 1999).

Continuous spike-waves are present from sleep onset, and are most often limited to slow wave sleep (disappearing or decreasing during REM sleep). There are several arguments for the view that CSWS are the result of secondary bilateral synchrony arising from one or several primary epileptic cortical foci which can be situated anywhere in the brain (see Tables 8.7 and 8.8). The CSWS pattern can be seen in idiopathic focal epilepsies without visible lesion or in symptomatic partial epilepsies of various etiologies, mainly those of pre- or perinatal origin (Roulet-Perez et al 1998). It has also been reported in children with shunted hydrocephalus of diverse causes (Veggiotti et al 1998), and more recently in children with thalamic lesions (Monteiro et al 2001).

TABLE 8.7
Main characteristics of the continuous spike-waves during slow sleep phenomenon

The variable age at which CSWS appear and finally stop, the spontaneous fluctuations and changes induced by drugs (disappearance or intensification), in addition to the difficulties in obtaining sleep EEGs, may explain why this EEG pattern and its clinical significance remained elusive for so long.

Onset during early mid-childhood (not in infancy)
Present from sleep onset, disappears or decreases during REM sleep
Can last for variable and long periods but remits before adulthood
Can be observed in idiopathic (functional) or lesional epilepsies
May be eliminated by diazepines and steroids and facilitated or provoked by some antiepileptic drugs (carbamazepine)
Marker of a very intense focal epileptic activity (bilateral synchrony). May play a direct negative role on cognitive functions
Physiopathology unclear but role of thalamic lesion recently emphasized

TABLE 8.8
The CSWS pattern is the manifestation of secondary bilateral synchrony: arguments

This table shows the data indicating why the CSWS phenomenon is considered as due to secondary bilateral synchrony from an initial cortical focus (Morrell et al 1995, Irwin et al 2001).

- CSWS may develop in the course of partial epilepsy with initially a cortical spike focus only
- A cortical epileptogenic focus can be found in the waking state or during REM sleep, or when CSWS decrease spontaneously or with drugs, and in the course of evolution
- The neurological 'epileptic' deficit is related to the location (function) of the cortical EEG focus
- Surgical treatment (multiple subpial transection or excision) of the epileptic focus eliminates the CSWS pattern

Since Monteiro et al published their study (Monteiro et al 2001), lesions of the thalamus on MRI have been found repeatedly in children with CSWS (Battaglia et al 2003, Kelemen et al 2003, Vanderlinden et al 2003). Considering the fact that most focal epilepsies do not show this striking EEG abnormality during sleep, there must be special factors to explain the CSWS phenomenon. Dysfunction of the thalamus, and not necessarily a lesion, might be a key condition for the generation of CSWS, in the presence of a cortical epileptogenic lesion. Experimentally, electroencephalographic patterns consisting of long sequences of continuous spike-waves resembling CSWS have been induced by bicuculline injected into the cortex of cats with unilateral thalamectomy (Steriade and Contreras 1998).

Despite this intense epileptic activity on the EEG during sleep, most children with CSWS do not, in general, suffer from sleep disturbances and do not, or very rarely, have recognizable seizures during sleep. During the day, epileptic seizures, which can be of various types, are rarely very severe or frequent. Sometimes the child has never had any seizures and, in rare cases, CSWS are discovered during a diagnostic work-up in a child with behavioural regression or learning problems.

The total amount of sleep occupied by CSWS is variable, and the percentage of sleep occupied by the spikes which may be clinically significant (85 per cent) is somewhat arbitrary. There are definite fluctuations in density of the EEG discharges, even during a single night (Deonna et al 1997) or between records obtained at short time intervals, and some antiepileptic drugs (mainly diazepines and ethosuximide) or corticosteroids can suppress them, whereas other drugs may increase them (Boel and Casaer 1989, Roulet-Perez 1995).

A striking phenomenon is the gradual decrease and final disappearance of CSWS with age, usually before adolescence. The condition is virtually never seen in adults (Tassinari et al 2000).

There are several reasons why it has been difficult to recognize the CSWS phenomenon and to prove the causal relationship between CSWS and cognitive dysfunction:

1 Sleep EEGs are often not done as a routine.
2 CSWS are usually discovered during a first sleep EEG, and it is not known how long this abnormality has been present.

3 It is in practice very difficult to document the evolution of this EEG pattern repeatedly during a prolonged period of childhood and correlate it with the clinical condition and therapy.
4 CSWS are usually not suppressed by conventional antiepileptic drugs, except with diazepines and in this case often only temporarily.
5 Steroids are often effective in suppressing CSWS, but frequently have side-effects.
6 Strict correlations between cognitive and EEG changes are difficult to make. First, there is the problem of obtaining reliable comparative cognitive and behavioural data in often very disturbed and uncooperative children. Second, and especially in the most severe and long-standing cases of cognitive regression or aphasia, the recovery under therapy is rarely rapid and often not closely related chronologically to the EEG improvement. For unclear reasons, the deterioration can start slowly and insidiously but at a later period become quite rapid, so that natural dynamics of the disease may hide or delay the recognition of a beneficial effect of therapy.

Despite all these difficulties, there are now sufficient available data to reach some conclusions and make a working hypothesis. The cognitive deficit is first of all related to the location (i.e. function) of the primary epileptic focus at the time it becomes active, with possible local (intrahemispheric) extension or bilateral spread, CSWS being mainly the marker of the severity of the epileptic activity (Robinson et al 2001). If the epileptic process affects an area directly implicated in cognitive processes, or starts at a period of active organization of specific neuronal networks (critical period for a given function), it may prevent their stabilization or consolidation, with major cognitive consequences. On the other hand, if the epileptic focus becomes active in an area which has already completed its maturation and has no major role in cognitive processes, and if the epileptic process is not very severe and of short duration, no or minimal consequences will ensue.

However, the CSWS phenomenon may contribute to the deficit by impairing the consolidation of newly learned skills (see Chapter 5, section 5.4 on sleep and epilepsy). The age at onset, severity of epileptic dysfunction and duration (months, years) will influence the final outcome. It is thus not surprising that the clinical correlate of CSWS is extremely variable, both in severity and type of deficit involved (Deonna et al 1997).

In the last few years, several centres with an interest in this area, and facilities for sleep EEGs, have been conducting a systematic search for CSWS in cases with unexplained cognitive or behavioural regression with 'mild' epilepsy or even sometimes without epilepsy at all. These studies have revealed an enlarged spectrum of disabilities in these children (Table 8.9).

Among the many diverse epileptic neurobehavioural syndromes seen in these partial epilepsies with CSWS, the most severe, catastrophic situation is that seen in children with a primary focus in the prefrontal region, because of its combination of cognitive regression and major behavioural problems whose co-occurrence, combination and evolution are very difficult to interpret and document. It is the prototype of the direct psychiatric manifestations of epilepsy, and indeed some of these children may initially be diagnosed and treated as having primarily a psychiatric disorder, namely a psychosis (Kyllerman et al 1996, Deonna et al 2003) (see below).

TABLE 8.9
Types of cognitive dysfunctions which have been reported to be associated with CSWS

This table shows the main types of neuropsychological deficits in relation to the site of main epileptic focus reported in the literature, in which a clear relationship with the CSWS activity has been demonstrated in longitudinal studies. Because the age at onset, severity and duration of the epilepsy, and focal brain areas preferentially affected are extremely variable between different children (and even in the same child at different periods), one may see an obvious loss of acquired skills or only a gradual stagnation, which may take a long time to be recognized, or the non-development of a given function. Similar cases have been described as acquired epileptic psychosis (Hirsch et al 1990, Kyllerman et al 1996).

Main acquired deficit	Localization of main focus (EEG)	Comments and references
Deficit in verbal and nonverbal reasoning, time concept, severe behavioural disorders	Frontal (left and/or right)	Uni-/bilateral frontal (see text)
Aphasia (different types)	Perisylvian (bilateral)	In verbal auditory agnosia (most frequent) focus in superior temporal gyrus = auditory cortex (Morrell et al 1995)
Drooling, speech arrest, swallowing difficulties	Rolandic	1 case, epileptic 'opercular syndrome' (Colamaria et al 1991)
Mild dysphasic signs, dysfluency, slow learning	Left parietal (main); left frontal (occasional)	1 case, arachnoid cyst in the left sylvian fissure. More subtle dysfunction (Deonna et al 1997)
Dyslexia, dyscalculia, global dyspraxia	Left temporo-occipital	1 case, acquired 'Gerstmann syndrome' (Badinand et al 1995)
Navigational and visuospatial disorder, left hemineglect	Right hemisphere	2 cases, right hemispheric dysfunction, language considered normal (Zaiwalla and Stores 1995)
Visual agnosia	Occipital bilateral, parietal right, temporal left	1 case, visuoverbal dysconnection, visual perception, language and praxis normal (Pavao Martins et al 1993) 1 case, visual agnosia with CSWS (Eriksson et al 2003)

8.4.1 Acquired Epileptic Frontal Syndrome with CSWS: The Prototype of Epileptic Dementia or Epileptic Psychosis

In 1993, we reported four boys followed longitudinally for several years with a cryptogenic partial epilepsy, a frontal epileptic focus and continuous spike-waves during sleep (CSWS) on the EEG (Roulet-Perez et al 1993). All had repeated cognitive and neuropsychological evaluations coupled with whole-night EEG recordings. Cognitive and behavioural regression followed by a variable degree of recovery could be documented in all cases, which correlated with the severity of the epilepsy measured by the intensity of epileptic activity on the EEG during sleep. The neuropsychological and behavioural regression were both very severe, and the boys' overall clinical profile seemed to be unique. The behavioural symptoms could not be explained by a psychological reaction to the cognitive loss and did not correspond to a known psychopathological syndrome.

The relative severity and interplay between behavioural and cognitive symptoms varied greatly during the course of the illness. The unique clinical and EEG profile of these children suggested a frontal dysfunction, which we termed 'acquired epileptic frontal syndrome'. Given the multiple functions of the prefrontal lobes in cognition and emotions and their increasingly important role as the child grows older, one should expect a complex mixture of cognitive and psychiatric problems, which were indeed difficult to pin-point and analyse. The four children we described are probably exceptional in so far as: (1) they were quite normal up to the age of 3–5 years, when much normal development had already taken place; (2) they became very severely affected; (3) they were followed in great detail and frequently, and during the active epilepsy phase; (4) they showed sufficient improvement (with medication) to allow a separate study of cognitive, linguistic and behavioural disturbances at different periods.

We feel that they probably presented a severe and relatively pure sample of an epilepsy involving the prefrontal regions for which no focal lesion could be found. This idiopathic form of frontal epilepsy is probably quite rare, since frontal epilepsies are more often found to be lesional, unlike the perisylvian epilepsies such as acquired epileptic aphasia. The syndromes of partial epilepsy with CSWS and acquired epileptic aphasia are often considered as different but extreme manifestations of the spectrum of 'benign' partial epilepsies with focal sharp waves, but when making this analogy, care has to be taken to include only idiopathic forms of epilepsy with CSWS.

A new recent case, described below – a boy whom we could follow in detail before the deterioration and before the onset of CSWS – illustrates in a spectacular fashion many of the important issues related to this particular epileptic situation.

Case T.G.

T.G. was first seen at the age of 4 years 2 months following a first nocturnal seizure. In the preceding months, his mother had noticed brief episodes of sudden arrest of activity without eye deviation or movement, which had also been seen in the kindergarten. His first EEG showed focal sharp waves in the right occipital area. His cognitive development had been normal, but some features of his behaviour worried the family (tendency to repetitive behaviours and to remain alone), although this was not considered clearly pathological when we first saw him, except that he was hyperactive and inattentive and became increasingly so. A repeat EEG was then done at 5 years 3 months and showed bilateral focal sharp waves in the frontal region with almost continuous diffuse spike-waves during sleep (CSWS). He underwent his first detailed neuropsychological examination at 5 years 5 months. This was repeated two to four times a year until 9 years 6 months, with repeat sleep EEGs depending on the clinical evolution and antiepileptic drug changes (see Figs. 8.7 and 8.8).

At around 7 years he developed a severe behavioural disorder of 'frontal type' and a dysexecutive syndrome. At this age, he was unable to learn anything and had to be taken out of school. At his worst, he had perseverations (activities, games), stereotypies (verbal, gestural), aberrant repetitive behaviours (looking at running water, alignments, spinning of objects, interest in mechanical toys), dependence on environment ('stimulus-bound'), abnormal verbal and non-verbal communication, absence of initiative and play, thought disturbances (occurrence of unrelated perseverative thoughts and themes in conversation), and lack of social interests. A detailed questionnaire about social and emotional behaviour at his worst period showed that, despite qualitative impairments in emotional behaviour, he was able to

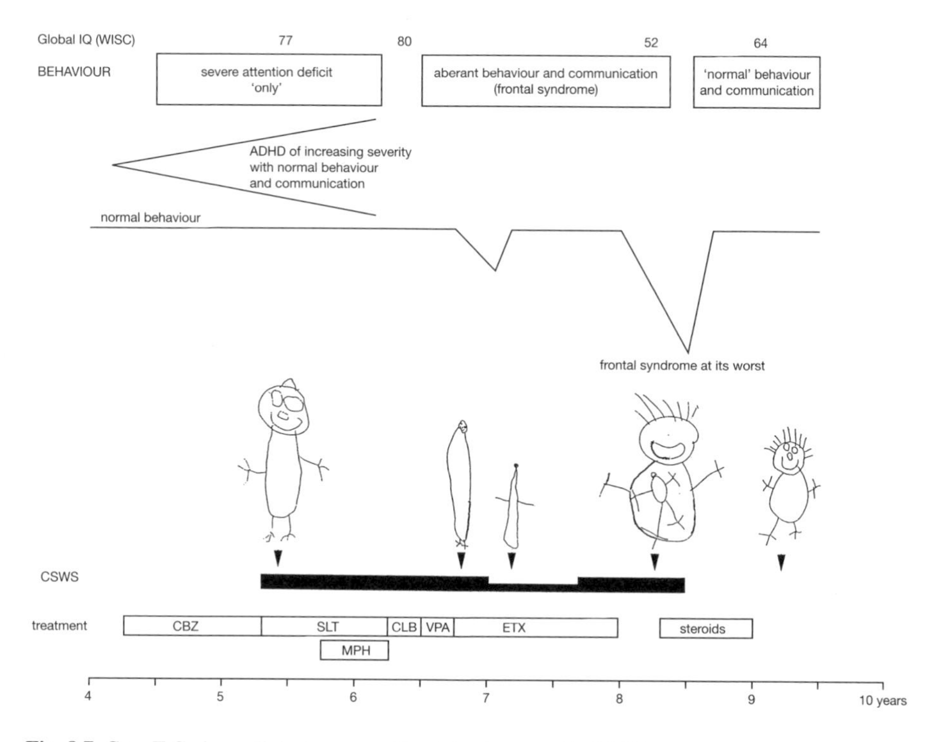

Fig. 8.7 Case T.G., boy: clinical course of frontal epilepsy with CSWS.

This figure shows the insidious evolution of behavioural-cognitive regression of psychotic type with cryptogenic frontal epilepsy and CSWS. A temporary improvement was seen with ethosuximide and a marked clinical and EEG improvement (disappearance of CSWS) occurred on prednisone. Note that there was initially an increasingly severe attention deficit disorder for about 18 months, but without cognitive regression at that stage. The cognitive regression occurred later, with a severe dysexecutive syndrome, stereotypies, aberrant behaviours and a thought disorder. (CBZ: carbamazepine, SLT: sulthiame, CLB: clobazam, VPA: valproate, ETX: ethosuximide, MPH: methylphenidate).

The figure also shows the child's drawing of a man at successive periods of the disease from 5 to 9 years. There was a regression in the quality of drawing during the worst phase of the disease, with recovery to the initial level but no significant progress during the four years of the disease.

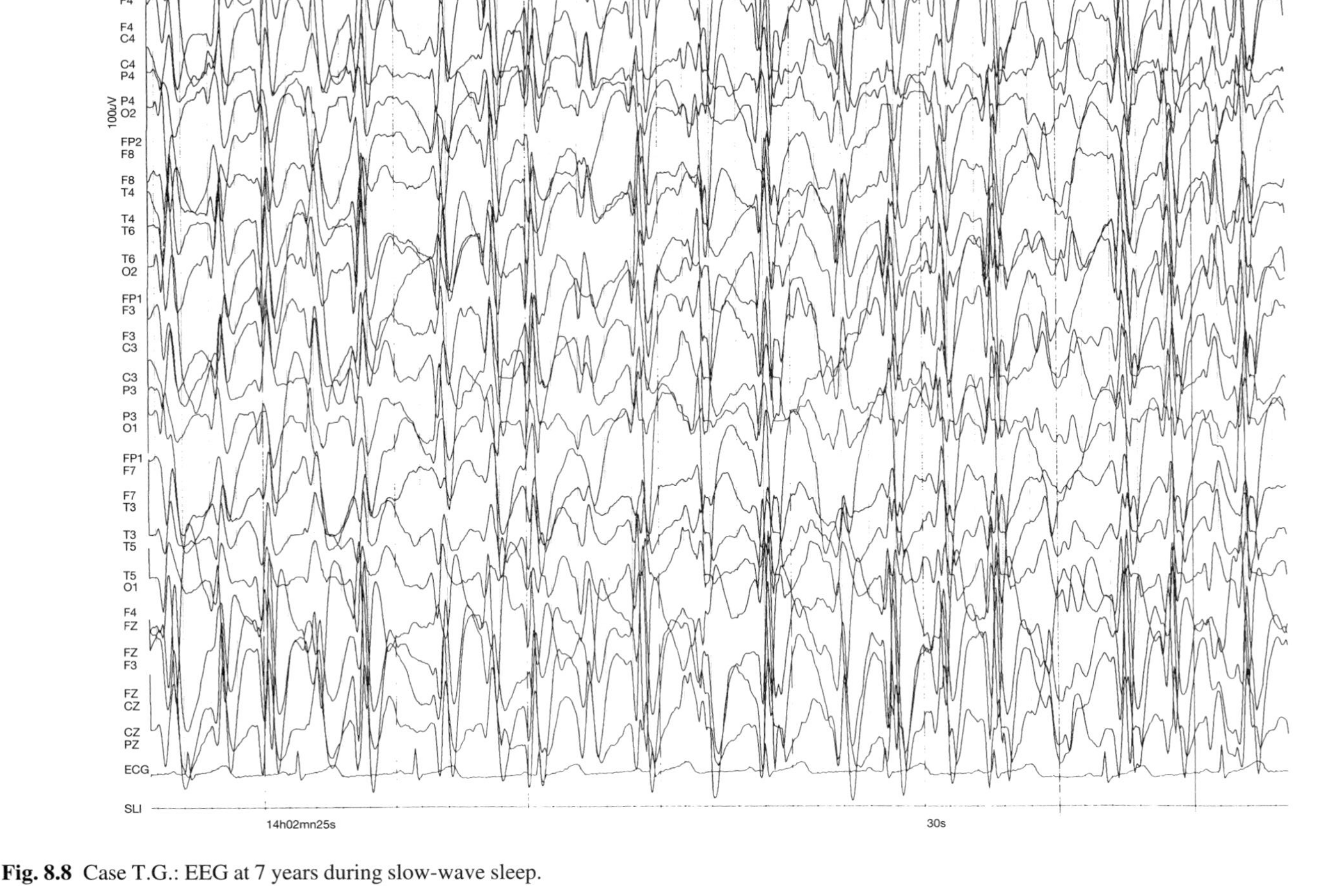

Fig. 8.8 Case T.G.: EEG at 7 years during slow-wave sleep.

Sleep EEG obtained shortly before treatment with prednisone was started, showing diffuse continuous spike-waves (typical CSWS pattern). During the waking state and the rare moments of less intense CSWS a bilateral but predominantly right frontal spike focus could be seen (not shown).

feel and express primary (sadness, happiness) and social emotions (pride, guilt). The emotions of a more cognitive nature (e.g. humour, worries, confidence) were the most impaired.

Ethosuximide led to some temporary clinical improvement and decrease of CSWS. Prednisone (which had initially been refused by the parents at 7 years 2 months) was started at 8 years 4 months, with spectacular clinical improvement and disappearance of CSWS within two months. Behaviour almost normalized, cognitive abilities began to recover, and, as the mother wrote to us, 'he started to learn for the first time in four years'. Prednisone was maintained for about a year, but decrease of the dose was followed by rapid relapse of CSWS and a new regression, though much less severe than the first one (the relapse is not shown in Fig. 8.7).

This remarkable case history and the data displayed in Fig. 8.7 about child T.G. deserve comment. This boy developed a most dramatic cognitive decline which had all the features of a severe executive disorder with massive behavioural-emotional disturbances, all due to a special partial epilepsy characterized by bifrontal epilepsy and CSWS. Importantly, we could document the progression from an increasingly severe but still isolated attention deficit disorder with hyperactivity to psychotic behaviour. With effective therapy and disappearance of CSWS, a marked improvement was seen both in his behaviour and in his cognitive abilities. At his worst, his behaviour had some 'autistic' characteristics such as marked stereotypies, repetitive behaviours and aberrant social communication. However, the late age at regression, the preservation of some emotional abilities and the florid thought disorder were features that distinguished this condition from autism, and were consistent on a behavioural level with a diagnosis of psychosis (see Chapter 12, section 12.4.4).

The behaviour problems in this child during the first year or two after onset of his epilepsy and before the full-blown frontal syndrome became manifest suggest that less severely affected children, whose epilepsy does not progress or in whom therapy is rapidly effective, may show only a mild cognitive stagnation, hyperactivity and attentional problems, but no major psychopathology or regression. This is a most important and challenging possibility because one is dealing with an epilepsy which directly interferes with attentional mechanisms and higher cortical functions, but this is difficult to prove. The attentional-behavioural symptoms are quite non-specific and can be due to different causes, such as drug effects, whereas the more complex psychological disturbances may be interpreted as reactive phenomena or the exacerbation of innate traits (Deonna et al 2002).

Within the spectrum of these cognitive-behavioural partial epilepsy syndromes, there are, or must be, even more complex situations, with a combination of a specific linguistic deficit, a general cognitive regression and behavioural problems of psychotic nature occurring together or successively. We suspect that these are not being reported because the tendency of neurologists and neuropsychologists is to look for and report pure neuropsychological syndromes.

One must be aware, of course, that besides partial epilepsy of prefrontal origin with CSWS, any epilepsy of whatever etiology which causes a prolonged or recurrent epileptic dysfunction in the prefrontal regions (from an epileptic focus in this region or by spread) can cause similar symptoms. This is shown in the case presented in Chapter 4 (R.A., newly diagnosed epilepsy). Such symptoms can also occur in epilepsy syndromes of genetic origin, namely epilepsy associated with ring chromosome 20, in which an acquired progressive epileptic cognitive regression with frontal nocturnal seizures was recently reported (Augustijn et al 2001).

Prognostic factors in partial epilepsies with CSWS

The prognostic factors are listed in Table 8.10. The table shows that CSWS in themselves are mainly the 'signature' of the activity of the disease and that a number of more important variables must be taken into account. In some situations, there might be no or minimal consequences, whereas in others the consequences can be devastating. One particularly unpredictable factor is how long the epileptic disease will last and whether a durably tolerable and effective antiepileptic therapy can be found. The duration of the disease may be related to the etiology, that is, whether there is a structural (but not always recognizable) focal lesion (i.e. a dysplasia) or whether the disorder is purely functional.

It must be noted that most studies on epilepsy with CSWS are not longitudinal and give only limited data on therapy and correlative EEG and clinical findings. There have been detailed single case observations where antiepileptic therapy, started very late after a delayed diagnosis and years of severe disability, was clearly effective, with spectacular improvement (Veggiotti et al 2001). How hard, how long and with how many different drugs one should persist in trying to suppress CSWS in late-recognized cases with severe cognitive delay or regression is open to question. It is a race against time, because CSWS will eventually disappear. Treatment with subpial transections, which has been used in acquired epileptic

TABLE 8.10
Important prognostic factors in partial epilepsies with CSWS

Factors	Comments
Location (function) of primary epileptic focus	Deficit is more specific if it affects a zone which has completed its maturation (before or after organization of relevant networks)
Age of appearance of CSWS	Before, during or after critical learning period for function concerned
Duration of activity of CSWS (months, years before diagnosis)	Continuous epileptic dysfunction (network cannot be used) or intermittent periods of normal function during the whole duration of epilepsy
Severity (intensity of epileptic process during active period)	Network cannot be used and/or function cannot be consolidated
Efficacy of therapy	Persistent or only temporary suppression of discharges with drugs (or surgery – multiple subpial transection) with tolerable side-effects

aphasia (Morrell et al 1995, Irwin et al 2001), has not to our knowledge been applied to other situations with partial epilepsy and CSWS, although in theory the basic epilepsy problem is the same (see Chapter 14).

8.5 West syndrome

Infants who present with the clinical syndrome of epileptic spasms (infantile spasms) with hypsarrhythmia on EEG (West syndrome) usually show a stagnation or regression in development corresponding to the onset but sometimes preceding the first recognized spasms.

Infantile spasms are now seen as an age-related generalized epileptic manifestation related to focal or more diffuse cortical lesions of any nature and location. It is customary to distinguish babies who were normal developmentally prior to the onset of the epilepsy, and in whom no etiology is found (cryptogenic cases), from those who already had a developmental delay (symptomatic cases), the majority of the former having normal long-term outcome (Gaily et al 1999). A global lack of interest in surroundings, irritability, sleep disturbances, and poor and fluctuating visual attention, sometimes presenting as blindness, are commonly noted in the acute phase, which is sometimes described as autistic. This particular aspect is discussed in Chapter 12, section 12.4.3).

West syndrome illustrates in a paradigmatic fashion how a continuous paroxysmal epileptic anomaly (seen on the EEG), and not the seizures themselves, which are brief, can present in an insidious way as a developmental arrest or regression. The spectacular improvement of behaviour and development when the EEG normalizes with therapy provides a clear illustration of the role of epilepsy. This is sometimes obscured by the behavioural side-effects seen with the classical treatment with ACTH. Since vigabatrin emerged as the first alternative effective therapy and is now quite often used as the initial drug, with no or minimal side-effects, this improvement is much more obvious and easy to see. The epileptic regression can be partially or totally reversible depending on the effective control of the epilepsy, but also on the etiology of the disorder. Many factors will influence the final prognosis, among others the duration of the epileptic syndrome, which depends on early diagnosis and successful treatment.

In babies who did not have a diffuse encephalopathy or severe developmental delay prior to the onset of epilepsy, the nature, location, extent and function of the brain area(s) involved have an influence on the early clinical manifestations and the long-term sequelae, in addition to the direct effect of the epilepsy. Babies with focal ischemic lesions in the sylvian region or congenital tumours who present with West syndrome may have a very good developmental prognosis. In babies with ultimately severe mental retardation and autistic features, functional imaging has shown bilateral pathology in the temporal lobes (Chugani et al 1996).

Few precise neuropsychological studies at the early stage of the disorder have examined whether specific aspects of early cognitive-perceptual development can be particularly involved (Guzzetta et al 1993). Focal paroxysmal EEG abnormalities, in addition to the diffuse hypsarrhythmia, are more often found in the posterior regions in babies with West syndrome (Koo and Hwang 1996), possibly because these regions mature earlier and faster than other cortical areas and can express the epileptic disorder earlier. Visual inattention that may indicate a specific dysfunction of the visual system is indeed an early and major sign in babies with West syndrome.

In a prospective study of high-risk babies with various perinatal lesions whose visual attention was systematically studied (using a special paradigm of attention shift) Guzzetta et al (2002) identified a few children who developed West syndrome. The evolution of their visual attention could be studied and compared before, during and after recovery from the epileptic syndrome. In one child, visual attention, which was normal initially, decreased with the onset of spasms but did not recover after remission. Whether this reflects a general attentional problem or a more specific alteration within the visual system is open to question, because other co-occurring developmental dimensions were not studied. Such studies, which are very difficult to carry out, show that the effects of early epilepsy may now be approached with new paradigms developed by experimental psychologists.

Children with late onset epileptic spasms are discussed in Chapter 12.

8.6 Epilepsy with absence seizures

It is not unusual to encounter children with very frequent and long-standing absences before the diagnosis of epilepsy is made who do not seem to have suffered any cognitive or behavioural consequences. This indicates that very brief interruptions of cognitive activity may be well tolerated and that cognitive capacities may not be altered beyond these brief periods. On the other hand, others become inattentive, fail in school or have behaviour problems shortly after the disorder starts, or even before the diagnosis is made, and improve very much on medication which suppresses the absences. This suggests important differences between absences which on the clinical level appear typical.

During the typical 3 c/s spike-wave discharge, there is a momentary interruption of the capacity to carry out or initiate a voluntary action (motor arrest), in addition to a disturbance in conscious awareness (Gloor 1986). It is thus not possible to find out directly if any sensory perception or other kind of information processing has occurred or can occur. The term ‘loss of consciousness’ supposes that there is an inability to assimilate any information during an absence. In fact, one should rather speak of loss of conscious awareness (Gloor 1991, Damasio 1999), because forced choice experiments and other evidence suggest that, in some absences, information can be processed but cannot be retrieved voluntarily. There is also experimental evidence in conditioned rats carrying the genetic spike-wave trait that information processing can occur during spike-wave discharges (Drinkenburg et al 2003).

The clinical data and the EEG correlates, which often show a frontal predominance, are calling into question whether even typical absences with apparently generalized spike-wave discharges are not in fact ‘focal’ in the sense that they involve a specific but distributed thalamocortical circuit. The normal function of this circuit is essential for motor initiation and/or conscious awareness to be present (van Emde Boas et al 2003).

Children are usually unaware that they have had an absence. They learn that a discontinuity in an ongoing activity or an unexplainable change in the world means that they have had one, but in ordinary life this is not a sure guide. A high degree of vigilance is usually a protective factor against absences and rarely a provoking one (Matsuoka et al 2000). We have seen two children whose absences were increased by demanding tasks or triggered by specific activities (cognitive or physical), so that factors other than attentional ones may play a role.

Typical childhood petit mal absence epilepsy seems to be the ideal situation to study the possible cognitive consequences of the basic genetic trait responsible for primary generalized epilepsy. It is a well-delineated clinical syndrome and it is easy to rule out that the patient is having even a minimal seizure at time of testing. Despite this, there are very few studies which have addressed this question. As the differences from the controls are likely to be small, any confounding factor or individual characteristic of the case has to be taken into account. In a recent study on neuropsychological assessment in children with absence epilepsy, Pavone et al (2001) studied 16 subjects and controls. All subjects were on antiepileptic therapy (three with two drugs). There were marked interindividual differences in IQ (total, verbal and performance) in the group with absences (up to 40 points), indicating that other variables apart from the epilepsy were playing a role.

8.7 Non-convulsive status epilepticus

The fact that mental changes of prolonged duration can be the sole manifestation of epilepsy has been a historical landmark in the recognition of the cognitive-behavioural aspects of epilepsy (Putnam 1941, Bornstein et al 1956, Goldensohn and Gold 1960).

Non-convulsive status epilepticus is a general term to describe prolonged episodes of altered mental state without obvious motor manifestations. These are associated with more or less continuous epileptic activity on the EEG. The prototype is the so-called absence status (petit mal status, status pycnolepticus, spike-wave stupor) in primary generalized epilepsy (Andermann and Robb 1972), but non-convulsive status epilepticus can have a focal origin (non-convulsive status epilepticus of frontal or temporal origin (Engel et al 1986, Thomas et al 1999)), even though the surface EEG may show diffuse abnormalities.

During non-convulsive status epilepticus, the behaviour of the children is described as 'apathetic', 'slow', 'somnolent', 'inattentive', 'amnesic', with 'absence of initiative' and 'reduced speech' (Manning and Rosenbloom 1987). What these descriptions mean in terms of affected cognitive systems is rarely if ever studied in detail and can probably be quite variable. Indeed, clinical experience suggests that different cognitive abilities can be preserved or altered during such episodes and that it is not an 'all or nothing' situation. Only detailed studies during the ictal state can answer these questions (Matsuoka et al 1986, Gloor 1991, Thomas et al 1999).

A unique and recently described situation is epilepsy associated with ring chromosome 20, in which there are frequent and refractory episodes of non-convulsive status epilepticus. Although it has been known for some time that a severe epilepsy can occur in this syndrome, it is only in the past few years that the special and unique electroclinical manifestations of this syndrome with refractory episodes of non-convulsive status epilepticus have been recognized (Inoue et al 1997, Roubertie et al 2000). These episodes of non-convulsive status epilepticus are clinically different from a classical petit mal or temporal lobe status, and the ictal EEG shows bursts of rhythmic theta or notched slow waves with frontal predominance. Frontal lobe ictal onset was found in one patient during presurgical evaluation (Inoue et al

1997). Because of the frequency of episodes, it is possible to carry out ictal neuropsychological studies with some specific questions in mind, as shown in the following case.

Case K.C.:
Non-convulsive status epilepticus associated with ring chromosome 20

This girl's epilepsy started at the age of 8 years and has always been refractory, but she has remained cognitively and behaviourally normal. At 18 years a videoEEG and some neuropsychological tests were done before, during and just after the end of an episode of non-convulsive status epilepticus lasting 12 minutes (triggered by hyperventilation), and six weeks later. During the seizure, the young woman could understand, speak, have access to old memories, and learn some new material (although not normally), and she was able after a delay of six weeks to recall some of the material she was exposed to during the seizure. Memory functions were thus remarkably preserved during the seizure which mainly affected initiative and speed of cognitive processing. It was interpreted as a transient dysexecutive state, consistent with the predominant frontal epileptic activity on EEG.

8.8 Febrile seizures

For a long time, there has been concern that repeated febrile seizures could lead to minor damage to the brain which might result in cognitive disadvantage in the long term. Older studies had suggested that this might be the case. However, these studies did not or could not always exclude children with a pre-existing brain pathology or an epileptic tendency manifesting initially with seizures during febrile episodes, either (or both) of which could have affected cognitive development. In fact, there is no evidence that even frequent typical febrile seizures have any impact on cognitive development. A carefully controlled and prospective British study of a large sample of children with simple febrile seizures followed up to the age of 10 years did not show any differences compared to controls. This study has, in our opinion, definitively settled the matter (Verity et al 1998, Baram 2003).

In the last few years, families with members having either febrile seizures and/or generalized non-febrile seizures (grand mal epilepsy) in several generations have been reported, the so-called GEFS+ (generalized epilepsy with febrile seizures plus) (Scheffer et al 1995, Scheffer and Berkovic 1997). In some of these families, children with either myoclonic-astatic epilepsy or severe myoclonic epilepsy of infancy (or Dravet syndrome) have also been reported, and these genetic epilepsies are now increasingly found to be related to various ion channel mutations. Myoclonic-astatic epilepsy and severe myoclonic epilepsy of infancy are discussed in Chapter 11 on mental retardation and 'epileptic encephalopathies' (section 11.3.2).

9 EPILEPTIC COGNITIVE DYSFUNCTION IN SOME SPECIFIC BRAIN PATHOLOGIES

We have seen that the epilepsies or epileptic syndromes that have the most important cognitive impact can be 'non-lesional' epilepsies. The cognitive disorders are related to functional bioelectric abnormalities without demonstrable brain pathology.

However, there are special developmental or acquired brain anomalies which are interesting models for one aspect or the other of the cognition–epilepsy relationship. New techniques of brain imaging, data from epilepsy surgery, neuropathology, neuropsychology and genetics are increasingly showing that not all epileptic pathologies affect brain excitability and brain function in the same way, so that different cognitive consequences (or none) can be seen. The most relevant examples are briefly reviewed here.

9.1 Malformations

9.1.1 Focal Cortical Dysplasias

Focal dysplasias are often very epileptogenic, although not always so and sometimes only after many years. It is not unusual to diagnose on MRI a large area of dysplasia in an older perfectly normal child being evaluated after a first epileptic seizure. By definition, those who are diagnosed and draw the most attention are those who present with epilepsy which often turns out to be refractory.

The nature of disturbed local brain excitability within and around an area of dysplasia and the local and distant circuits with which the dysplasia might be connected probably represents a unique epileptic situation, which differs from what is seen with an ischemic lesion or a tumour, for example (Sisodiya et al 1995). Even with high resolution MRI, focal cortical dysplasias may remain undetected and only be found on histopathological examination after surgery. There is often an overlap with normal neural tissue, and a specific function normally ascribed to an affected region may persist in its neighbourhood, sometimes in a modified manner. The transfer of function to the contralateral 'normal' hemisphere, which is seen with a large hemispheric ischemic lesion of prenatal or early postnatal onset, does not seem to occur with dysplasia (Duchowny et al 1996, Roulet-Perez et al 1998).

Case G.S.

This boy had suffered complex partial seizures and severe language, cognitive and behavioural deterioration from the age of 3 years 6 months, with a left frontotemporal EEG focus and continuous spike-waves during sleep. After a long relative remission of his epilepsy, seizures became intractable and he had epilepsy surgery at the age of 25 years. Cortical stimulation over the left lateral frontal area elicited speech and reading arrest, and the remembrance of a similar experience of spontaneous intermittent speech difficulties as a young child. Histology after surgery revealed cortical dysplasia not visible on MRI (Roulet-Perez et al 1998).

This observation suggests that, despite early onset and many years of continuous epileptic activity originating from an extensive area of his left frontal lobe, the language functions had been maintained on that side, at least partially.

9.1.2 The Special Case of Tuberous Sclerosis Complex

Tuberous sclerosis is a remarkable but insufficiently studied model for the study of the cognitive effects of epilepsy. Affected children may be fully normal, mildly or severely mentally retarded, or present autistic features, independently of epilepsy. This depends on the severity of the disease as determined, at least in part, by the size, location and number of tubers (Curatolo 2003).

Contrary to previous beliefs, a proportion of children with tuberous sclerosis complex have normal intelligence. Bourneville, a pioneer in the care of people with mental retardation, first described this condition as a physician in institutions for mental diseases in Paris. He was not in a position to see the spectrum of the disease (Gateaux-Mennecier 1989).

Because of its extreme epileptogenicity and possible onset from any brain area, tuberous sclerosis may cause any sort of epilepsy, starting at any age, often very early, presenting typically as West syndrome. Children with West syndrome due to tuberous sclerosis complex usually have massive regression and severe permanent mental retardation, but some recover and may have a normal or near normal outcome. Acquired but reversible autistic behaviour associated with complex partial seizures of temporal origin has also been observed (Deonna et al 1993b).

In children with tuberous sclerosis and mental retardation, epilepsy may be a major additional factor in the cognitive disability. A highly epileptogenic tuber may have a direct impact on cognition, depending on the area involved and the spread of the epileptic activity. This has practical implications for therapy, including the possibility of surgery in selected cases (Guerreiro et al 1998).

Case M.K.

This girl presented at 7 weeks with numerous focal seizures. Cerebral imaging showed a large calcified dysplastic lesion in the left occipito-parietal region and multiple additional cortical lesions typical of tuberous sclerosis. Seizures were refractory to treatment. Presurgical work-up showed that all were originating in the large left posterior calcified tuber, which was removed surgically at 14 months. Unfortunately seizures relapsed three months after surgery, this time originating from foci in the right parietal and left frontal areas. Control was finally obtained at 4 years 4 months with a combination of topiramate and lamotrigine. Developmental evaluations showed complete stagnation for several months before surgery, with slow progress thereafter. A second episode of stagnation occurred at the period of a severe seizure relapse. At the age of 5 years, after eight months without seizures, there was a significant global cognitive deficit (DQ 32), with short attention span and some repetitive behaviours. The child had good social skills, however, and was able to speak in short sentences of two to three words. Apart from a well-compensated hemianopia, there were no visual problems. This evolution illustrates the important additive role of an active epilepsy, responsible here for cognitive stagnation related to an underlying multifocal cortical pathology that had already limited her potential for development.

The overall importance of epilepsy in the cognitive disability of children with tuberous sclerosis is variable. Epilepsy is certainly only one factor, because there are many normally intelligent children with tuberous sclerosis complex who have epilepsy. Children with mental retardation with tuberous sclerosis all have epilepsy but they also have many tubers in various locations which are the main cause of their intellectual disability. However, there may be children with tuberous sclerosis whose epilepsy is the primary factor responsible for mental retardation or an autistic spectrum disorder. This depends on the age at onset, type, site of origin, spread and, importantly, the severity of the epilepsy (Gillberg et al 1996, Curatolo 2003). The role of epilepsy arising in the temporal lobes in children with tuberous sclerosis and associated autism has recently been suggested in an important study by Bolton et al (2002) (see Chapter 12, section 12.4.3).

9.1.3 Hypothalamic Hamartoma

Hypothalamic hamartoma with gelastic seizures (i.e. seizures characterized by an abnormal laugh as the ictal manifestation) and precocious puberty is now a well-recognized phenomenon (Berkovic et al 1997). Epilepsy is of early onset and often refractory, and affected children almost always develop severe behavioural-cognitive changes over the years. It is now accepted that this is in direct relationship to the activity of the epilepsy originating in the dysplastic tissue and spreading to frontal cortex, amygdala and limbic structures.

It is a remarkable model for studying the effects of an early epilepsy originating from and spreading to areas which are fundamentally important for emotional and cognitive development (Berkovic 2003). There are very few detailed neuropsychological and psychiatric studies on this topic (Dusser 1992, Deonna and Ziegler 2000, Frattali et al 2001, Weissenberger et al 2001, Perez-Jimenez et al 2003).

In recent years, medically refractory cases have benefited from new surgical techniques (gamma-knife therapy, disconnection of the tumour) or other techniques (vagal nerve stimulation), with seemingly good results, not only for the epilepsy but also for behaviour. There are now unique opportunities to carry out detailed studies before and after surgery on the cognitive, mainly psychiatric consequences of this dramatic condition.

9.1.4 Double Cortex Syndrome (Subcortical Band Heterotopias)

In this brain malformation, which belongs to the recently recognized agyria-pachygyria-band spectrum (Barkovich et al 1996), cognitive development is usually moderately affected, although some affected women have cognitive functions in the normal range. Epilepsy is very frequent and sometimes severe. There have been a few neuropsychological studies in patients with double cortex (Jacobs et al 2001), but to our knowledge no follow-up studies have raised the question of whether epilepsy could be an additional or important factor in the cognitive disability. In a young girl with double cortex and moderately severe epilepsy, who never had status epilepticus or multiple drugs and whom we followed from 5 to 16 years, we could document a stagnation in cognitive abilities over the years. Although this evolution does not prove a direct causal role of epilepsy, it raises this important possibility. Epilepsy should be considered as a possible direct contributing factor to cognitive dysfunction even in conditions where the basic pathology seems a sufficient explanation (see Chapter 11 on mental retardation).

9.2 Acquired lesions

Any acquired cortical lesion, of whatever cause, may become epileptogenic and lead to a chronic focal epilepsy, but two situations stand out from the point of view of severity, chronicity, or impact on cognitive functions and behaviour.

9.2.1 Focal Vascular Ischemic Lesions of Prenatal Origin

Ischemic lesions of vascular origin (mainly middle cerebral artery infarction of the perisylvian region of prenatal or perinatal origin) are a common cause of hemiplegic cerebral palsy. Epilepsy occurs in about 50 per cent of the cases and epileptic discharges on the affected hemisphere are an almost constant feature, even when there are no clinical seizures. A subgroup of children with this pathology have a severe intractable epilepsy with major cognitive and behavioural problems for which hemispherectomy is a very effective procedure. In these cases, the ischemic pathology usually had a prenatal onset, and such difficult epilepsies do not, or only very exceptionally, occur after a stroke sustained in the perinatal period.

Other types of prenatal lesions, such as focal or unilateral hemispheral polymicrogyria due to ischemic damage sustained in the second trimester of pregnancy (but also sometimes of developmental origin), can be the cause of severe partial epilepsies with diffuse continuous epileptic activity during sleep (CSWS) and cognitive regression. In a study of 12 children (age range 5 to 13 years) with epilepsy, congenital hemiplegia and unilateral polymicrogyria, Caraballo et al (1999) noted a deterioration of cognitive performance during the active phase of the epilepsy, characterized mainly by atonic seizures and frequent bilateral epileptic discharges and CSWS. Cognitive performance returned to its previous mildly to moderately retarded level after seizure control. In these cases, an unexpected remission of the epilepsy was obtained with medical treatment, despite the severe initial course.

9.2.2 Hippocampal Sclerosis

Hippocampal sclerosis is the most frequent pathology in children with refractory temporal lobe epilepsy. Remarkably, however, despite the occasional local propagation of the epileptic discharges to other parts of the limbic system (Avanzini 2001, Wennberg et al 2002) and the frequent spread to homotopic areas of the contralateral hemisphere, the affected children usually have normal cognitive development, and a relatively good memory, suggesting that an enormous plasticity must exist in this system. They must rely entirely on an intact contralateral homologous region or a reorganization elsewhere on the same side, because surgical ablation of the hippocampus and amygdala (or whole anterior temporal lobe) on the affected side does not affect, or only minimally, memory functions when there is significant pathology in these structures (Hermann et al 1997, Mabbott and Smith 2003).

One of the reasons why cognitive functions and in particular memory may be relatively unaffected is that the onset of the epilepsy is often relatively late in childhood. In these cases, where the brain pathology has been acquired early, before it became epileptogenic, an efficient reorganization is more likely to have occurred (see Chapter 7, section 7.3.2 on memory).

10
EPILEPSY SURGERY IN CHILDREN: AN OPPORTUNITY TO STUDY THE DIRECT ROLE OF EPILEPSY IN COGNITIVE DISTURBANCES

In the final section of the famous book, *Epilepsy and the Functional Anatomy of the Human Brain* (Penfield and Jasper 1954), entitled 'Case examples', Penfield, the father of epilepsy surgery, chose to describe in detail three patients. Two of these were children at the time of surgery and all had a congenital or early acquired ischemic focal brain pathology.

'Among patients who have large areas of abnormality of one hemisphere, abnormality of behavior may appear, together with advancing mental retardation. The behavior abnormality is often a more important complaint than the seizures themselves.' Penfield coined the dramatic term 'nociferous cortex': 'Radical complete excision may stop the seizures, may correct the abnormality of behavior, and may allow improvement of the mental state' (Penfield and Jasper 1954: 841).

The surgical removal of the epileptic source (and of its spreading to the healthy functional areas of the same hemisphere or to the contralateral unaffected side) was considered the most important cause of the behavioural improvement. It was assumed that the removed hemisphere played no useful function and that the cognitive improvement after cessation of the seizures was proof of the deleterious role of the epilepsy.

Fifty years later, and despite many refinements in diagnostic methods and surgical techniques, we are still struggling to document and understand precisely how this 'nociferous cortex' is responsible for the cognitive and behavioural symptoms which Penfield clearly recognized as being directly related to the epileptic activity. It still remains difficult to separate the roles of all the different factors that contribute to the improvement (less time lost in seizures, fewer drugs, better mood, independence, etc.).

We will now review the new and unique clinical opportunities offered by the development of epilepsy surgery for understanding the direct role of epilepsy in cognitive development and behaviour in a great variety of epileptic situations. Data obtained during presurgical work-up and the clinical changes that may be seen after total and immediate cessation of seizures with successful epilepsy surgery can be a unique source of information on the role of epilepsy on cognition and behaviour.

10.1 Documentation of cognitive-behavioural manifestations during seizures and during the postictal state

During presurgical work-up, electroclinical seizures are recorded, often after partial or total drug withdrawal. The patient is in hospital and can be constantly observed. Although it is an unnatural situation, the behaviour of the child and the alteration or the maintenance of cognitive capacities during the seizure and the postictal state can be repeatedly documented. It is a unique opportunity, too often neglected, to study the cognitive-behavioural manifestations of epilepsy. These can be very variable from one seizure to the other, or between patients with an apparently similar epileptic syndrome or the same type of seizures (Gloor 1991). Good previous knowledge of the case can lead to a hypothesis as to what exactly happens during seizures, and determine which cognitive domain should receive priority for testing during the limited time available and be retested at different moments in the same episode or during successive ones.

10.2 Pre- per- and postoperative recordings

Peroperative electrocorticographic recordings and simultaneous surface EEG recordings can indicate the main source and local extension of the epileptic focus and its spread to the same or opposite hemisphere. Disappearance of the epileptic activity after surgery is an important indication of what has been achieved.

In epileptic syndromes with language and/or cognitive regression and continuous diffuse epileptic activity on the surface EEG (mainly during the so-called continuous spike-waves during slow wave sleep), electrocorticographic studies have been very important in confirming that symptoms are indeed related to a primary focus with secondary diffusion, and such studies have greatly contributed to the understanding of these syndromes (Morrell et al 1995).

10.3 Correlation of function/location using direct stimulation studies

Cortical stimulation of language zones with simultaneous language testing, which has been done extensively in adults (Penfield and Jasper 1954, Ojeman 1983, Lesser et al 1994), has now been applied to children. This has helped in understanding in which types of focal epileptic pathology (and its location and extension) there is a shift of language to the contralateral hemisphere or other reorganizations of function (Duchowny et al 1996).

10.4 Successful surgical removal of epileptogenic zone and cessation of seizures

Depending on the situation and type of surgery, the spread of abnormal epileptic activity is interrupted without damage because the diseased epileptogenic zone was non-functional, but sometimes an unknown amount of healthy tissue has to be removed. Any or all of these factors may contribute to the effect of epilepsy surgery on cognitive functions. When a marked improvement occurs rapidly after control of seizures without any negative effect on development or worsening of any cognitive function, this clearly shows the predominant deleterious role of epilepsy and the negligible role of the tissue removal (Caplan et al 1992b, Chugani and Muller 1999).

10.5 Hemispherectomy in childhood epilepsy and its importance for developmental neuropsychology

10.5.1 What Can We Learn from Hemispherectomy?

A single healthy hemisphere, when the contralateral one has been damaged early on in life or has been surgically removed or disconnected, may support practically all mental functions. This situation is also sometimes compatible with normal intelligence. It has been and still is a source of amazement (Battros 2000). Children who have to undergo hemispherectomy for intractable epilepsy are a potential source of information on important questions regarding brain organization and some aspects of plasticity in the case of early brain lesions and in epilepsy.

Hemispherectomy is one of the classical models showing that the right hemisphere can support language, because in cases where the usually dominant but severely damaged left hemisphere has been surgically removed or disconnected, the removal does not affect language at all (Bishop and Mogford 1988, Vargha-Khadem and Mishkin 1997).

Table 10.1 shows some of the neuropsychological questions which have been addressed in children who were treated by hemispherectomy for their epilepsy.

Language recovery may occur rapidly when the epileptogenic left hemisphere is disconnected, suggesting that the right hemisphere which had taken up language before epilepsy started had been relieved from epileptic inhibition (Rosenblatt et al 1998).

It should be emphasized that the above conclusions are derived from a very few cases. The specific clinical and neuropathological characteristics of each case have to be available and brought to the attention of the neuropsychologists who undertake such studies and usually do the theorizing, because the results may be influenced by any of these factors. These are summarized in Table 10.2. Studies using hemispherectomy cases are especially valuable when a specific paradigm (e.g. language lateralization on functional imaging) is chosen. Precise longitudinal documentation of clinical changes at frequent determined intervals can be undertaken shortly before and after surgery.

TABLE 10.1
Questions raised and data obtained in studies of children undergoing hemispherectomy

This table lists some important neuropsychological findings which have been obtained from studies of single, or a few, cases of children with refractory epilepsy who have undergone hemispherectomy.

- A single hemisphere can support most cognitive functions and this situation is compatible with normal language and at least low-normal or borderline intelligence
- The right hemisphere has an innate capacity for many receptive linguistic capacities (Boatman et al 1999)
- The right hemisphere can develop significant language even after the early years (up to puberty?) provided that the pathology of the left hemisphere occurred early (Vargha-Khadem and Mishkin 1997, Boatman et al 1999, Hertz-Pannier et al 2002)
- Language recovery may occur rapidly when the epileptogenic left hemisphere is disconnected, suggesting that right hemisphere language has been relieved from epileptic inhibition (Rosenblatt et al 1998)

TABLE 10.2
Hemispherectomy for intractable epilepsy:
important factors in the interpretation of neuropsychological findings

This table shows the important variables that need to be taken into account in the interpretation of neuropsychological studies in cases of hemispherectomy (Villemure and Rasmussen 1993, Vining et al 1997, Devlin et al 2003).

- Age at onset (prenatal, perinatal, postnatal), extent, location and side of lesion causing epilepsy (e.g. stroke)
- Integrity of contralateral hemisphere (absence of epileptogenic and other lesions)
- Nature of brain pathology (static or progressive*)
- Age at onset of epilepsy
- Duration of active epilepsy prior to therapy (hemispherectomy)
- Spread of epilepsy from original site(s), homolateral and contralateral
- Age (chronological) at the time of hemispherectomy
- Postoperative epilepsy variables (total control, antiepileptic drugs)

* Sturge–Weber syndrome and Rasmussen's encephalitis are examples of progressive pathologies with intractable epilepsy for which hemispherectomy is performed.

10.5.2 Language After Hemispherectomy of the Dominant Hemisphere

The studies below illustrate two important questions which have been studied in children undergoing hemispherectomy of the dominant hemisphere.

Shift in hemispheric dominance for language: documentation with functional imaging (Hertz-Pannier et al 2002)

Fig. 10.1 shows a case report of a boy with left Rasmussen syndrome, who was ambidextrous. Onset of seizures was at 5 years 5 months. The boy was tested at 6 years 9 months and had normal language. A first (f)MRI at 6 years 10 months showed left lateralization of language networks. Subpial transection of the left motor strip at 7 years 2 months, followed by resection of the left paracentral lobule at 7 years 4 months for intractable seizures, were both unsuccessful. An attempted (f)MRI at 7 years 8 months failed. A left hemispherectomy was performed at 9 years. After surgery there was complete mutism with loss of reading and counting (there was no detailed language testing prior to the procedure, but there was no obvious aphasia). Three months after surgery, the boy's semantic comprehension scored at a 6-year-old level. Eighteen months after surgery, he could construct short sentences and read some words. At that time the repeat (f)MRI showed right-sided activated networks for language tasks. These results suggest that the right hemisphere had progressively taken over language function between 7 and 10 years 6 months, possibly partly before surgery and partly afterwards.

Dynamics of language progression after hemispherectomy

When a rapid specific improvement occurs after surgery, a direct role of epilepsy (either suppression of spread of discharges, or alleviation of inhibition to the healthy hemisphere) can be considered. Table 10.3 has been compiled on the basis of the information provided in two single case studies which give good longitudinal data.

In these two cases, there was a remarkable improvement in language acquisition postoperatively after years of very slow and limited progress. However, the dynamics of

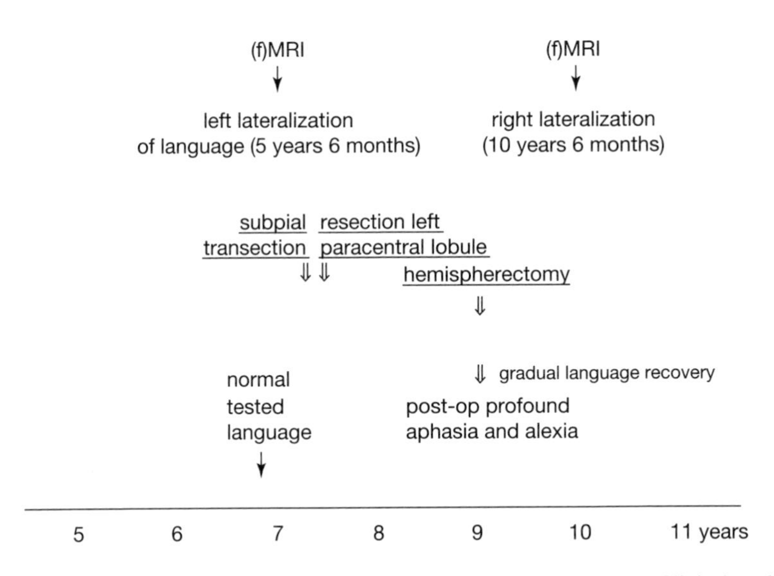

Fig. 10.1 Late plasticity for language in a child's non-dominant hemisphere. Clinical evolution and timing of investigations in a child reported by Hertz-Pannier, constructed from case report (Hertz-Pannier et al 2002).

The figure shows the history, timing and type of investigations in the remarkable case study of Hertz-Pannier et al, who were able to document with functional imaging the shift in dominance for language after hemispherectomy in a child with a progressive epileptogenic pathology in the language areas of the left hemisphere (see text).

TABLE 10.3
Dynamics of language development after hemispherectomy for epilepsy

	Vargha-Khadem et al (*Brain* 1997a)	**Rosenblatt et al (*Epilepsia* 1998)**
Underlying epileptogenic pathology	Sturge–Weber, left	Prenatal middle cerebral artery infarction, left
Age at hemispherectomy	8 years 6 months	3 years 8 months
Indication for hemispherectomy	Intractable epilepsy	Continuous epileptic discharges on the damaged hemisphere with developmental stagnation
Language before hemispherectomy	8 years 2 months: expressive speech: 'nearly non-existent' (unable to score); receptive vocabulary: ~ 4 years, 1 month	3 years 5 months: 35 words
Language after hemispherectomy	9 years: no change in expressive speech From 9 years 4 months on: 'within several months dramatic breakthrough, producing full sentences. At 10 years could converse with copious and appropriate speech'	Within nine months 'postoperatively' expressive speech improved from 35 to 750 words. At 3 years 9 months: mean length utterances: 4. At 7 years 6 months: mean length utterances: 8

'recovery' was quite different in the two cases. In Varga-Khadem et al's case (1997b), there was practically no change in speech until about one year after surgery, with surprisingly rapid progress thereafter. In Rosenblatt et al's case (1998), speech improvement was much more rapid, apparently from the time of surgery, but quantified comparative measures were given only after nine months. If the relief of an inhibitory effect of epileptic discharges on the healthy hemisphere is the possible main reason for the rapid improvement in Rosenblatt et al's patient, this was not the case in Varga-Khadem et al's patient. Factors such as the nature of the underlying pathology (i.e. whether it was 'sufficient' to provoke a shift to the healthy hemisphere), age at surgery and duration of 'bombardment' of the healthy hemisphere are probably major variables which contribute to the rapidity and amount of improvement after epilepsy surgery. Further studies with frequent enough follow-ups to evaluate the dynamics of the changes in similar cases will be important.

10.5.3 Cognitive-Behavioural Regression Due to Spread Distant from the Epileptic Activity: Improvement After Hemispherotomy

Case C.R.

We have studied a child with right congenital hemiplegia due to a left prenatal middle cerebral artery infarction, who developed epilepsy with CSWS, and massive cognitive and behavioural regression, with a typical frontal syndrome, between the ages of 4 and 5 years (Kallay 2005). Preoperative EEG recordings showed spread of the epileptic discharges from the left centroparietal to homolateral and contralateral frontal areas, which stopped immediately after functional hemispherotomy. Follow-up showed a rapid disappearance of the frontal symptoms. In this case, the spread of the epileptic activity to the 'healthy' frontal region caused the main clinical picture.

The new possibilities offered by the extensive presurgical study of the localization of the epileptic activity and corticographic peroperative recordings, coupled with precise developmental and neuropsychological pre- and postoperative evaluations, offer unique opportunities to relate the type of cognitive-behavioural problems to the main site of the epileptic dysfunction. These evaluations may also help in understanding the causes of persistent mental disability in children whose epilepsy has been successfully treated.

10.6 Epilepsy surgery in very young children

Infants with refractory epilepsy submitted to surgical therapy often have severe developmental delay and poor developmental prognosis due to their basic brain pathology, so that the aggravating role of epilepsy is difficult to judge. However, this need not always be the case. Some young children with focal dysplasias or Sturge–Weber syndrome may have a period of normal early development prior to onset of epilepsy and a good cognitive potential. In these cases, the dynamics of development after surgery when seizures have stopped is an important source of information. It may, for example, show whether developmental programmes which could not unfold due to frequent epileptic seizures can do so at a later date, or whether a critical period of development has been missed irretrievably. Detailed prospective studies of the dynamics and nature of developmental changes pre- and post-operatively over a prolonged period may be able to confirm or refute some of the hypotheses put forward on the direct role of epilepsy in these situations.

Case A.G. (Fig. 10.2)

This baby with a normal prenatal and perinatal history had numerous intractable complex partial and left focal motor seizures from the first weeks of life. MRI showed a large single area of right parietooccipitotemporal dysplasia. At 9 months of age epilepsy surgery consisting of disconnection of the dysplasia from the adjacent cortex and right temporal lobectomy (Daniel et al 2004) was performed, with immediate cessation of seizures. Using the Bayley developmental scale, evaluations were made at 6 months of age and postoperatively at 11 months, 15 months, 22 months and 39 months. A very rapid developmental gain was seen in the first two months following surgery, whereas progress was much slower in the following months. The rapid gain was not due to antiepileptic drug withdrawal and there was no recurrence of epilepsy (clinical or EEG) later on. The rapid initial improvement was probably directly related to the cessation of the almost continuous ictal and postictal states, allowing whatever development had taken place before surgery to become manifest.

Before surgery, the true level of development was indeed difficult to quantify with tests because of frequent seizures when the child was seen, but the mother had noticed moments of better social interaction, vocalization, reaching for objects and smiling during the rare hours or days without seizures, suggesting that some development was taking place despite the almost continuous epilepsy. The later much slower rate of development reflects the child's basic potential, which may be limited by his brain malformation and the possible additional brain damage from very early severe epilepsy and from the antiepileptic drugs.

Further and longer follow-up of this child and similar cases will be necessary to document the dynamics of development and the possible direct contribution of the ongoing seizures themselves. In this child, if seizures do not recur, it is possible that later-occurring repair-compensatory phenomena will allow better and faster developmental progress than has been seen in the last two years.

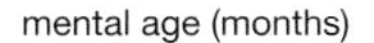

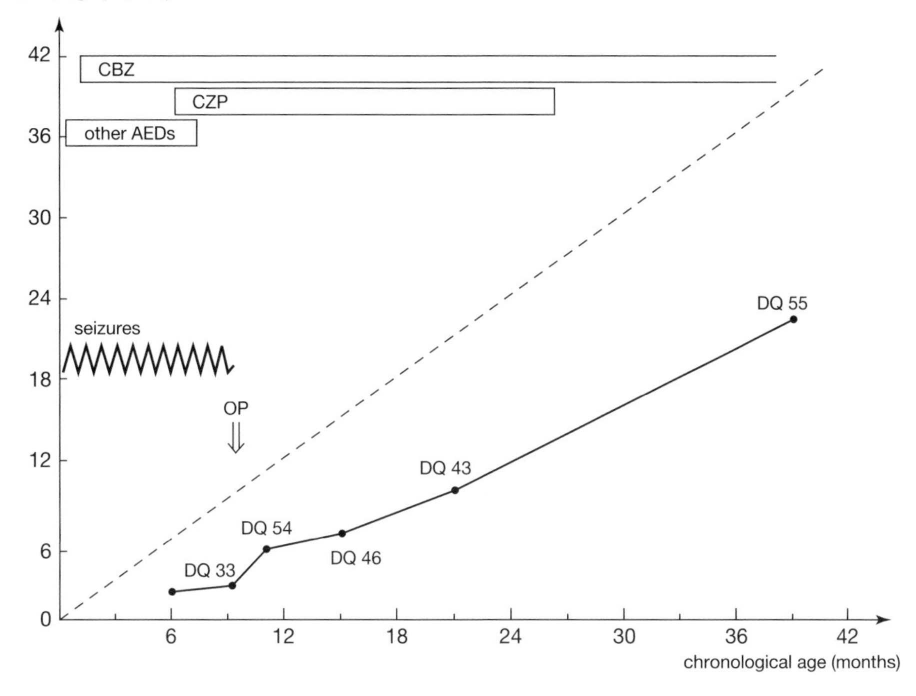

Fig. 10.2 Case A.G.: intractable epilepsy with onset in infancy.

This figure shows a pre- and postoperative longitudinal developmental study (Bayley scale) in a young child with intractable partial epilepsy from the first few weeks of life due to a large focal dysplasia, operated on at 9 months of age (see case history). (CBZ: carbamazepine, CZP: clonazepam, AEDs: antiepileptic drugs, OP: surgery, DQ: developmental quotient (Bayley).)

10.7 Early epilepsy surgery: optimizing the developmental potential?

An increasing number of severe, early onset epilepsies are now found to be caused by focal lesions that are amenable to epilepsy surgery. The impact of epilepsy on development can be major and there is an increasing tendency to offer earlier surgery, not only to treat seizures but in the hope of preserving the child's developmental potential. Epilepsy surgery can probably contribute to achieving this in some situations. In cases with rapid mental deterioration of an autistic type associated with uncontrolled epilepsy, some even consider it an emergency situation (Neville et al 1997). The relative importance of epilepsy itself and that of the primary disease causing the epilepsy in accounting for the developmental delay in an individual child is, however, very variable. Some children who become completely seizure-free after surgery do not improve cognitively, or do so minimally. We do not yet know enough to make generally valid guidelines in this area. Claiming that seizures are always bad for a developing brain and should be stopped rapidly, with early surgery if feasible, has to be tempered by our ignorance of the many variables which will determine outcomes in such situations. The study of the dynamics of development, looking for developmental stagnation or regression and for fluctuations in abilities in correlation with the activity of the epilepsy, can help in identifying the role of epilepsy and in deciding on early epilepsy surgery.

11
EPILEPSY AND MENTAL RETARDATION*: THE ROLE OF EPILEPSY

11.1 Introduction

Epilepsy is a frequent additional disability in many congenital or acquired brain diseases causing primarily mental retardation and/or cerebral palsy. However, certain diseases are invariably associated with severe and often early epilepsy, whereas in others epilepsy rarely occurs or, if it does, is only a minor aspect of the child's disability. Some genetic diseases involve genes implicated in some aspect of neurotransmission and lead to highly epileptogenic brain disorders such as Angelman syndrome and 15q duplication syndromes (Gurrieri et al 1999). An increasing number of different chromosomal disorders are now being found to be associated with epilepsy and variably severe mental retardation and dysmorphism, but some children may have a normal phenotype and intelligence (Schinzel and Niedrist 2001). In other genetic disorders, interestingly, epilepsy is rarely if ever a problem, such as in Prader–Willi syndrome and in the majority of children with Down syndrome. Epilepsy, usually mild, is not rare in fragile-X syndrome and, interestingly, the EEG shows a pattern similar to the idiopathic focal epilepsies with focal sharp waves (Berry-Kravis 2002).

It is probable that an increasing number of families will be discovered in which epilepsy and various degrees of mental retardation co-occur in the absence of abnormalities of the phenotype or identifiable brain malformations (Guerrini and Aicardi 2003). In such families, which have come to attention because of epilepsy, the question naturally arises whether the mental retardation could be secondary or at least partly attributable to the epilepsy rather than being a separate consequence of the gene disorder. With better knowledge of the existence of such families, the significance of the epilepsy in relation to the cognitive disability will be able to be evaluated. How strongly the severity of the epilepsy and mental retardation are linked, or dissociated, in different members, will be an important feature to examine.

When epilepsy is severe or has had an early onset, it is of course difficult to know what part of the mental disability is due to the basic brain disorder and what can be attributed to a direct additional effect of epilepsy. In a long-term follow-up study of children with epilepsy, Huttenlocher and Hapke (1990) found that a majority of those with intractable seizures were mentally retarded and that most of the latter (73 per cent) had seizure onset before the age of 2 years. These results suggest that young age at onset of epilepsy is a risk factor for mental retardation, but do not establish whether this is due to an underlying diffuse

* Equivalent UK usage: learning disability.

brain pathology or to the effects of the epilepsy itself. By including only individuals (n = 100) with intractable epilepsy and a lesion restricted to one lobe of the brain, Vasconcellos et al were able to show that the risk for mental retardation based on early age of onset was independent of the underlying etiology. This risk persisted within subgroups of different etiologies (for example, malformations of cortical development and benign tumours), and was greatest with daily seizures that occurred within the first 24 months of life (65 per cent of subjects had an IQ <70) (Vasconcellos et al 2001).

Regression in development, fluctuations in cognitive abilities and new behavioural problems, sometimes without overt seizures but with severe paroxysmal EEG abnormalities, all potentially reversible, can certainly be observed as a direct effect of epilepsy, even in children with a very low cognitive level, such as in Angelman syndrome (Laan et al 1997).

However, there are neurodegenerative, neurometabolic diseases or neurogenetic disorders where one may erroneously think that the epilepsy (or paroxysmal EEG abnormalities) is the cause of the regression when there are still no clear clues for the diagnosis. In Rett syndrome, for example, the typical developmental regression which occurs more or less rapidly some time in the first two to three years of life is sometimes associated with clinical seizures (early seizure variant) or with severe paroxysmal EEG abnormalities without evident clinical seizures (see section 11.5 for further discussion).

Case E.S.

This girl was first seen by a paediatric neurologist at the age of 2 years 10 months, with a history of stagnation and possible regression between the ages of 1 and 2 years. Neurological examination, head growth and behaviour did not suggest a particular diagnosis and she appeared mentally retarded without clear autistic features. MRI was normal. The EEG showed bilateral centrotemporal sharp wave foci with brief generalized discharges but no clinical seizures (Niedermeyer and Naidu 1990). She was considered to have cognitive delay and deterioration, possibly due to the EEG epileptic activity. She was given valproate and later clonazepam, with some improvement but no change in the EEG, and she was also given steroids, with some improvement but again without EEG changes. She was lost to neurological follow-up for two years. From the age of 4 years she developed hand stereotypies, and episodes of 'panic' with tachycardia. At 6 years of age she was seen again for neurological evaluation of a diagnosis of autism which had been made elsewhere. Her head circumference was at the 3rd percentile (10th percentile at 3 years), and she was markedly mentally retarded, with absence of language, autistic behaviours but good eye contact, and 'hand washing' and other stereotypies typical of Rett syndrome. The absence of microcephaly or significant head growth deceleration, the late onset of stereotypies and other typical behaviours (panic attacks), and the apparent improvement with antiepileptic drugs all contributed to the late diagnosis.

11.2 Cognitive decline due to epilepsy in children with chronic mental retardation or other neurological disabilities

In a child with moderate long-standing and apparently stable mental retardation and chronic epilepsy who shows stagnation, regression or new cognitive problems, the question is often raised whether epilepsy could be the cause, or whether both symptoms are due to the basic condition which is getting worse.

The same principles and reasoning apply here as they would with a child with epilepsy without mental or neurological disability. Epilepsy may be a major aggravating factor in relation to the basic cognitive disability and this possibility should be explored. New behavioural problems, loss of independence, or loss of laboriously acquired skills and increasing difficulty with new learning can be a direct and probably underestimated consequence of epilepsy.

It is reasonable to think that the cognitive consequences of epilepsy are less well tolerated and less likely to be reversible in a child whose brain function is already significantly compromised. In practice, however, the difficulties in obtaining a proper EEG and documenting cognitive fluctuations or regression in a child with mental retardation can be major. In addition, the tolerance and regular use of antiepileptic drugs in people with intellectual disability pose special problems (Alvarez et al 1998). Finally, some physicians doubt that recognition and treatment of possible cognitive effects of epilepsy will make a real difference to the child's well-being or level of function. There are no hard data on this topic, although such problems should logically occur more often in children with mental retardation than in otherwise normal children with epilepsy.

11.3 Mental deterioration of epileptic origin leading to permanent mental retardation

11.3.1 Partial Epilepsy of Prefrontal Origin

Progressive mental deterioration as a direct effect of epilepsy can occur in epilepsies involving prefrontal regions. Even after the epilepsy stabilizes, a more or less severe chronic and stable mental retardation can ensue. This can occur in the syndrome of partial epilepsy with CSWS when it is unrecognized and untreated or is refractory to treatment (Roulet-Perez et al 1993, Hommet et al 2000, Veggiotti et al 2001) (see Chapter 8, section 8.4.1 and Chapter 12, section 12.4.7). In this situation, epilepsy itself, which impinges for durable periods on brain systems which are crucial for higher cognitive functions such as attention, planning, inhibition and memory organization, is the direct cause of mental retardation. Partial epilepsies in other brain areas, even if extremely severe, do not lead to mental deterioration, unless there is sustained propagation to frontal areas.

11.3.2 Epileptic Encephalopathies

Epileptic encephalopathies are 'conditions in which deterioration results mainly from epileptic activity' (Dulac 2001: 23), with the exclusion of progressive neurodegenerative diseases. In this wide definition, many different forms of severe epilepsies of infancy or early childhood are included (West syndrome, severe polymorphic epilepsy of infancy, myoclonic-astatic epilepsy, Lennox–Gastaut syndrome), but also epileptic syndromes occurring later, in which the epileptic activity is only or mainly seen on the EEG, but has a severe cognitive impact (Landau–Kleffner syndrome, epilepsy with CSWS). These situations are so diverse that grouping them together is not really helpful in understanding the probably diverse underlying pathologies and the specific role of the epilepsy on cognitive development, among the other variables. The term 'epileptic encephalopathies' is justified only to draw attention to special epilepsies which have a direct impact on neurological development and cognition, as opposed to others which do not.

The prototype of these so-called epileptic encephalopathies is Lennox–Gastaut syndrome, characterized by frequent seizures of multiple types (mainly myoclonic, tonic, astatic), which are usually refractory to medical therapy. The course is characterized by a very uneven development, with phases of satisfactory progress followed by stagnation or regression, which fluctuate in relation to the activity of the epilepsy and the response to therapy. There is no etiological specificity. Some children are normal at onset, but most already have a cognitive delay. The severe epilepsy, protracted over many years, creates additional brain damage or dysfunction on top of that which was responsible for the basic disorder. If the child has had normal early cognitive development, their mental development stagnates and they gradually score in the mentally retarded range and do not improve, or only minimally, even if seizures remit at a later age. After some years, there is non-specific mental retardation, indistinguishable from that due to other causes. There are many interrelated 'epileptic' variables in these situations (frequent seizures, status epilepticus, multiple drugs, seizures during sleep, and 'subclinical' EEG discharges) which can account for the cognitive deterioration, and it is rarely possible to identify which is the predominant one (Oguni et al 1996).

There are two severe epileptic syndromes of early childhood considered as typical examples of 'epileptic encephalopathies', namely myoclonic-astatic epilepsy (Doose and Völzke 1979) and severe polymorphic epilepsy of infancy, in which sodium ion channel mutations ('channelopathies') have recently been discovered. Aside from causing disturbed excitability, this pathology could possibly affect other developing neuronal functions and this could contribute to the progressive mental retardation. In this sense, these syndromes would be 'true' instances of epileptic encephalopathies (Guerrini and Aicardi 2003).

There are very few, if any, detailed longitudinal neuropsychological studies on the early phases and on the course of these epileptic syndromes.

Myoclonic-astatic epilepsy

Table 11.1 shows the course of cognitive development in three children, who were studied longitudinally from early on in the course of their severe myoclonic-astatic epilepsy, and the problems of interpretation of the neuropsychological findings. These three children had a history of completely normal development prior to their epilepsy. All had normal phenotypes and neurological examination and normal cerebral MRI. They had frequent myoclonic and astatic seizures (but no tonic seizures), with generalized major convulsive episodes and typical EEGs, which necessitated several combined antiepileptic drugs. Common features in their neuropsychological examination (under polytherapy) were:

TABLE 11.1
Myoclonic-astatic epilepsy (Doose syndrome): longitudinal study of three cases

See case description. This table shows the results of longitudinal cognitive, language and behaviour evaluations in three previously normal children with severe myoclonic-astatic epilepsy.

Age at onset of epilepsy	Cognitive age evaluation (medication)	Language testing	Behaviour
H.L. (girl) 3 years 2 months	3 years 6 months PIQ: 94 (valproate, clobazam, lamotrigine)	normal	attention deficit ++, perseveration (verbal and motor), impulsivity
	5 years 1 month TIQ: 76, VIQ: 88, PIQ: 68 (clobazam, lamotrigine, ethosuximide)	normal	unchanged
F.M. (boy) 2 years 7 months	3 years 6 months TIQ: 76, VIQ: 85, PIQ: 72 (topiramate, sulthiame, clonazepam valproate)	phonological immaturity only	attention deficit +++, perseveration (verbal and motor), clumsiness
Z.L. (boy) 2 years 8 months	3 years 4 months TIQ: 79, VIQ: 88, PIQ: 79 (topiramate, clonazepam, valproate)	speech and language delay	attention deficit +++, perseveration (verbal and motor), impulsivity, clumsiness
	4 years 6 months TIQ: 61 VIQ: 73 PIQ: 54 (lamotrigine valproate topiramate)	specific language impairment (phonologic-syntactic) and dysarthria	increasing attention deficit, oppositional, rage, perseverations, clumsiness

TIQ: total IQ
VIQ: verbal IQ
PIQ: performance IQ

marked attentional deficit, impulsivity, perseverations, borderline results on formal cognitive testing. Significantly lower results were observed on the non-verbal items, whereas language development was normal or showed only minor difficulties.

It is not possible to say if this particular profile reflects the dysfunction of specific systems or if it is related to the effects of antiepileptic therapy. Only prospective studies of cases in whom control of seizures or remission allowed less or no medication could help to answer this question more precisely and ascertain whether these deficits are potentially reversible. In practice, one has to try to suppress or limit these very incapacitating seizures, and one always hesitates to undertake drug withdrawal when improvement is obtained. However, there is no doubt that during the periods of exacerbation of the epilepsy, attention capacities, quality of speech and motor coordination deteriorate and there is a stagnation in development, independently of changes in therapy. This shows a direct effect of epilepsy which is, at least partially, reversible.

Severe myoclonic epilepsy of infancy (or severe polymorphic epilepsy of infancy)
This is perhaps the most catastrophic situation, in which a child with normal early development shows an insidious stagnation in cognitive development during the second year of life, corresponding to the aggravation of the epilepsy together with a mild non-progressive ataxia. Even if epilepsy stabilizes or becomes less severe after a few years, there is permanent severe mental retardation, sometimes with autistic features (Cassé-Perrot et al 2001). It is not clear what accounts for this course in the absence of any progressive brain disorder in the classical sense.

Case B.A.

This girl presented with frequent febrile and afebrile episodes of alternating mainly left-sided or generalized convulsive status epilepticus from the age of 6 months. Her personal and family history was negative. The first brain CT, done at 9 months, was normal, but at 14 months a brain MRI done after a prolonged episode of status epilepticus revealed an atrophy of the whole right hemisphere, including hippocampal sclerosis. The first developmental examination at 15 months showed only mild language delay and her global developmental quotient was 82. The epilepsy was very difficult to treat, with persisting episodes of status epilepticus, axial atonic and complex partial seizures. The EEGs were normal until 12 months of age, but later showed multifocal predominantly right-sided spikes and generalized discharges with a slow background rhythm on the right hemisphere. A diagnosis of severe myoclonic epilepsy of infancy (Dravet syndrome) was considered on clinical grounds. Cognitive stagnation was documented between 15 and 37 months (DQ = 47 at 37 months). At the age of 40 months, severe acute motor and mental regression occurred after an episode of generalized status epilepticus. At this time, a slight swelling of the left hippocampus was found, which evolved into a mild left hippocampal sclerosis on repeat MRI one year later. During this year the child recovered to her previously delayed level, but made no further acquisitions despite major improvement of her epilepsy. At the last evaluation at 4 years, her DQ was 36 and she had mild autistic features.

This case illustrates the complexity of so-called epileptic encephalopathy, here 'severe myoclonic epilepsy of infancy': the underlying (probably genetic) cause of this child's epilepsy was responsible for the developmental delay (which was not congenital), which was still mild at 15 months, despite seizure onset at 6 months. Stagnation and regression clearly coincided with the worsening of the epilepsy and the occurrence of bilateral postepileptic lesions (right and later left hippocampal sclerosis) which probably contributed to the very limited potential for recovery. Severe myoclonic epilepsy of infancy, a condition characterized by recurrent prolonged febrile and afebrile focal status epilepticus of early onset, may be one among other epileptic situations in which bilateral hippocampal sclerosis (DeLong and Heinz 1997) could develop, although this has not been looked for systematically.

11.3.3 Other Situations: Unexplained Acquired Mental Retardation in Childhood Epilepsy (Excluding 'Epileptic Encephalopathies' and Progressive Encephalopathies)

Progressive school delay and falling IQ scores, reaching the mentally retarded range, are sometimes found in children whose epilepsy is neither severe nor necessitates multiple drugs, and in whom there is no evidence of a progressive disease. In such cases, it is difficult to pin-point any particular factor, and it is only after a long period that one realizes that the child has not remained in the normal range – an outcome that had not been expected at onset of the disorder. Such cases are never studied in detail prospectively and remain a frustrating experience for the clinician in charge. It is probable that several different factors act insidiously and in a cumulative fashion throughout the years, possibly among them the involvement of frontal circuits, as a result of a spread of the epileptic activity, which has gone unnoticed in the absence of sleep recordings or repeat tracings. However, this is purely speculative and remains an open area for research.

In some cases, however, a gradual improvement is seen, and the child, who has functioned for a long time in the retarded range, gradually 'recovers' to a normal or subnormal level. This has been recognized for a long time, as described below.

> Attention is drawn to certain cases who improve after long periods of apparent deterioration and a hypothesis is put forward that some form of 'subclinical' epilepsy may be partly responsible for deterioration which is not a true dementia.
>
> (Chaudhry and Pond 1961: 219)

11.4 Mental retardation (dementia) from chronic antiepileptic drug intoxication or intolerance

Dementia due to chronic intoxication with phenobarbital or hydantoines is well known in the early literature, but has been described more recently with newer antiepileptic drugs such as valproate and topiramate. It is usually reversible after drug withdrawal. Importantly, it can occur without other signs of intoxication, and even with a normal or low dose and blood levels of the drug.

11.5 Mental deterioration and epilepsy as the only sign of neurometabolic and degenerative diseases

When a previously normal child presents with epilepsy and mental regression without other neurological or brain imaging abnormalities, the question always arises whether these could be the first and only manifestations of a progressive inflammatory, neurometabolic or neurodegenerative disease. At an early stage, the severe epilepsy that develops in Lafora disease, ceroid-lipofuchsinosis, subacute sclerosing panencephalitis or Rasmussen's encephalitis may wrongly be blamed as the causal factor in the regression, but this is exceptional. Usually, mental regression precedes the onset of epilepsy and there are other associated neurological signs such as ataxia or visual disorders. Detailed analysis of the seizure semiology and EEG findings should alert one to the special nature of these epilepsies.

Rett syndrome is a special case in point, especially the 'early-seizure' variant. Infantile spasms or a mixed seizure disorder may occur in the first one to two years of life, before or at the same time as the mental regression is starting, and long before the typical neurological features of the disorder have developed. It can aggravate the downhill course of the disorder. Alternatively, when a young girl is evaluated because of slow development or suspected stagnation or even regression, there may be nothing to point to a precise diagnosis, but the EEG can already show marked epileptic abnormalities. In such circumstances, the suspicion that epilepsy is the main or an important cause of the symptoms can be entertained for some time. This is all the more likely when some or many of the features considered typical are still absent (see case S.E. in Chapter 11, section 11.1).

These situations raise the question of how much and for how long one should pursue the diagnostic work-up for metabolic disease when a child presents with epilepsy as the only symptom. When known genetic epileptic syndromes and investigation for a static epileptogenic lesion are negative, a period of observation without further investigation is justified. The onset of new types of seizures (especially myoclonic), poor or no response to antiepileptic drugs, stagnation or regression in development, and, of course, the presence of special clinical (e.g. ophthalmic, cutaneous, visceral) or neurological features (e.g. ataxia) may give essential clues for a specific classical or a new neurometabolic disease. For instance, children with inborn defects in creatine synthesis, whose clinical phenotype appears much more varied than originally reported, may have prominent epilepsy quite early on (De Grauw et al 2002).

In infants in whom symptomatic epilepsies are more frequent and EEG abnormalities less specific than in older children, a more 'aggressive' work-up is justified when unexplained seizures do not respond to treatment. For instance, a new metabolic disease, glucose-transporter deficiency (GT1), is a cause of severe early seizures and fluctuating motor and cognitive abilities, which improve dramatically when the children are put on a ketogenic diet (Klepper 2004). Besides pyridoxine dependency and biotinidase dependency, it is one of the rare known neurometabolic diseases in which early epilepsy is the main or only symptom, but it is likely that a metabolic origin will increasingly be discovered in children with a combination of epilepsy and some form of cognitive delay (Baxter 1999).

How often and for how long epilepsy can be the first and only symptom of such neurometabolic diseases remains to be studied.

12
DEVELOPMENTAL DISORDERS AND EPILEPSY

12.1 Can epilepsy be the cause of some developmental disorders, and in which situations?

The recognition, in the last 10 to 20 years, that epilepsy can manifest mainly in the cognitive or behavioural sphere, from a very early age and sometimes without 'visible' seizures, has led to an increasing amount of research trying to find evidence of 'hidden' epilepsy in children with developmental disorders, especially those with a history of stagnation, regression or fluctuations in development. This possibility is entertained mainly in children with developmental disorders of language or communication (pervasive developmental disorders, autistic spectrum disorders) and less so in children with 'simple' cognitive delay. Although there is a definite increased incidence of epilepsy (clinical and/or EEG) in these populations, it has proved very difficult to know in an individual case if it represents simply a 'marker' of the brain pathology rather than a causal factor (Ballaban-Gil and Tuchman 2000).

Case M.F.

A 6-year-old child was seen for evaluation of developmental and language retardation. He had practically no verbal comprehension, strange verbal stereotypies, almost no communicative intention, autistic behaviour and marked cognitive delay. There had apparently been no concern about his development until elementary school. At that time deafness had been suspected, but a stagnation or regression could not be proven, although it was strongly suspected. Several EEGs showed sustained independent left temporal and right temporooccipital focal epileptic discharges during waking and sleep. A trial of sulthiame was not convincing and was not pursued. Progress was minimal for about two years. Over the last year, his comprehension has markedly improved, and he can form small sentences and use gestures. Autistic features are also much decreased. He can repeat correctly strings of complex sentences but has marked verbal semantic difficulties. This dissociated language pattern, the early developmental course and unexpected late improvement are unusual and very suggestive of functional brain disorder, probably of epileptic origin, as a significant component.

We have seen several such cases, and so have many others, but almost never with sufficient convincing and quantifiable EEG and clinical data to warrant publication. The developmental course and clinical profile are unlike those seen in known early brain disorders, static or progressive, and the children do not turn out at later ages to have diagnosable metabolic or other unsuspected disorders. Only long-term follow-up can sometimes show these very surprising and unexpected outcomes (for the better or for the worse), suggesting that a very unusual type of brain dysfunction is operative. Clinical and EEG follow-ups over prolonged periods of time are necessary, particularly because these bioelectric disorders typically have a tendency to exacerbate and remit unpredictably during childhood.

Despite all the difficulties in evaluating the possible role of epilepsy in some developmental disorders, there are several important clinical facts which should be kept in mind and which justify further attention to this problem:

1 Congenital brain disorders have many different etiologies and varying prognoses. When known epileptogenic disorders such as genetic syndromes, brain malformations, congenital tumours and rare early metabolic brain diseases have been excluded, one is still left with many undiagnosed children with clinical epilepsy (or epileptic EEG abnormalities), the role of which in the child's altered development remains uncertain but possible.
2 Unusual dynamics of development, including regression, stagnation and fluctuations of acquisitions or behaviour, has many possible causes. Whereas fluctuations/regressions do not necessarily mean epilepsy, epilepsy remains an important possible factor. The rapidity of clinical change (worsening or improvement) in some epileptic situations can be very variable at different periods and even in the same child (Neville et al 2001).
3 Some early epilepsies (first year of life) can present with developmental and sometimes reversible regressions of various types, often with autistic features, outside the well-known situation of West syndrome. In these situations, complex partial seizures of frontal or temporal origin are usually found and are often refractory. In some children, seizures may be subtle and go unrecognized, or are falsely interpreted as purposeful repetitive movements, i.e. stereotypies (see cases B.A., section 12.4.5, and D.A., section 12.4.7, and Deonna et al 2002).
4 Intense epileptic activity can occur in a young child's brain without obvious surface EEG abnormality (Acharya et al 1997) or even visible clinical seizures. In addition, very epileptogenic brain pathologies such as focal cortical dysplasias are not always easily diagnosed with MRI in the first months of life (Neville et al 1997), and in some cases the examination, which was initially considered normal, has to be repeated.

Case R.E.

A 13-month-old girl was referred because of developmental delay and suspected autism. On examination she had a developmental level below 6 months of age and had no active communication and emotional reactivity. The parents gave a history of episodes strongly suggestive of infantile spasms at the age of 3, 6 and 8 months, with regression and improvement in between. An EEG done two days after the consultation was normal and the rest of the neurological work-up was non-diagnostic. Two months later, her communication, surprisingly, had very much improved. At this time, review of the videofilm made during the initial consultation showed a typical axial myoclonic seizure which had been overlooked. Follow-up showed a steady catch-up with transient language delay and a performance IQ of 84 (WPPSI-R) at 4 years 8 months. Such an outcome was totally unexpected and difficult to explain, except as being due to temporary epilepsy (epileptic spasms), which could only be demonstrated clinically (the family refused a repeat EEG after the 'spontaneous ' recovery).

5 Rare but well-documented cases have been reported in whom a marked rapid cognitive/ behavioural improvement and developmental catch-up could be correlated with antiepileptic therapy and suppression of EEG discharges (Deonna et al 1995, Uldall et al 2000). The positive clinical response to an antiepileptic drug may be considered as a psychotropic effect of the drug (e.g. valproate, carbamazepine) on the affective component of the disorder (Di Martino and Tuchman 2001). This should be kept in mind, but appears unlikely, especially when the change is very rapid or if a return of epileptic discharges and relapse of the behavioural disorder can be seen while the child is on the same drug.
6 Failure of antiepileptic therapy (or even worsening as a result) is not proof that epilepsy is not an important causal factor.

12.2 Familial disorders featuring epilepsy (or paroxysmal EEG abnormalities) and developmental problems: role of epilepsy?

In the last 10 to 20 years, an enormous amount of data on the genetics of various epilepsies has appeared. An increasing number of individual families are being described with associated epilepsy and developmental problems in siblings or in successive generations (Temple 1997, Roubertie et al 2003). The epilepsy and the cognitive disorder can be due to the same abnormal gene(s) but constitute independent consequences. It is also possible that the epilepsy itself, in some instances, could be responsible for the cognitive-behavioural disorder (or part of it). These situations typically exemplify the problem of the interrelationship between the cognitive disorder and epilepsy, the latter sometimes appearing to be a major aggravating or the main factor. Here are some examples.

12.2.1 Families with Rolandic Epilepsies or with Focal Sharp Waves and CSWS

In the same family, some members remain fully normal cognitively, some have minor and transient cognitive changes during the active epilepsy phase, and some have severe progressive and prolonged language and/or cognitive regression with sequelae (Weise et al 1995). This suggests that epilepsy plays a variable role in the neurological or cognitive deficit (Fig. 12.1).

12.2.2 Families with 'Autosomal Dominant Speech Dyspraxia'

A large family with 'autosomal dominant speech dyspraxia with rolandic epilepsy' was first reported by Scheffer et al (1995), but other families have been observed since. Scheffer et al suggested that the speech dyspraxia and the epilepsy are different manifestations of the same gene with a phenomenon of anticipation. They did not consider that the speech defect could be a consequence of early epilepsy in the opercular region. In some of the

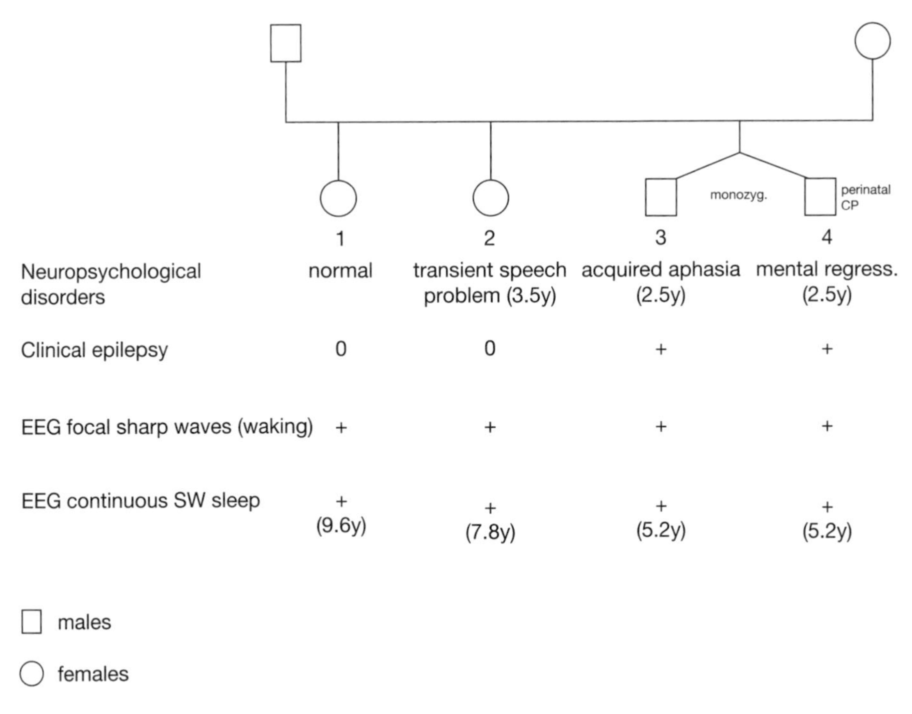

Fig. 12.1 Family with an epileptic disorder characterized by focal sharp waves on the EEG and CSWS (Ors, Lund, Sweden, 2003).

This family has been studied by Dr Marianne Ors and colleagues (unpublished, 2003, reproduced with kind permission) in Lund, Sweden. Note the variability of clinical symptoms despite EEG abnormalities present in all children. One of the monozygotic twins had a perinatal brain lesion with cerebral palsy (CP), possibly explaining the different clinical manifestations of the two twins.

affected children, however, there was deterioration of speech and other functions when epilepsy was severe, suggesting that at least one component of the deficit was functional in origin. Prats et al (1998) reported a family in which the father and three children had an opercular epileptic syndrome in the context of benign partial epilepsy with rolandic spikes. The children had an acquired (at 4 years), fluctuant and difficult to treat oromotor dysfunction with sequelae 15 years later. These observations are very important because the oromotor and speech dysfunction was largely acquired and of functional epileptic origin. This epileptic syndrome is a relatively 'simple' model illustrating that in these familial disorders with epilepsy, a strong dichotomy between epilepsy being either the primary cause of the disorder or an associated manifestation is not justified. Further family studies and identification of the type and functions of the genes involved in these disorders may provide a better understanding of the relative role of epilepsy and that of a focal structural developmental anomaly of the cerebral cortex.

12.2.3 Developmental Disorders in Siblings Associated with Paroxysmal EEG Abnormalities (Mainly During Sleep) Not Further Diagnosed

With the increasingly frequent practice of performing EEG recordings in children with unexplained developmental disorders, it is not unusual to find siblings with a combination of a variably severe developmental disorder (mental retardation and/or autistic disorder) and paroxysmal EEG abnormalities or clinical epilepsy, who do not belong to a known syndrome (for instance, fragile X syndrome). We know of many such families from discussion with colleagues, but they are rarely if ever published or studied in detail. This is an important field of research because in some families there can be a regression or fluctuations which are directly caused by the epilepsy (Temple 1997, Roubertie et al 2003).

Table 12.1 shows two unrelated families (each with two affected siblings) that we have followed over a prolonged period. In each family, one of the two children had a regressive and fluctuating course with significant late improvement, which we believe was related, at least partially, to the epileptic activity (the girl in family D.C. is reported in detail in section 12.3.2 below on developmental language disorders).

12.3 Developmental language disorders and the role of epilepsy

There is no good evidence that epilepsy is ever (except in exceptional cases) the only or main cause of the language problems in children who present with an isolated specific developmental language impairment, that is, with normal cognitive level, absence of other developmental or behavioural problems, and a positive family history. According to Bishop (1997), there may be a subgroup of children with specific developmental language impairment who have a history of early regression, but this has never been systematically studied. In EEG studies of children with developmental language disorders, very different percentages of paroxysmal EEG abnormalities are found, depending on which children with developmental language disorders are chosen for study (Maccario et al 1982, Echenne et al 1992, Duvelleroy-Hommel et al 1995, Parry-Fielder et al 1997, Picard et al 1998).

TABLE 12.1
Familial development disorder and paroxysmal interictal focal epileptic EEG abnormalities: two unrelated families with affected siblings

The table shows the clinical characteristics in sibling pairs from two unrelated families studied personally for several years. Note that one sibling in each family had a developmental course and EEG evolution (one with clinical seizures) suggesting some direct role of epilepsy in his/her developmental problem. The girl in family D.C. is the patient reported as D.C.M. in the section on developmental language disorder and epilepsy.

Family D.C.			**Family J.**	
Age at first consultation	**Girl, 5 years**	**Boy, 3 years**	**Girl, 3 years, 6 months**	**Girl, 7 years**
Duration of follow-up	5 years	3 years	8–9 years	—
Developmental problem (at presentation)	Severe developmental language delay, mild cognitive delay	Severe developmental language delay, severe hyperactivity	Mild developmental delay, dyspraxia	Moderate developmental delay, severe speech impairment
Other family data	No other siblings, father with possibility of developmental language delay		No other siblings, father with mild developmental general and language delay	
Phenotype and physical growth parameters	Normal	Normal	Normal	Normal
Genetic findings	X fragile negative	Normal karyotype X fragile negative		Normal karyotype X fragile negative
Clinical epilepsy	No	No	Rare 'absences' at 3–4 years	No
Evolution/ fluctuation documented	Regression, partial recovery	Very slow progress	Cognitive stagnation (7 years); late progress (11 years)	Slow progress
EEG abnormality	Bitemporal focal sharp-waves (no CSWS)	Frontal and temporal multifocal spikes increased in sleep	Multifocal spikes, CSWS	Multifocal spikes, no CSWS (one EEG at 7 years)
Effect of antiepileptic drugs (steroids) on cognition and EEG (documented)	Partial positive effect of sulthiame and steroids	No change (sulthiame, clobazam, valproate, methylphenidate, levetiracetam)	No clear effect (clinical and on EEG discharges) of valproate and lamotrigine	Not tried

12.3.1 Developmental Dysphasia vs Early Forms of Acquired Epileptic Aphasia (Fig. 12.2)

Children with acquired epileptic aphasia (Landau–Kleffner syndrome) sometimes have a history of delayed language development, but in other cases there is a very early loss of language (before 2 years) in a child who had developed normally or even precociously

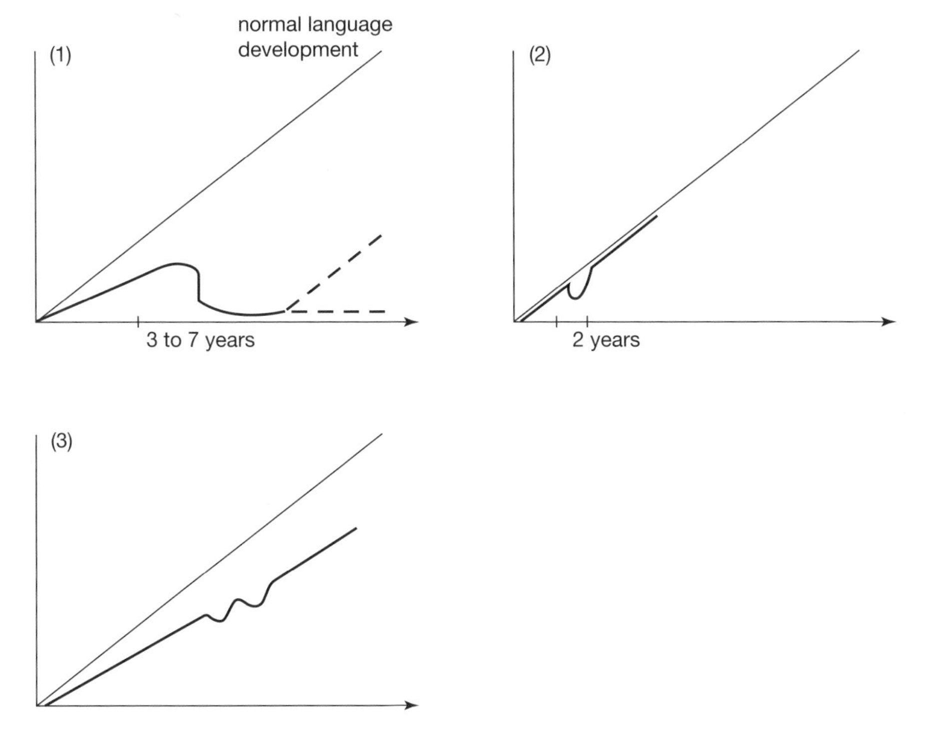

1 The child has significant language delay but makes regular progress and the aphasia occurs much later in the course after significant language has developed (Yung et al 2000, case 1).
2 The child has normal early language or prelanguage development but the loss of language occurs quite early (at less than 2 years or even at 15 months), after which there is a significant or complete recovery (Uldall et al 2000, Mayor Dubois et al 2004).
3 The child has developmental language delay, makes limited progress and may show fluctuations in language abilities or a questionable regression, but not a clear history of loss (Maccario et al 1982).

Fig. 12.2 Developmental language disorder versus early acquired dysphasia.

This figure shows the possible effect of epilepsy on early language development. The situations in (1) and (2) have been well documented, whereas that in (3) certainly occurs but is more difficult to relate directly to the epilepsy (see text).

in that domain before the regression (Uldall et al 2000). There are, of course, no truly prospective studies of such children, but from a review of the few sufficiently well-described case reports, three types of situation have been encountered (see Fig. 12.2).

In the first two situations, a good correlation has been found between, on the one hand, the language delay, loss and recovery and, on the other, the clinical seizure or paroxysmal EEG activity. In the third situation, the role of epilepsy remains difficult to prove.

Of course, there may be either a coincidence of two unrelated pathologies – developmental language delay and an epileptogenic brain disorder – or the same genetic disorder causing both independently.

12.3.2 Other Patterns of Aberrant Language Development

Other even more complex patterns of abnormal language development with recurrent language regression at different stages of language acquisition do sometimes occur, causing aberrant and probably unique language profiles, as illustrated by the following case.

Case D.C.M. (family D.C. in Table 12.1 and Fig. 12.3)

This girl was first seen for evaluation of developmental delay at the age of 5 years 3 months. Her younger brother was later found to also have developmental delay, with severe attention deficit disorder and paroxysmal multifocal EEG discharges increased during sleep (see Table 12.1, family D.C.). Neither of them ever had recognized clinical seizures.

On examination at 5 years 3 months, the girl had limited understanding of speech, said a few isolated words and was at times echolalic with surprisingly good articulation. She was withdrawn but clinically not autistic. Her overall performances were delayed, but much more so in verbal language. Non-verbal development corresponded to that of a child aged 3 years 6 months (DQ 68), whereas language was at a level of approximately 2 years. Language was characterized by production of single words or rare short utterances (2–4 words). Phonological skills were superior to lexical and syntactic abilities. Comprehension was limited, but designation of body parts, objects and actions using pictures was possible. She was able to repeat isolated words correctly. She could repeat sentences of up to three elements, but in this case only part of each word was repeated correctly.

These features were quite unusual for a specific developmental language impairment, and resembled transcortical sensory aphasia, as described in adults but almost never in children (Rapin and Allen 1988, Jambaqué et al 1998). The surprisingly late recognition of this severe clinical picture suggested a possible early acquired condition and this is what prompted an EEG. This showed, during sleep, frequent bilateral right frontotemporal and left temporooccipital focal sharp waves, but no continuous spike-waves during sleep (CSWS). Brain MRI was normal.

The developmental history was then reviewed again with the help of questionnaires on early language development and the paediatrician's notes. She vocalized a lot as a baby and was very communicative. Between 1 and 2 years, she became 'very agitated', 'hyperactive', 'nervous' and 'did not understand what she was told'. She said her first words at 2 years, 2 months, but did not use them appropriately (mama for papa). Between 2 and 3 years, her mother noted that her behaviour was different from that of other children (play, constructions). She did not turn when called 'as if she did not hear or did not understand' and 'she said words that had nothing to do with context'. She did not learn new words between 2 and 3 years. She was, however, sociable, and had no special habits, except hand biting when angry.

	5y 3m	5y 6m	6y	6y 5m
verbal stereotypies	none	maximum	less	none
echolalia	+	+++	++	none
comprehension of simple questions	a little	no	no	yes
pointing to objects*	60%	variable	100%	100%
expressive language	words	words + jargon	words + jargon	phrases conjugated verbs

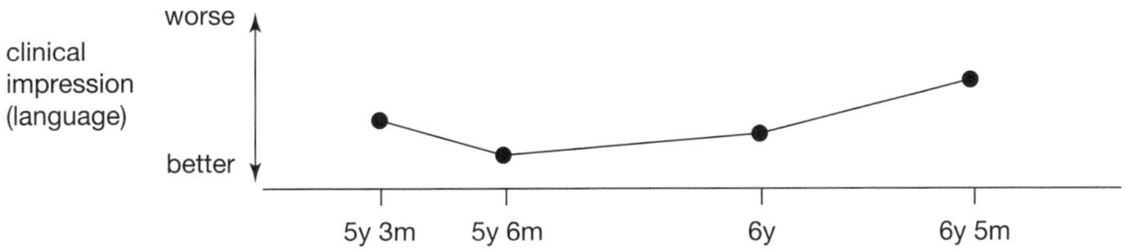

clinical impression (language)

worse

better

5y 3m 5y 6m 6y 6y 5m

*% rate of 'correctly pointed to' objects

Fig. 12.3 Case D.C.M., girl: evolution of abnormal verbal behaviours from 5 years 3 months to 6 years 5 months.

This figure shows the fluctuations in very striking abnormalities in language behaviour (echolalia and verbal stereotypies: 'mamamama'). Their presence and intensity were in fact the marker of the language deterioration and improvement. They correlated clinically with the language deterioration and improvement (and paroxysmal EEG activity) at a time when formal language tests were impossible.

At 2 years 6 months, she 'pinched her nail' on the right hand and after that became left-handed, whereas she had always used her right hand preferentially before. In retrospect, this suggested a shift in hand dominance related to an active brain dysfunction, and the 'accident' was probably coincidental.

Three months after the first consultation (5 years 6 months), a clear deterioration was noted: echolalia became more prominent, she had verbal perseverations (mama mama . . .) and she used an incomprehensible jargon with pseudowords. During the session she seemed to have fluctuations in comprehension, being able to point in turn correctly and incorrectly at the same pictures or objects.

Antiepileptic therapy with sulthiame was started, and a gradual clinical and EEG improvement was noted within the next six months, with first a decrease of the fluctuations in comprehension, decreased verbal perseverations and echolalia, and disappearance of jargon and neologisms, with a parallel decrease of her overall language output ('speaks less'). However, what she produced was more appropriate, and for the first time significant comprehension beyond a few simple words could be documented.

Improvement continued for 18 months up to the age of 7 years 2 months, when a new stagnation and decline were gradually noted. On formal language testing, a complete stagnation or regression in most language dimensions, especially in phonology, was noted, together with a worsening of the EEG discharges. Prednisone was given, with definite clinical and EEG improvement for a few months, but with a plateau in acquisitions during the gradual withdrawal. A new increase of prednisone was tried, but this time was inconclusive and was stopped. She is now 13 years old and has slowly progressed over the years. She has functional, although quite delayed, language and moderate global mental retardation (performance IQ: 68).

The long follow-up study from the age of 5 years 6 months and the retrospective inquiry indicated a very early language regression around 1 year of age followed by aberrant language development thereafter and two further late regressions documented at 6 and 7 years of age, with fluctuations which correlated with the EEG paroxysmal activity. Her very unusual language profile and language behaviour were unlike what is seen with any developmental language disorder and suggest a disruption and partial recovery of different language systems in the course of development, best explainable by fluctuating epileptic activity.

12.3.3 Indication for an EEG in a Child with a Developmental Language Disorder

In practice, the question is often raised whether and when an EEG should be done in a child presenting with a developmental language disorder. In view of the above discussion and data from the literature, an EEG should be considered in the situations summarized in Table 12.2.

TABLE 12.2
Indication of a possible role of epilepsy and for performing an EEG in a child with a developmental language disorder

This table lists the situations in which epilepsy could be suspected to play a role in a child with a developmental language disorder. In these situations an EEG (including a sleep recording) should be considered.

- Predominance of receptive language disturbance
- Stagnation in language development
- Loss of previously acquired words followed by lack of progress
- Regression after good progress in a child with a developmental language delay
- Presence of a sibling with atypical language impairment
- History of past or present paroxysmal phenomena of possible epileptic origin

12.4 Pervasive developmental disorders, autism, 'autistic regression' and the role of epilepsy

12.4.1 Overview: The Relationship Between Autistic Disorders and Epilepsy

The relationship between autistic disorders and epilepsy will be discussed in detail not only because epilepsy is more frequent in autism than in other developmental disorders but also because regression in development often occurs in these situations and in some instances a direct role of epilepsy may be suspected.

Autism is a behavioural phenotype that manifests with impairment in social interaction and in verbal and non-verbal communication, and a restricted repertoire of activities and interests. Some authors, including ourselves, prefer the term 'autistic spectrum disorders' (or pervasive developmental disorders), acknowledging the fact that there is a continuum in severity between those with 'typical' autism (according to ICD-10 1992/DSM-IV 1994, for example), and those who present most but not all classical features, or only in a mild way.

The same child may have autism and mental retardation or a specific developmental language problem, such as phonologic-syntactic deficit or verbal apraxia, in addition to delayed and aberrant language use (Rapin and Dunn 2003). The different components of the disability may improve at their own rate – or recover completely or almost completely – so that, depending on the age at which the child is seen, a different clinical diagnosis could be given. The tendency now to consider developmental disorders using qualitative dimensions rather than a categorical approach has emerged as a result of observations of these variable features and overlapping clinical pictures, as well as evolution over time (Bishop 2000).

The clinical overlap between autistic spectrum disorder, language disability and mental retardation is probably due to abnormalities in different brain systems, with one single or several underlying etiologies. The same pathology may account for the involvement of several systems, but different pathologies may coexist in the same child. The basic etiology responsible for the disorder may also cause epilepsy, or epilepsy may have an independent cause (e.g. genetic). Epilepsy arising in part of an already abnormal system (e.g. limbic system) at a particular age may have major consequences for specific aspects of development, for example in the domain of emotions, memory or communication, leading or contributing to an autistic phenotype. These relationships and the possible significance of epilepsy in these situations are summarized in Table 12.3.

The orbitofrontal cortex, the anterior cingulate gyrus and the amygdala are structures belonging to the complex limbic networks that are involved in emotions and adapted social behaviour (Avanzini 2001). They have all been suspected to be dysfunctional in autistic disorders and have been shown, at least in adults, to be the site of onset of focal epilepsies with emotional and behavioural manifestations.

In addition, the clinical consequences of a dysfunction in another system (for instance, the sound perception system responsible for auditory agnosia), even if not directly related to the emotional and social behaviour processing systems, may lead to major disability in

TABLE 12.3
Autistic spectrum and related developmental disorders (developmental language disorder and mental retardation): levels of study and possible role of epilepsy

This table shows the different explanatory levels which have to be considered (etiological, brain system involved) when looking for the 'cause' of developmental language disability, autistic spectrum disorder or mental retardation in a given child. The possible significance of epilepsy in this context is indicated (see also text).

Etiological level	Structural (network) level	Clinical level (resulting behavioural phenotype)
The same etiology (e.g. tuberous sclerosis) may disrupt the function of one or several systems Different etiologies in the same child (e.g. one genetic, one acquired lesion) may account for the dysfunction of different brain systems Epilepsy *per se* due to above etiologies or unrelated	One or several structures (networks) involved Epilepsy may start in one or several of these dysfunctional structures (networks) at successive times and cause additional dysfunction	Autistic disorder with or without associated specific language disability and mental retardation Abnormal behaviours due to verbal language problems or mental retardation may contribute to the autistic phenotype Dysfunction in one system (e.g. sound perception system) with auditory agnosia may lead to an autistic-like withdrawal

communication and reactive behavioural problems (withdrawal or lack of interest in contact and stereotypies), as observed in autism. The existence of an associated genetic predisposition for developmental disorders or the presence of adverse environmental factors can probably be important contributors to an autistic phenotype in these children, especially during the first two to five years of life.

12.4.2 Epilepsy and Autism: Possible Reasons for Co-occurrence

Autism may be due to many different brain disorders (Gillberg and Coleman 2000). Epilepsy and autism can co-occur for several reasons:

1 Autism and epilepsy are totally independent.
2 The same underlying pathology is the origin of an autistic phenotype and epilepsy, both being independent consequences of the same disorder.
3 The epileptic process interferes with the function of specific brain networks involved in communication and social behaviours (orbitofrontal cortex, anterior cingulate gyrus and mesiotemporal structures).
4 A focal or multifocal pathology (e.g. tuberous sclerosis) that involves frontal and mesiotemporal structures can be the origin of an autistic phenotype as well as trigger epilepsy which can aggravate the autistic symptoms (Deonna et al 1993b).
5 An autistic phenotype may be due to a withdrawal reaction in a vulnerable individual when an epileptic process interferes with a specific sensory or cognitive function.

There are several reviews on the association between epilepsy and autism: on the type of seizures, age at onset, prognosis, and therapy with antiepileptic drugs (Olsson et al 1988, Volkmar and Nelson 1990, Tuchman 2000, Tuchman and Rapin 2002). This literature, usually based on large groups of children with different etiologies, is not really pertinent to the question of the possible direct effect of epilepsy in causing an autistic syndrome. The incidence of epilepsy is higher in autistic children with mental retardation than in the more 'high-functioning' ones, probably reflecting the severity of the underlying brain disorder.

12.4.3 Epilepsy as a Possible Direct Cause of an Autistic Spectrum Disorder

There are several clinical situations in which the possibility of epilepsy being the main cause or an important contributing factor to the autistic behaviour has been considered.

Early epilepsies starting in the first or second year of life, such as infantile spasms with hypsarrhythmia (West syndrome) or complex partial epilepsies (frontal and limbic), characteristically lead to developmental regression which has some autistic characteristics (Gillberg and Schaumann 1983, Dalla Bernardina et al 1994, Deonna et al 1995, Gillberg et al 1996).

The probable importance of the specific localization of an epileptogenic lesion in children with autistic features is highlighted by the study of Taylor who examined 98 children before epilepsy surgery from the psychiatric point of view (Taylor et al 1999). Eleven out of 98 children were found to have an autistic spectrum disorder, associated in 9/11 with mental retardation. Remarkably, 9/11 had either cortical dysplasia or a congenital tumour in the right temporal lobe, with onset of epilepsy before 12 months of age. Surgical outcome of the epilepsy and impact on development are unfortunately not known in this particular subgroup, except for one case who was published separately and who showed some improvement in communication.

Recently, Bolton et al (2002) have shown in a large number of children with tuberous sclerosis that the co-occurence of temporal lobe tubers and an early onset epilepsy originating in the temporal lobes was strongly associated with an autistic spectrum disorder. The presence of temporal lobe tubers alone, regardless of extent, or severe epilepsy by itself, did not correlate with an autistic disorder. These data, although retrospective and incomplete from the EEG description and seizure semiology viewpoint, clearly point to the role of early epilepsy arising in developing temporal networks as being the determining factor. Together with the rare individual longitudinal studies in which epileptic activity and autistic behaviour in children with tuberous sclerosis could be correlated directly (Deonna et al 1993b, Gillberg et al 1996), these data provide strong evidence that early epilepsy in specific networks important for social development can contribute to an autistic spectrum disorder. In these situations, outcome could be positively influenced by appropriate early antiepileptic therapy.

West syndrome and autism: the history of a long association

This association is interesting to review, not only because it was one of the first proposed examples of a neurobiologic etiology for autism at a time when psychogenic theories were still flourishing, but also because it illustrates in a remarkable way the evolving thinking and ideas about the relationships between epilepsy, brain dysfunction and autism. Table 12.4 summarizes the key stages in this association. Obviously these retrospective data cannot inform us on the possible direct role of epilepsy in this situation. The underlying brain pathology may be responsible for both epilepsy and autism. The bilateral pathology in the temporal lobes found at a late stage in such cases on PET-scan is not surprising considering the brain systems thought to be implicated in autism (Chugani et al 1996).

Babies in the acute phase of West syndrome show a regression in development which has sometimes been described as autistic because inattention and loss of smiling and social contact are prominent features. Table 12.5 shows the possible explanations given for these behaviours.

When there are very frequent or continuous seizures or epileptic discharges (status epilepticus) the child is disconnected from all afferent inputs and has no initiative and affect. The child can thus appear autistic. However, for an epileptic state to give rise to a truly autistic syndrome, one has to demonstrate that social interaction and verbal and non-verbal communication are predominantly affected whereas other cognitive competences are preserved (e.g. visuospatial).

Jambaqué et al, following observations made in babies in the acute phase of the syndrome, have suggested that the visual inattentiveness and autistic behaviour could be explained by an epileptic dysfunction of the visual cortex, with a central visual impairment

TABLE 12.4
West syndrome and autism: summary of historical landmarks

This table summarizes the different clinical situations in which an association between West syndrome and autism has been recognized.

- A small but significant number of children diagnosed with autism have a history of infantile spasms in infancy (Taft and Cohen 1971)
- Children with autism who had infantile spasms also have associated mental retardation (no or very few high-functioning individuals among these children)
- Children with autism with mental retardation who had infantile spasms continue to have a severe persistent epilepsy with multiple seizure types, mainly Lennox–Gastaut syndrome
- Tuberous sclerosis complex is a typical etiology for infantile spasms followed by autism and mental retardation, but many other etiologies exist
- Some children with autism with mental retardation who had infantile spasms, who were studied by PET at a late stage, show bilateral temporal hypometabolism (Chugani et al 1996)

TABLE 12.5
Explanations given for autistic-like behavioural regression in West syndrome (infantile spasms with hypsarrhythmia)

- The constant epileptic activity (hypsarrhythmia) with cognitive status epilepticus precludes interpersonal communication and initiative
- A specific dysfunction of posterior cortical areas with complex visual problems (central visual impairment) prevents the recognition of emotional clues essential for development (Jambaqué et al 2001)
- A cortical dysfunction in specific brain systems necessary for early emotional development and social aspects of cognition (frontotemporal) can lead to an autistic syndrome

preventing the recognition of emotional clues essential for development ('by an early perceptual visual impairment that prevents face and emotion perception' (Jambaqué et al 1993b: 181). This idea was supported by the fact that functional imaging (SPECT) had shown a predominant hypoperfusion in the posterior cortical areas in these babies. Children with congenital peripheral blindness or central visual impairment may have some autistic features, probably related to their visual disability (Hobson 1995), but this is certainly not the fundamental cause of permanent autism.

Some children can develop autistic behaviour as the major symptom in the context of complex partial epilepsies of early onset, or in the context of so-called late infantile spasms.

Late infantile spasms

Some children with late infantile spasms have already developed high competencies in social and emotional communication prior to the onset of epilepsy. The nature of the regression, with the loss of this aspect of development, is then striking and can be analysed along with other autistic characteristics. If recovery occurs, this is very suggestive of a true autistic epileptic phase. This is probably not simply a prolonged seizure (status epilepticus) or postictal state but continuous brain dysfunction, either due to recurrent seizures without any possibility of complete functional recovery in between or due to some other mechanism. Focal EEG discharges (after the generalized discharges have subsided) are seen predominantly in the frontal or frontotemporal areas in children with late infantile spasms who have regression of autistic type (Bednarek et al 1998). Interestingly, one recent EEG study performed in older autistic children has found epileptic foci in the frontal regions. This is probably only a marker of the dysfunctional cortex involved, but one can speculate whether early unrecognized epilepsy in some specific networks implicating the frontal lobes could have been the cause of the autistic disorder in some of these children (Hashimoto et al 2001).

TABLE 12.6
Arguments for a possible direct role of epilepsy in causing an autistic phenotype in children with 'late infantile spasms' (1–3 years)

This table lists some of the reasons why children with late infantile spasms may be a good model to study the nature of epileptic regression and its autistic features.

- Typical infantile spasms can occur later than the usual period (3 to 7 months) and are called 'late spasms' (1–3 years)
- These late spasms are usually associated with other seizure types (complex partial)
- There may be other associated paroxysmal phenomena (stereotypic movements) which may be unusual seizure manifestations suggesting involvement of the mesiofrontal cortex (i.e. anterior cingulate)
- Some of these children had reached an adequate level of cognitive, social and emotional development before the epilepsy started
- Regression (and recovery) in these children is easier to document because of the level of development these children had already achieved
- The regression in development may have many autistic features
- The regression may persist after acute seizures have subsided but disappearance of the autistic state may be seen later if epilepsy is controlled
- Focal EEG discharges (after generalized discharges have subsided) are seen predominantly in the frontal or frontotemporal areas

The case illustrated below shows that early partial epilepsy in frontotemporal areas (manifesting as epileptic spasms) can lead to true autistic regression which is potentially reversible (see case report and Fig. 12.4).

Case D.G.T.

A 28-month-old boy was referred for acute onset of abnormal head movements. The history revealed an insidious regression in behaviour and communication over several months. Head and shoulder 'spasms' with alteration of awareness and on one occasion ictal laughter were seen. The EEG showed repeated bursts of brief generalized poly-spikes and spike-waves during the spasms, followed by flattening, a pattern which never recurred after treatment. Review of family videos showed a single 'minor' identical seizure six months previously. MRI was normal. Valproate was ineffective, but clonazepam brought immediate cessation of seizures, normalization of the EEG and simultaneous spectacular improvement in communication, mood and language.

Follow-up over the next 10 months showed a new insidious regression without reported seizures, although numerous ones were seen during the videotaped neuropsychological examination, when stereotyped subtle brief paroxysmal changes in posture and behaviour could be studied in slow motion and compared to 'prototypical' initial ones. The EEG showed predominant rare left-sided frontotemporal discharges. Clonazepam was changed to carbamazepine, with marked improvement in behaviour, language and cognition, which has been continuous. He has had no seizures since the age of 5 years and carbamazepine was stopped at the age of 9 years, at which time his EEG was normal.

In summary, this boy had late onset epileptic spasms, subtle complex partial seizures (laughter, alteration of awareness), and an initial reversible epileptic autistic syndrome followed by a later insidious regression which could be directly related to his epileptic disease. This epileptic disease was a partial cryptogenic epilepsy (dysplasia?) and was revealed by epileptic spasms in the second year of life but had a likely earlier onset. Videotaped home observations allowed the documentation of striking variations in social interaction and play of autistic type in relation to the epileptic activity. (For details of the symptomatology and methodology used for this case study, see Deonna et al 1995.)

12.4.4 Regression in Classical Autism and Disintegrative Disorder: Does Epilepsy Play a Role? (Fig. 12.5)

A history of unexplained regression after a seemingly normal early development is reported before the second year of life in up to one-third of children later diagnosed as suffering

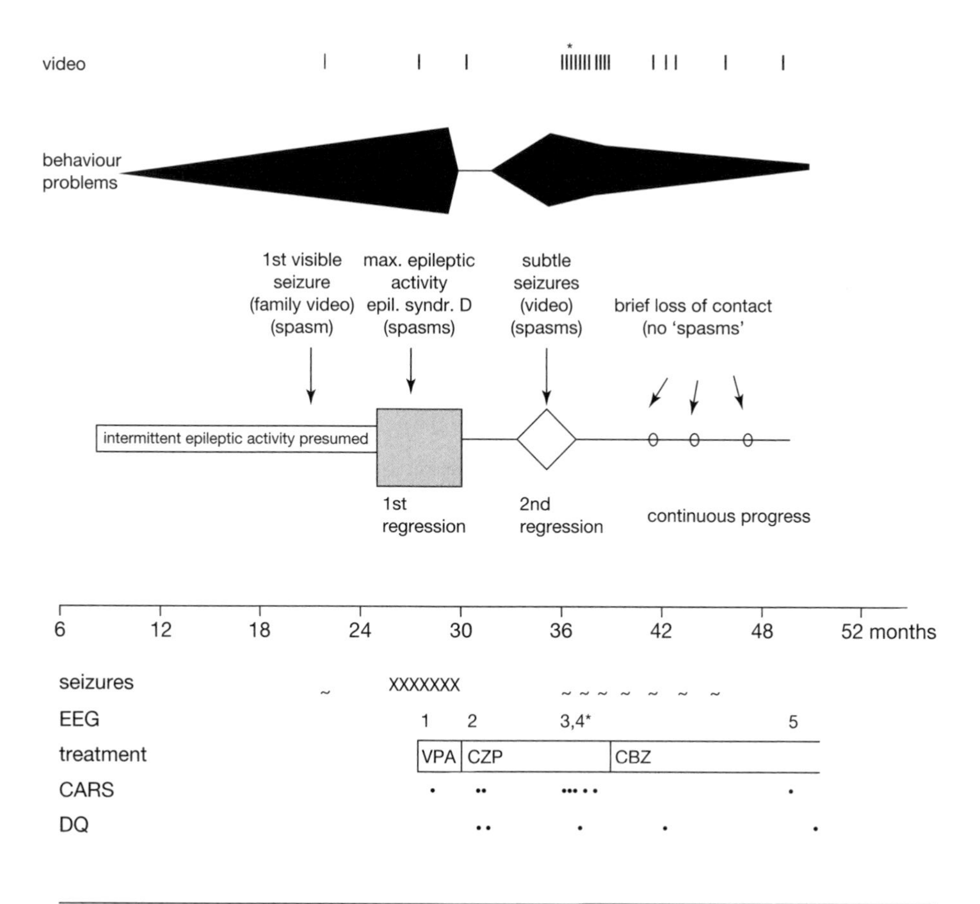

Fig. 12.4 Case D.G.T.: late spasms and complex partial epilepsy with reversible autistic regression.

This figure shows the clinical course, type and timing of longitudinal investigations (for details see Deonna et al 1995). Seizures were recognized on family videos six months prior to initial deterioration and diagnosis of epilepsy. The second regression was insidious and not rapidly recognized as epileptic, although subtle seizures could be seen on repeat videos done by the psychologist. EEG 1 showed brief generalized bursts of high voltage polyspikes and spike-waves followed by flattening. EEG 2 two months later showed no discharges. EEG 3 after six months showed isolated infrequent small amplitude spikes and spike-wave discharges in the left frontotemporal area. EEG 4* (continuous videorecording) showed no discharges. EEG 5 showed rare left frontotemporal spikes. (Modified from Deonna et al 1995.)

from typical autism (Rapin 1991). Sometimes, the regression occurs later, usually after the third year when language has fully developed, a situation referred to as disintegrative disorder or childhood disintegrative disorder (also called disintegrative psychosis) (Evans-Jones and Rosenbloom 1978, Hill and Rosenbloom 1986, Mouridsen et al 1999).

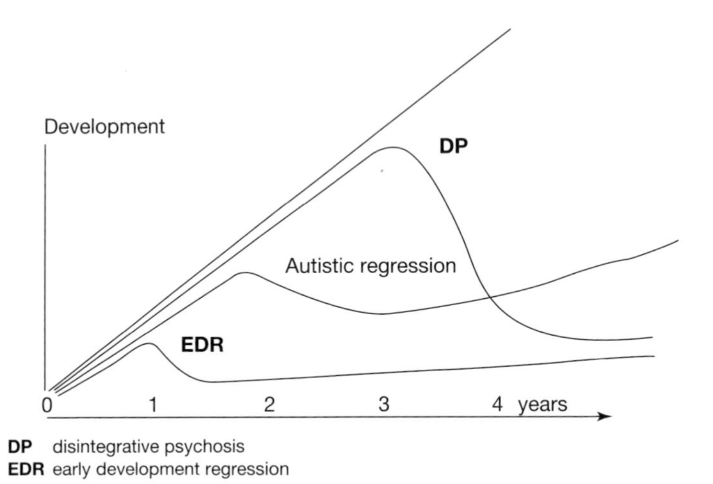

Fig. 12.5 Onset and course of some autistic spectrum disorders.

Age at onset of regression and course in children with typical autism, disintegrative psychosis and early developmental regression with autistic features (EDR). EDR may be due to various diseases, for instance Rett syndrome or epileptic disorders of early onset. These may start after a period of normal or already delayed development.

The terminological distinction between autism and disintegrative disorder is based only on the age at regression and says nothing about the etiology of the underlying disorder. In disintegrative disorder, the children had acquired normal verbal language prior to the regression. In some children, a rare neurometabolic or neurodegenerative disease may be found, but most of the time the cause remains unknown. In the older literature, these children were diagnosed as suffering from Heller's dementia (Heller 1930, Rapin 1965). As a group, children with disintegrative disorder have a greater incidence of epilepsy and a more severe long-term evolution, although the latter point is controversial.

Rett syndrome, now recognized as a specific genetic disease, is one possible cause of regression in development, which usually starts earlier than in children with typical autism, but there can be some overlap. Some girls with Rett syndrome have severe early seizures ('early seizure variant'). The loss of language and communication in affected girls who had reached that level of development sometimes leads to an initial diagnosis of autism, although the maintenance of eye contact and social smiling, and the loss of purposeful hand movements, as well as other neurological features, give a clinical picture clearly different from that seen in children with typical autism.

As previously discussed, epilepsies or epilepsy syndromes of various causes presenting with infantile spasms and/or complex partial seizures may be accompanied by early developmental regression after normal or delayed development.

12.4.5 Autistic Regression of Epileptic Origin? Evidence from the Literature

The high incidence of epilepsy in autism and the possibility of a direct causal link, as discussed above, has led many centres to include EEG recordings (sometimes with sleep studies) as part of the systematic modern neurobiological diagnostic work-up of autism (Tuchman et al 1991, Rapin 1995). Many such children have paroxysmal EEG abnormalities of epileptic type (whether or not they have had clinical seizures). Several therapeutic studies with antiepileptic drugs, steroids and even surgery (subpial transsections) (Lewine et al 1999, Nass et al 1999) have been performed with the aim of ameliorating the autistic symptoms. The results are difficult to interpret but on the whole have been rather disappointing (Kanner 2000).

Another approach to evaluating the possible direct role of epilepsy has been to see whether children with autism and a history of regression had more epileptic EEG abnormalities than those who did not have such a history. The results showed no significant statistical differences (Tuchman and Rapin 1997, Baird and Robinson 2000), and it now appears clear that the autistic regression found in about one-third of children later diagnosed as suffering from typical autism is not related to an epileptic dysfunction.

Arguments for a direct link between epilepsy and autism can only come from studies in which a close time correlation between the epileptic variables and the clinical autistic syndrome has been demonstrated. We have thus looked at this matter in detail. We first chose to review all papers whose title claimed an epileptic origin for the autistic behaviour. We then analysed those studies that were longitudinal (usually single case studies or studies of a few cases) in which we felt some attempt had been made to directly correlate the behaviour and its changes with the epileptic activity (clinical, EEG, and effects of therapy (antiepileptic medication or epilepsy surgery)). This obviously implies some bias and possibly does not do justice to all publications. Large group studies (e.g. Lewine et al 1999) have not been included, because these do not give enough clinical details in each case at close enough time intervals to make a judgement about the direct role of epilepsy. The results are summarized in Table 12.7.

The rapid and spectacular improvement in close correlation with the activity of the epilepsy documented in some of the cases offers good evidence for a true autistic epileptic regression. In others, one cannot rule out the possibility that the observed changes are due to the natural improvement of the autistic syndrome, possibly temporarily delayed because of the epilepsy.

Despite the often limited follow-up and lack of specific etiologic diagnosis in the majority of the published cases, it does not seem that the regression was due to another type of acquired disease, which reinforces the idea of a direct role of epilepsy.

Finally, this review shows how difficult it is to obtain hard data in this domain and how uncertain many of the conclusions remain, despite all the efforts made.

Illustrative case from literature review

A particularly striking case found in this review is case B, reported by Gillberg and Schaumann (1983), which is worth summarizing.

TABLE 12.7
Published longitudinal case studies in which authors claimed to have documented that the autistic behaviour or the autistic regression was of epileptic origin*

Note that the age at onset of the regression, seizure types, epileptic syndromes, specific etiology of the epilepsy and mode of therapy (medical and surgical) are extremely variable. Note also that the largest study (Lewine et al 1999) on this topic has been omitted from this table (see text).

Number of studies reviewed: 11; number of cases: 24
Regression in development mentioned: 19 (3 had a second phase of regression or stagnation)
Age at regression: 7 months to 5 years 9 months
Duration of follow-up: 1–2 years: 9; 2–5 years: 8; >5 years: 4
Prospective documentation of situation: 15/24
Specific brain disease diagnosed: 8 (tuberous sclerosis: 4; congenital tumour: 3; cortical dysplasia: 1)
Epileptic syndrome diagnosis given: early Landau–Kleffner syndrome: 7
Seizure types: infantile spasms: 4; others: 12; possible seizures: 3; no seizures: 5
VideoEEG documented fluctuations of 'autistic behaviour': 0 (several had videoEEG mentioned, but not further analysed)
Surgical therapy of epilepsy: 14
Authors' basis for judgement of improvement: clinical impression only: 7; with tests and questionnaires also: 17
Direct relationship between behaviour and epileptic activity: clear: 8; probable or possible: 6; doubtful: 10

* Dalla Bernardina et al 1994
Deonna et al 1993b
Deonna et al 1995
Gillberg and Schaumann 1983
Gillberg et al 1996
Hoon and Reiss 1992
Jacobs et al 2001
Nass et al 1999
Neville et al 1997
Plioplys 1994
Szabò et al 1999

This boy was born preterm (35 weeks, 2260 g) and had some neonatal problems (24 days in hospital), but was first seen by the authors at the age of 8 years when he was admitted to an inpatient psychiatry unit. At this age, 'a preliminary diagnosis of autism and mental retardation was made' (performance IQ: 60). His EEG showed continuous 3 c/s spike and wave activity lasting 15–20 seconds with free intervals of 5–10 seconds. A diagnosis of petit mal was made and he was put on ethosuximide. Three months later the EEG showed only sporadic bursts of sharp waves in the left frontotemporal leads, and he had made marked progress in speech and socialization. At 11 years, he was transferred to an ordinary school for children with mild disability. His mother considered it to be a miracle. The detailed description of his development (obtained retrospectively) indeed showed major problems in the areas of speech, socialization and behaviour, consistent with an autistic spectrum disorder. Interestingly, at the age of 4 years an EEG had been planned but in the end had not been done because of his difficult behaviour.

It appears that this child in fact had frontotemporal epilepsy with secondary generalization rather than true childhood absences (there was no sleep EEG, so that the possible presence of CSWS is not known). It presented as a developmental disorder in the autistic spectrum with a remarkable late 'recovery' under antiepileptic treatment. In the absence of prospective observations and detailed psychiatric data, it is difficult to be more precise about the nature of his psychiatric disorder. Prefrontal epilepsy with CSWS may cause a severe behavioural disorder with several autistic features but not typical autism (see case T.G., Chapter 8, section 8.4.1).

The following personal case, first seen at the age of 13 months because of epilepsy, allowed us to document prospectively the autistic regression and recovery.

Case B.A. (see also Fig. 12.6)

This boy has been followed prospectively from the age of 13 months when his epilepsy was first diagnosed and treated (in retrospect he had had seizures for at least three months before, mainly sudden 'fatigue', 'eye rubbing'). A videoEEG showed intermittent diffuse spike-waves accompanied by transient loss of contact. After initial therapy with valproate, the diffuse spike-waves disappeared and he had an intermittent left frontal focus. A brain MRI was normal.

The main objective of our follow-up was to see if there would be a 'catch-up' in development (he had a mild delay) after treatment of his epilepsy. Progress was noted for a few months, followed by an insidious regression in communication and play reported by the parents and by the educational specialist during home visits: 'he is busy with himself without the need of others; his games become too systematic', 'his behaviour resembles autism'. This regression worsened quite rapidly at around 25 months, with development of epileptic stereotypies and late onset spasms (for details of this semiology, see Deonna et al 2002), and his behaviour became typically autistic. His communication improved rapidly with prednisone. While at his worst, he was not lethargic but rather hyperactive, and he was able to 'fit' shapes with ease, showing a clear dissociation between his very regressed communicative abilities and preserved visuospatial capacities. This observation is unusual because the regression developed 'under our eyes' and could be documented prospectively.

12.4.6 Early Onset Landau–Kleffner Syndrome with Autistic Symptoms: Linguistic vs Autistic Regression?

In a young child who presents with behavioural regression and loss of verbal language, the question is often raised whether the child could suffer from an early form of Landau–Kleffner syndrome (Tuchman 1995). The children in whom the diagnosis of Landau–Kleffner

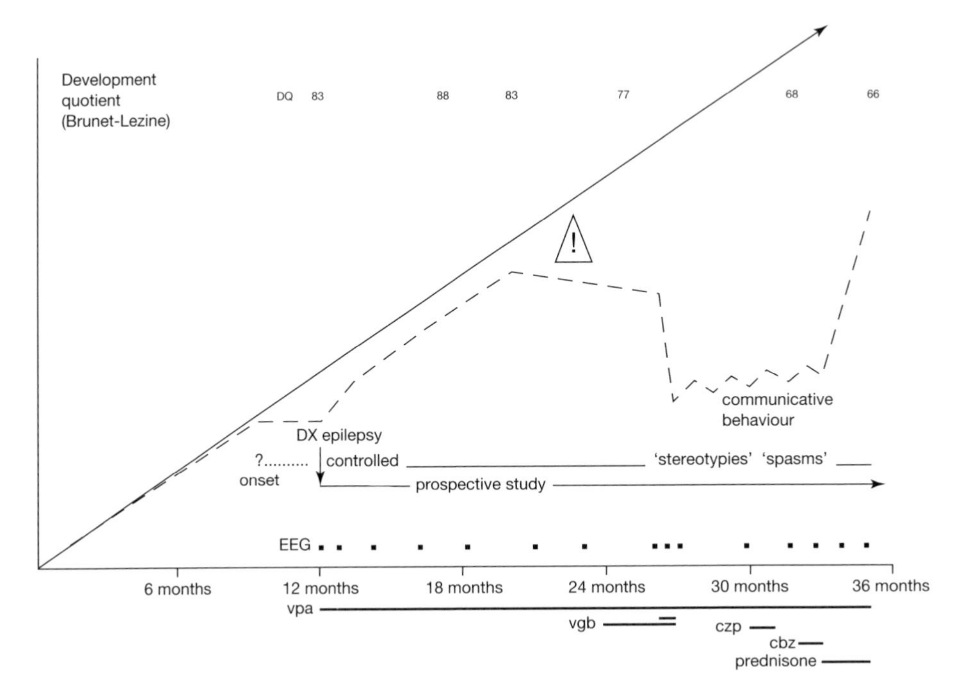

Fig. 12.6 Case B.A., boy: early autistic epileptic regression.

See case description. This figure shows the timing of clinical and EEG observations: progress could be documented for several months (Brunet-Lezine test) before the 'autistic' regression, which started first insidiously and later became more rapid. Regular home visits and videos were made at 13, 14, 16, 21, 23, 25, 28 and 36 months. (VPA: valproate, VGB: vigabatrin, CBZ: clobazam, CZP: carbamazepine.) (Modified from Nehlig et al 1999.)

syndrome is finally made but who present initially with many autistic symptoms or have even been diagnosed as suffering from typical autism are a challenge (Mantovani 2000). The suggestive cases published had an autistic spectrum disorder or pervasive developmental disorder. The improvement they showed on antiepileptic treatment or steroids was the main reason why they were considered as variants of Landau–Kleffner syndrome. It is difficult to know from the descriptions of these cases if they ever had behaviour consistent with classical autism (Stefanatos et al 1995, Uldall et al 2000). Review of the case histories published and our own experience suggest that they are probably only exceptionally this severe and do not present all the signs found in children diagnosed as suffering from typical autism, in whom a history of regression in development is often obtained. In the latter, in fact, the EEG, including sleep recordings, although often showing paroxysmal epileptic EEG abnormalities, rarely if ever show the typical temporal focal sharp waves and CSWS seen in Landau–Kleffner and related partial epilepsies (Lewine et al 1999).

In Kurita's classic study (Kurita 1985) on speech loss in autistic children before 30 months of age (mean age at onset of speech loss was18 months), only expressive vocabulary was documented and there was no mention of earlier lack of attention to sounds or understanding of words. It is thus difficult to ascertain if both verbal and other communicative behaviours regress together, even by studying family videos (Adrien et al 1993). It is not known whether and for how long early language regression, as a result of focal epilepsy in developing language areas for example, can affect oral language comprehension specifically, leaving other communicative abilities intact. Children with early language regression are practically never investigated by specialists close to the time of the regression, but only months or years later (Shinnar et al 2001). The remarkable case below, studied by Dr A. Chilosi and Professor R. Guerrini in Pisa, Italy – a boy whom we also had the opportunity to examine personally, and we also reviewed several videos – may be an exception. This case illustrates the difficulties, but also some of the possibilities, in documenting these situations. The boy was seen shortly after the onset of the deterioration (15 months) and the data given by the parents (who are both paediatricians) were of exceptional quality.

Case F.M.

This boy had normal early development (including prelanguage and communication) until the age of 15 months. The initial symptoms predominated in the domain of verbal comprehension and later extended to expression (intermittent at onset). The boy's auditory attention was fluctuating and this aspect appeared disproportionately more severe than the other non-verbal and social communication skills. This latter aspect was clearly abnormal when the child was first examined at 25 months and was consistent with the diagnosis of autism. At the very beginning, however, the child still seemed to have normal emotional-social behaviour, at least for a while.

The EEG showed an intense left parietal focus with generalized spike-waves which disappeared with ACTH therapy, along with marked improvement in language and autistic behaviour. This was studied with language questionnaires, video observations and precise documentation of autistic symptoms. There were subsequent relapses in the following years, which responded to several courses of ACTH therapy. At the second regression, verbal comprehension problems were again the predominant early symptom. In the subsequent regressions, it was not possible to say which component in his overall communication was more affected.

In this case, the data were of sufficient quality to show that verbal and other communicative dimensions were differentially affected by the epileptic activity, the former aspect being the first involved.

12.4.7 Epileptic Frontal Syndrome with CSWS: A Cause of Autistic Regression or Childhood Disintegrative Disorder?

Children with so-called 'partial frontal epilepsy with CSWS' may present with an acquired severe behavioural disorder of the psychotic type, with cognitive arrest or dementia but preserved verbal language (Deonna et al 2003). In the most severe form, they present a unique combination of aberrant emotional and cognitive behaviour compatible with a prefrontal dysfunction, which we have ourselves termed 'acquired epileptic frontal syndrome' (Roulet-Perez et al 1993; see Chapter 8, section 8.4.1).

In some of these children, the initial regression occurred without clinical epilepsy (or possibly with subtle seizures which had remained unrecognized), and the 'epileptic' sleep EEG was the only marker of the disorder. We wondered at this point whether some children diagnosed as having a disintegrative disorder could be suffering from this special epileptic syndrome. We may have given rise to undue hope in some families who had a child with disintegrative psychosis (Catalano 1998), as there is a strong incidence of epilepsy and epileptic EEG abnormalities in the reported series of children with disintegrative psychosis (Evans-Johns and Rosenbloom 1978, Mouridsen et al 1999).

Although we have not found in any of these series a case whose epilepsy course had the typical pattern of partial epilepsy with CSWS on the EEG, this is certainly a possible etiology. Children with a descriptive diagnosis of disintegrative psychosis in whom epilepsy is found to be the cause, and who recover, would not be reported and published as such. There are also cases of prefrontal epilepsy other than the 'partial epilepsy with CSWS' who may present initially with a behaviour disorder and regression descriptively compatible with an incipient disintegrative psychosis before the diagnosis of epilepsy is made and before recovery takes place.

Case D.A.

A previously normal 3-year-old boy was evaluated because of mood changes, disturbed communication and loss of play of one-month duration, all symptoms being of fluctuating severity. Repeat videotaped observations showed abnormal language use and non-verbal communication, repetitive play, attentional difficulties and marked mood changes, perseverations and fascinations. He also had bizarre paroxysmal movements and gestures ('as if wants to push away flies', 'gesticulates like a clown').

Extensive work-up was negative, apart from the EEG which showed a few paroxysmal rhythmic high voltage slow waves in the frontal region, more on the right side. An incipient disintegrative psychosis was considered or, alternatively, an unusual frontal epilepsy. Carbamazepine was introduced. A spectacular rapid behavioural improvement was seen within days and the stereotyped gestures disappeared. Comparative videotaped observations of behaviour and language, as well as ad hoc questionnaires, before and after recovery, confirmed the clinical impression (Deonna 1995).

The boy had a single brief recurrence of symptoms a few months later during a febrile episode. Developmentally, he progressed normally with slight language delay and significant hyperactivity, but he could attend a normal school. When last seen at

14 years a formal neuropsychological examination and EEG were normal and he had no behaviour or personality problems. Drug withdrawal, which had been considered for some years, was finally accepted by the mother.

The early behavioural-communicative regression and abnormal motor symptoms were considered as unusual epileptic manifestations of an early idiopathic frontal epilepsy with a self-limited course.

Another extremely severe and probably exceptional case was observed by Dr Mary King in Dublin and was seen personally on two occasions by one of the authors (TD).

Case B.P.

A boy, born 28.1.88, presented at the age of 4 years 10 months with massive behavioural and cognitive regression that occurred within a period of two to four weeks: loss of all communication with mutism, purposeless motor activity, absence of self-initiated actions and disturbed sleep, all needing constant supervision, were reported and observed. Only basic sensory, vegetative and motor functions were preserved. A descriptive diagnosis of childhood disintegrative disorder was made.

Extensive work-up gave no support for a toxic, metabolic or infectious etiology. He gradually recovered over a four- to five-month period. The only abnormal laboratory finding was a sleep EEG with a right frontotemporal epileptic focus, on two occasions two months apart. He was then treated with carbamazepine and had no further relapses. The last EEG (waking and sleep) at 8 years was normal.

The developmental history and a neuropsychological work-up a few months after he had recovered showed normal cognitive functions, but his language had features of a moderate semantic pragmatic disorder. He gradually improved over the years and at the last follow-up at 14 years he was performing normally in secondary school (case of Dr Mary King, Children's University Hospital, Dublin).

The behaviour of children with the frontal epileptic syndrome and CSWS (or other types of prefrontal epilepsy) has some features seen in a child with autism, but of course this syndrome is an acquired late disorder (after 3 to 4 years). This acquired and reversible syndrome has not been looked at in detail by child psychiatrists, despite the fascinating clinical model that such cases present. The child reported in Chapter 8 (T.G.), whom we have followed prospectively from 4 to 9 years, who deteriorated massively under our eyes and 'recovered', had, at the worst period, some autistic features (repetitive behaviours, social indifference, lack of imaginative and creative activity, aberrant behaviours). However, he also had distorted thoughts, confusion between reality and his own ideas, hallucinations, and flattened and aberrant emotional reactions, and some high-level social emotions were preserved (see discussion of case T.G. in Chapter 8).

12.5 Conclusions

The main problems in this difficult issue of the role of epilepsy in causing some autistic spectrum disorders are summarized in Table 12.8.

Epilepsy is not the cause of clinical symptoms in children with typical autism, whether or not there is a history of regression. In such cases, especially those without significant mental retardation, an EEG investigation (which, if done, should include a sleep tracing) cannot be considered mandatory any longer. The children in whom this possibility exists have a combination of verbal language delay or regression, general cognitive impairment and deviant behaviours or patterns of communication and socialization, with one aspect having been, or presently being, in the forefront of the parents' concerns. The priority is not so much to try to push a child into one behavioural classification and to decide whether the child is more autistic, dysphasic or mentally retarded, but to document as precisely as possible all facets of the disorder for later comparison, and to try to find out whether there has actually been a stagnation or regression at any previous point in time, which, among other data, may suggest the possibility of epilepsy.

The follow-up of the child often enables differentiation between the components of a particular neuropsychological or behavioural profile. For instance, a child who presents without any communication whatsoever, can be found at a later time to have a specific linguistic problem, which was not or could not be recognized at an earlier age. These children are not usually included in systematic group studies by psychiatrists or psychologists, and are often in a no-man's land between child neurologists, child psychiatrists, developmental specialists and educators. Unless there is close cooperation between them, it is very difficult

TABLE 12.8
Autistic spectrum disorder with epilepsy (or paroxysmal epileptic EEG): association or causal link? Summary of the main problems

This table summarizes the major clinical and conceptual issues which make the problem of the possible direct relationship between autistic spectrum disorder and epilepsy so controversial and difficult.

- Epilepsy is not the cause of clinical symptoms in children with typical autism whether or not there was a history of regression
- Several epileptic disorders in the first years of life may cause behavioural–language regression of the autistic type (not only Landau–Kleffner syndrome)
- Epilepsy may be an aggravating factor and not the main cause of the brain dysfunction responsible for the autistic disorder
- A confusional-apathetic epileptic state in a young child should not be described as autistic unless communication, social interaction and play are severely altered while other skills (e.g. fine motor, visuospatial, etc.) are relatively preserved
- Children are sometimes evaluated long after epilepsy was active or before it becomes active, so that its possible role in causing autistic symptoms is difficult to clarify (importance of follow-up)

to get a clear picture of all facets of the disorder, its dynamics and the role of all therapeutic factors. According to one's model of reference, one may be tempted to attribute improvement or worsening to psychological rather than physiological factors (including epilepsy).

Several epileptic disorders in the first years of life may cause a behavioural–language regression with autistic features, and not only Landau–Kleffner syndrome (O'Regan et al 1998). The tendency to label any child with early regression, paroxysmal EEG abnormalities and no recognizable neurological disease as having an early form of Landau–Kleffner syndrome or variants (e.g. partial epilepsy with CSWS) is blurring the issue (Kanner 2000, Neville et al 2000). Recent studies in children with early autistic/language regression and paroxysmal EEG abnormalities show that they do not, or only exceptionally, have the typical perisylvian focal sharp waves and the CSWS pattern (Lewine et al 1999). Multifocal independent sources of epileptic activity can be found in the same child or in different children with regressive autistic spectrum disorders, outside the typical perisylvian/temporal region (Lewine et al 1999, Kanner 2000). Epilepsy may be an aggravating factor and not the main cause of the autistic disorder. Malformations, tumours or other pathologies affecting the limbic system, from which epilepsy may start, are typical examples. The case of tuberous sclerosis is particularly important here.

The description of the child's behaviour and the labelling of the behaviour as autistic are particularly difficult in an active epilepsy situation. A child with recurrent seizures, especially of the complex partial type, who is apathetic, with little or no social interaction and play, may be called autistic, but this is unjustified unless one can show that other cognitive skills (e.g. fine motor, visuospatial, etc.) are relatively preserved.

Finally, follow-up of these children is a crucial issue. Epilepsy, in a given case, may have been at one point, or will become later on, one important cause of the child's disability, but not at the time it is being evaluated. A rapid onset of symptoms and recovery, never seen in classical developmental autism or in autistic disorders due to specific genetic or other diseases in which acquisitions occur over a much longer time span, can occasionally be documented. Despite the disillusionment which has appeared after an initial excessive enthusiasm for an epileptic etiology in some of these cases, the possible role of epilepsy has to remain open. The difficulty of studying this clinical issue in a standard scientific manner, of presenting clinically convincing cases and finding efficacious antiepileptic drugs, remains a major issue.

13 NEUROPSYCHOLOGICAL EVALUATION OF COGNITIVE-BEHAVIOURAL EFFECTS OF EPILEPSY IN CHILDREN

(with Claire Mayor-Dubois)

> 'Why do you want to test him, you see that he cannot do anything.' And when the child recovered: 'You do not need tests, you see that he is all right now.'
>
> (Mother of a child with epilepsy)

> 'Comme s'il suffisait de pouvoir mesurer pour comprendre.'
>
> (Jeanne Hersch)

> 'What is important is hidden, the devil is in the details.'
>
> (anon.)

13.1 Introduction

The neuropsychological assessment of a child with epilepsy may have different objectives which need to be distinguished. First is a functional assessment of the general cognitive level and the identification of specific cognitive deficits and weaknesses and behavioural abnormalities, in order to differentiate these from primarily psychological problems and define needs for special remediation and schooling. This is what is done with any child with a suspected or known brain dysfunction. Second is the search for a focal neuropsychological deficit that can help to localize the site of the epileptic pathology. This is typically considered the role of neuropsychological evaluation in adult epilepsy surgery centres, but is much less a priority in young children in whom such correlations are often impossible or misleading. Finally, the neuropsychological evaluation is carried out to assess the current level of abilities and functioning, for follow-up and direct correlation with the epileptic disease and its treatment. This will be specifically discussed in this chapter.

In order to evaluate the cognitive and behavioural disorders observed in a child with epilepsy and to try to relate them to their many possible causes, and especially to the direct role of epilepsy, one has to take into account the unique characteristics of this condition, as opposed to other childhood brain disorders. Therefore, the following points have to be considered:

1 Indications for neuropsychological investigations in children with epilepsy, considering the clinical features of the child's specific epileptic condition and its cause (who).
2 Special problems in neuropsychological evaluation of children with cognitive/behavioural disturbances of suspected epileptic origin.
3 The appropriate timing in relation to the epileptic activity (when).
4 The appropriate site for investigations (where).
5 The cognitive functions to receive priority for evaluation (what and how).

These questions should be asked before embarking on a sometimes long and tedious testing procedure, the results of which may be irrelevant or uninterpretable, depending on the clinical context. Data are sometimes painstakingly obtained but useless, and this reduces the likelihood of good cooperation when really needed at a later time.

13.2 Indications for neuropsychological investigations in children with epilepsy (who)

The importance of identifying areas of specific cognitive deficit, or anticipating potential problems, is increasingly recognized by child neurologists in a variety of congenital or acquired brain disorders, especially in epilepsy which is the most frequent condition they deal with. In any epilepsy, seizures can be temporarily difficult to control, or drugs poorly tolerated. It is also difficult to foresee at the onset if and what cognitive and learning problems might later develop. For these reasons, especially for later comparison, a baseline neuropsychological evaluation always has to be considered, but poses some problems. First, this is not always locally available, or only in a limited way. Special expertise and time are needed and the results have to be integrated into the general epilepsy context of the child. It may also not be advisable in the first stage of diagnosis. When there are no problems apart from seizures, proposing a cognitive evaluation implies that problems might develop which often will not. One should not forget that the child who does well in school, is happy and who presents no behavioural problems at home and with friends has passed the most difficult of the psychological and cognitive tests, 'the life test'. Following this principle, most children with 'epilepsy only' will not need special cognitive tests unless there is an unexplained learning or behavioural problem which has to be clarified, or unless they are involved in a research project. However, the threshold for proposing a first evaluation when no or only subtle problems are identified may be lower in certain situations in which cognitive problems can develop. This applies to very active rolandic epilepsies, frontal or temporal lobe epilepsies and special syndromes such as epilepsy with CSWS. In such cases, the child may need a complete baseline evaluation even if he/she is presently having no problems, apart from seizures. In these cases, the cognitive dysfunction can occur insidiously and be protracted without necessarily being accompanied by new clinical seizures.

Limitations in terms of neuropsychological expertise, time, resources and other constraints mean that a complete examination in each child with suspected or anticipated cognitive and learning problems is not possible, and priorities have to be established. This situation may change with the development of quick clinical tools for screening acquired and developmental cognitive deficits (Ouvrier et al 1993, 1999, Billard et al 2002a, 2002b).

13.3 Special problems in neuropsychological evaluation of children with cognitive/behavioural disturbances of suspected epileptic origin

The general principles that have to be respected when performing a neuropsychological examination in a child of course apply to a child with epilepsy. However, there are special problems to be taken into consideration in these children before deciding on an investigation, and also when interpreting the results.

13.3.1 Alertness (Vigilance)

The level of the child's vigilance can be very different, depending on motivation, and whether a seizure has occurred shortly before testing. Antiepileptic drugs can also affect the degree of vigilance. In addition, seizures, sometimes subtle, or paroxysmal EEG discharges, tend to occur in states of decreased vigilance and can further worsen the child's performance. All these factors have to be taken into account when interpreting neuropsychological results, especially when the child's overall performance deteriorates or fluctuates during the course of testing.

13.3.2 Psychoaffective State and Behaviour of the Child During Testing

This factor is evidently very important in any testing situation but can be exacerbated in epilepsy. It cannot be quantified and its importance in the interpretation of the results of cognitive tests is always difficult to evaluate. It is often a source of disagreements between parents and professionals and between paediatric neurologists and psychiatrists, who may find the testing inappropriate or consider it a harassment of the sick child with epilepsy. Failure of the parents to comply with follow-ups, to accept repeated tests and to adhere to antiepileptic therapy is often the result of their own (or the caregiver's) interpretation of the problems and of their suffering and doubts about the cause of the problems (physiological versus psychological), and this is not sufficiently acknowledged. This psychoaffective dimension should thus be thought of at every level of diagnosis and therapy and when neuropsychological tests are requested and interpreted.

The 'untestable' and 'uncooperative' child

In some children, the behaviour is so disturbed (short attention span, irritability, low tolerance to frustration, refusal of any imposed task) that it seems to preclude the gathering of any reliable data: most of the time psychologists would not even attempt to expose the child to the constraints of the tests. They may feel that to document failure is useless or destructive to the child's self-image, or that any result obtained will be unreliable or not reflect the child's potential. The parents may feel the same way, and even more strongly. One has to take these factors into account and be reasonable in one's demands. However, if it is possible to document at least some preserved abilities (starting at a low level in order not to discourage the child), this may be a very useful basis for comparison in the future. The results obtained will show at least a minimum of preserved skills and also help to define the nature of the behavioural disorder (e.g. frontal syndrome). Besides sheer incapacity and lack of motivation (refusal, opposition), which often reflects the child's own intuition of loss of capacity as well as previous negative experiences, some behaviours in children with epilepsy can greatly affect the test results:

1 Inattention: this may be so prominent as to preclude either entering into the task or focusing on it for a sufficient length of time.
2 Perseverations, stereotypies, inappropriate use of the material: we have found these latter behaviours particularly in some children with epileptic frontal dysfunction.

13.4 Appropriate timing of neuropsychological investigations (when)

Considering that epilepsy is an unstable, dynamic condition, results at one point in time reflect one specific moment in a child's epilepsy history, which needs to be taken into account, or at least specified, depending on the question one is interested in. Fluctuations in performance may be due to a postictal state, lack of sleep, drug sedation or other unspecific factors. It should be remembered that the cognitive domain in which a child is least at ease is the most fragile, and likely to suffer from any situation which makes extra demands on the child's cognitive resources or weakens them.

The evaluation should be carried out in the period that is most likely to reveal a recent deficit or sudden gain in relation to the epilepsy. One may have to propose a test when a child appears at their worst or at their best, a period that intuitively one might not think to be the most appropriate (see the mother's comments above). This also requires that the psychologist is available on a kind of emergency basis and is ready to change his/her schedule and tempo of work – for instance, for testing the child at different moments in the same day.

13.4.1 Time After Epilepsy Onset

As previously discussed, children evaluated immediately after the onset of epilepsy (normal children with 'epilepsy only') may already show slight problems before any therapy. This could indicate a possible cognitive influence of epilepsy, already present at its onset (Schouten et al 2001). Such studies are complex to carry out and difficult to interpret because the observed differences, if any, are usually minimal.

13.4.2 Study During Interictal Period (Chronic Period)

This is a baseline which will be taken as the child's usual or 'normal' functioning. It will allow evaluation of progress over time and also a comparison with periods of acute deterioration possibly due to epileptic activity. The more severe the epilepsy, the more difficult it will be to 'catch' this period of supposedly best functioning. One needs to know when the last seizure was and if the parents feel their child is in a good period. In children whose epilepsy starts immediately with difficult to control, frequent seizures, obtaining a baseline evaluation is sometimes 'forgotten', because of the many other priorities, but later on, when the question of epilepsy-related or drug-related cognitive slowing or loss is raised, this essential information is missing.

13.4.3 Ictal–Postictal Period

In order to know which cognitive functions are altered or preserved during a partial seizure, it is necessary to interact with the child. This is not the usual approach of a physician, which would be to terminate the seizure with medication as soon as the diagnosis is made. Only a limited amount of cognitive function can be tested during the usually brief duration of a seizure and it is difficult to plan in advance what are the most pertinent data to obtain. When previous episodes have occurred and observations have already been made, one can plan in advance what should be tried if a new episode is witnessed in the hospital, ideally under EEG monitoring. These opportunities rarely occur, except in patients who undergo epilepsy surgery or those with frequent seizures. The simultaneous EEG monitoring allows one to determine what manifestations are ictal or postictal. However, even without this information, the purely clinical documentation of a deficit and its exact nature, followed by a comparison with the period after recovery, gives significant information. It allows one to judge whether the observed change can be explained in any other way but a temporary epileptic dysfunction (see case F.G. in Chapter 8).

The postictal period is often considered unrepresentative because the child is tired or bad-tempered. Nevertheless, it can be important to find out if it corresponds to a state or behaviour that parents have observed at times, possibly independently of visible seizures. If so, it may be an indication of cognitive or behavioural manifestations of the epilepsy, which had been unrecognized. The possibility of carrying out detailed testing during post-ictal states is of course variable, but often there is enough time to gather useful information.

13.4.4 Relationship to Antiepileptic Therapy (Before, Under, and Off Therapy)

If it is possible to obtain an evaluation before any antiepileptic therapy, this is of course the best option. It is very helpful if one can show that cognitive or behavioural problems had already been present before any treatment. Antiepileptic drugs are almost invariably blamed by parents, teachers or well-meaning acquaintances, at one point or another, as the cause of the problems. When the child is on therapy a serum drug level may be useful, especially when the child is on high doses or on polytherapy. In retrospect, one often regrets not having a serum drug level when a cognitive side-effect of the drug becomes apparent at a later period. When a drug which has been taken for a long time is stopped, one has to take into account the possible biological or psychological effects of the withdrawal in planning the evaluation.

13.4.5 Timing of the Evaluation in Relation to the Last EEG Recording

The ideal condition is to have the two examinations as closely related in time as possible. The paroxysmal EEG activity can change both in intensity and sometimes in location in short periods of time, especially in partial epilepsy syndromes with focal sharp waves. The interpretation of unusual neuropsychological findings will be impossible if no EEG was done at the same time. Testing under videomonitoring is rarely feasible in a busy EEG department, outside a research project, or has to be reserved for specific situations such as the documentation of transient cognitive impairment during EEG discharges. A repeat combined neuropsychological and EEG examination may sometimes have to be obtained again within a short period, to be sure of the interpretation of results and also sometimes to convince parents that an aggressive antiepileptic therapy is necessary.

13.5 Appropriate place(s) to evaluate children (where)

In older children without major behavioural problems, evaluation in a neutral, 'serious' and always similar setting, such as the hospital office, is preferable and may encourage the child to perform at their best level without being distracted as they would be at home. The situation is different for infants or young children for whom strange environments such as hospitals or laboratories cause a certain amount of discomfort or distress. This may alter the results of cognitive testing. The younger the child, the more important are the conditions in which a developmental examination is performed. A lack of sleep from travelling or a change in eating routines and an unfamiliar environment can greatly affect level of performance and cooperation. This is particularly important also because these early epilepsies are usually accompanied by severe behavioural problems which, even in the best circumstances, make precise evaluations difficult.

Clinical follow-up in difficult situations and research on developmental and behavioural consequences of epilepsies in infants and very young children sometimes require that the child be evaluated at home. We have been fortunate to have a paediatrician (Dr Anne-Lise Ziegler) specially trained in infant testing for these types of evaluations. The behavioural and other changes (including suspected abnormal paroxysmal phenomena), particularly at a young age, can thus be put into the context of the general infant development, health and home situation (Deonna et al 1995).

As major diagnostic and therapeutic investments (including epilepsy surgery) are now being made for these early epilepsies at increasingly younger ages, and the accurate evaluation of their consequences for cognitive development is a crucial issue for which precise data are desperately needed, it is surprising that home testing is apparently not a generally available resource in most centres. Developmental psychologists have been doing this for a long time, and it is an integral part of their routine research budget. This includes, among other things, travel expenses, mobile test material and video equipment. This is very important since repeated evaluations may be necessary to document changes that could occur quite rapidly in this early life period – that is, at closer intervals than those necessary for purely medical-neurological controls.

Testing of the children in their own school may also be a useful and practical option, and give a valuable insight into the child's general functioning, behaviour and school progress, as perceived by the teachers. In any case, the results of the neuropsychological tests, wherever they are done, should be available and ideally discussed personally with those, besides the parents, in charge of the child's education and teaching, and put into the context of the epileptic disease.

13.6 Neuropsychological evaluation (what and how) (see also Table 13.1)

13.6.1 History of Cognitive Development, Learning (School) and Behaviour

The first step is to obtain a detailed history of the course of early development, looking for age at emergence and progress in the different cognitive domains, and to review the child's school record, looking for possible stagnation, regression or fluctuations in the months or years prior to the first systematic evaluation. Even if a child has no problems when first seen, the dynamics of development and the documentation of prior difficulties, even if already addressed (e.g. early behaviour problems, or slow language development or reading acquisition), are important, but may have been forgotten or dismissed as non-relevant. Children sometimes come to the attention of specialists fairly late, so that it is difficult to document retrospectively a possible deterioration, stagnation or marked fluctuations in cognitive skills, behaviour and emotional competences. Yet, these may be crucial clues as to the time of onset, duration and type of manifestations of epilepsy (Shinnar et al 2001).

The ability of a child to learn and to follow the regular school curriculum is certainly a good index of cognitive functioning regardless of any test result. Of course, the child may not perform to their full potential even though they are not failing. It is not uncommon to find that the child had an insidious decline in average marks over the years (initially being one of the best students and gradually becoming one of the lowest) or was put in less demanding school groups.

In practice, the use of school reports to evaluate the dynamics of learning in a child who one suspects either stagnates because of epilepsy or, in the opposite case, catches up after successful epilepsy therapy or spontaneous remission, is difficult to include as a quantifiable variable, but it can be a useful clinical indicator. Changes are often too slow, and the different steps in the learning process have not been quantified and monitored at the appropriate time or evaluated by the same teachers, to be correlated precisely with the epilepsy variables. School achievement tests are available in some countries and may contain useful data for later comparison.

13.6.2 Neuropsychological Tests and Other Tools (see Table 13.1)

Standard neuropsychological tests, to evaluate general intelligence and specific functions, and questionnaires are the main tools, whereas computer-generated tests for direct EEG correlations or computerized clinical tests are less regularly used or only for special clinical purposes or research.

Evaluation in children with epilepsy should go beyond standard intelligence tests, because relatively hidden factors, for instance in the domains of attention, memory, executive functions and motor control, are frequent (Beckung and Uvebrant 1997, Culhane-Shelburne et al 2002).

The question that is sometimes asked is: what tests do you use in children with epilepsy? In fact, there are no tests that are specific to children with epilepsy, except those designed to assess very brief changes (seconds) in accuracy or speed of a given cognitive function. This could be slowness of response, no response or erroneous response while the child performs a continuous task that can be measured and directly correlated with electroencephalographic epileptic discharges. These are computer-generated tasks designed to search for the so-called 'transient cognitive impairment' (see Chapter 4).

Neuropsychological tests used in children with epilepsy are thus the same as those used in childhood neuropsychology in general, taking into account the necessary precautions and attention to the conditions which are uniquely relevant to these children, which have been discussed above. However, more than other brain dysfunctions, epilepsy can interfere with one or several very specific aspects of cognitive function simultaneously or at different periods (for instance, a specific language disturbance with an attention deficit). For these reasons, one has to choose and use the most appropriate tests developed and standardized for specific domains, or only a part of these, as indicated by a clinical suspicion or by previous tests.

Sometimes, it is necessary to identify rapidly the specific or main problem that could result from the epileptic dysfunction and to focus immediately on the seemingly most affected domain, without trying to obtain a basic intelligence test or carry out a systematic testing protocol, which can be done later. This allows documentation of an epileptic cognitive deficit which will have disappeared in a short period (for example, memory loss). The range of problems that can be encountered is as vast and rich as the range of possible deficits due to any acute focal brain lesion. The difference is that the epileptic deficit is dynamic and reflects the involvement of the epileptogenic zone but also that of distant zones due to seizure spread from the initial focus. Several foci can also be active at the same time or in close succession.

13.6.3 Methodological Problems Linked to Repeated Evaluations: Test-Retest Effects

Test-retest effects are a general problem in neuropsychology, but more important in epilepsy where one wants to repeat the same tests at close intervals to document rapid changes. Some items are not sensitive to a test-retest effect and may be repeated. For others, one may need to change the material used while addressing the same problems (e.g. use of different lists of words to read or write for comparison, but of the same phonological complexity). Test-retest effects have been studied and discussed by Aldenkamp et al (1990). Particular profiles are usually quite stable and are presumably due to the underlying brain disorder causing the epilepsy or to the direct effect of a chronic epileptic dysfunction (or both).

13.6.4 Neuropsychological Tests

Table 13.1 lists the main tests that we regularly or occasionally use in our practice and which have been applied to the children mentioned briefly in the case studies or in more detail in some of the clinical studies presented in the book. One must realize that there is and will be no test which will be fully appropriate for the myriad possible transient impairments that can be seen in epilepsy and which one wants to document precisely. One has to invent them 'ad hoc', or use tools that have been created for very different purposes (e.g. computerized analysis of handwriting developed by developmental psychologists who study the development of normal handwriting).

TABLE 13.1
List of neuropsychological tests and other tools

The reader will find source references for these tests in Appendix 1. Most of them are in current use in child neuropsychology and we have used them in the various case studies presented in the book.

Function	Name of test (age)	Characteristics and comments
General intelligence (IQ)	WISC-III* Wechsler intelligence scale (6–16 years)	Has a verbal and a nonverbal (performance) part. The verbal part is not a specific test of language
	WPPSI-R* Wechsler intelligence scale (3–7 years)	
	K-ABC* Kaufmann assessment battery for children (2 years 6 months–12 years 6 months)	Contains original tasks designed to distinguish simultaneous from sequential mode of processing. Individual tasks can reveal specific problems in different aspects of visual perception and prompt more detailed specific testing in these areas
	MacCarthy scale* (2 years 6 months–8 years 6 months)	Standardized from a very early age. Also contains tasks to test motor maturation (fine and gross motor)
	PMS/PMC* Raven's progressive matrices	Evaluation of logical reasoning on nonverbal material
Developmental scale (DQ)	BSID Bayley scale of infant development (0–42 months)	Developmental scale (mental and motor)
Language: *Oral language skills (production and comprehension)*	BEPL Batterie d'évaluation psycholinguistique (Chevrie) (3–4 years)	Analysis of phonological, lexical, syntactic level in expression and comprehension
	EEL/NEEL Epreuves pour l'examen du langage (Chevrie) (4–8 years) parlé	
	TLP Test de langage (5–10 years)	
	L2MA (Chevrie) (8–12 years)	Oral and written language
	Renfrew language scales (3–8 years)	Indication of level of grammatical competence, narrative skills and word-finding ability
	CELF-3 Clinical evaluation of language fundamentals (Semel)	Good discrimination between children with and without language impairment
	Preschool language scale (Zimmerman) (0–6 years)	For very young children
	Test of language development: primary (Newcomer) (4–8 years)	Norms for 4–8 years
Oral comprehension	EVIP** (2–16 years) Peabody vocabulary test–R	Lexical comprehension
	ECOSSE*** Epreuve de comprehension syntaxique-sémantique (4–12 years)	Semantic-syntactic comprehension
	TROG (Bishop)	
	O–52 (Khomsi)	
Written language	BELEC Batterie d'évaluation du langage écrit et de ses troubles	Words and pseudowords, reading with control for frequency, complexity and length. Regular and irregular words. Allows assessment of phonological and lexical routes to reading

	LOBROT	Reading skills and orthographic skills
Communication	ESCS Early social communication scale (2–22 months) ECSP Evaluation de la comunication sociale précoce	Early interactional competencies of infants. Measures of joint attention, social interaction and behaviour regulation
Play	Belsky (7–21 months)	Infant free play behaviour
	Lowe & Costello (12–36 months)	Symbolic play test, standardized
Visual gnosic skills	TVPS Test of visual-perceptive skills (4–12 years) Hooper (from 5 years) BORB Birmingham object recognition battery Subtest of K-ABC	Tests of visual perception, associative and integrative functions
Constructive praxis	Subtest WISC-III: cubes RCFT Rey complex figure test	
Memory:		
Short-term memory	Digit span (WISC-III)	Short-term auditory memory
	CBTT* Corsi-block tapping test	Short-term visuospatial memory
Anterograde memory	CMS Children memory scale (5–16 years) RAVLT Rey's auditory verbal learning test CVLT* California verbal learning test Rey's visual design learning test BEM Batterie d'efficience mnésique (8–12 years) RCFT Rey complex figure test	Evaluation of anterograde memory. Tests of visual and/or verbal modalities, with analysis of processes of encoding, recall and recognition
Episodic memory	RBMT Rivermead behavioural memory test (5–10 years)	Ecological test, good correlation with daily life memory
Attention	CPT Conners' continuous peformance test	Computerized test with analysis of vigilance, sustained attention, index of inattention, impulsivity
	D2 Test D2 d'attention concentrée Corkum Z2B Test des 2 barrages Subtest WISC-III: code	Task with paper and pencil, detection of targets among distractors
Executive functions	Stroop colour-word test	Inhibition of automatic responses (verbal)
	Go–no go	Inhibition of automatic responses (motor)
	Verbal and figural fluency tests	Creativity in verbal and nonverbal modalities
	TMT Trail-making test	Planification and mental flexibility
	Wisconsin card-sorting test	Mental flexibility
	Hanoi tower	Planification
	Mazes	Visuospatial planification
Others	BREV Batterie rapide d'évaluation (4–8 years)	Screening of cognitive difficulties (see discussion in Chapter 13)
	FePsy Multiple domain battery	Composite battery of computerized tests with evaluation of several cognitive functions
	Purdue Test of manual dexterity	Left and right and bimanual speed and coordination
	Dichotic listening	Language lateralization

TABLE 13.1 *continued*

Function	Name of test (age)	Characteristics and comments
Questionnaires	BRIEF Behaviour rating inventory of executive functions	Questionnaire on behaviours presumed to be associated with prefrontal dysfunction
	CARS Childhood autism rating scale (Schopler) (from 3 years)	
	CBCL Child behaviour checklist (Achenbach)	
	CCC Children's communication checklist (Bishop)	Questionnaire on language use (pragmatics)
	Index of hyperactivity (Conners)	Questionnaire on hyperactivity
	ERC-N Evaluation résumée du comportement – nourrisson (Sauvage) (0–3 years)	Early detection of autism in infants

* These tests have an adapted version in French
** French equivalent of Peabody vocabulary test
*** French equivalent of TROG (Bishop)

Standard intelligence tests such as the WISC or K-ABC may serve as a standard baseline for later comparison, depending on evolution. These tests cover different aspects of cognitive functioning (verbal, visuospatial, attention tasks) and may give hints for particular weaknesses, which may be looked at more closely with other tests of specific domains (i.e. language, visuospatial, memory, motor). This may be guided by the history or school reports, or by a hypothesis generated by EEG, seizure history, general IQ tests, brain imaging or other neurological data. The testing of the many different components of attention (see also Chapter 8) is complex and particularly important in epilepsy because attentional problems can be the causal factor of school failure in otherwise normally intelligent children with epilepsy. There are several standardized tests of attention (computerized and clinical), in which stimulus and response demands of increasing complexity are given. These tests can sometimes be failed for reasons other than poor attention, when the modality in which it is tested is already a problem for the child (visual or auditory).

Mental efficiency (processing) is a special issue which is difficult to address directly. Current life demands and school curricula require a child to do things at a certain speed and with other constraints (e.g. with background noise, two things at a time, one subject after another) which are different from those of a testing situation. This can exceed the capacity of the child's nervous system, especially if the child has a brain injury or dysfunction, whatever its cause, and even when the child has otherwise normal or above-average intelligence. In children with epilepsy, this may be due to the disease which caused the epilepsy, or to side-effects of drugs, but it can also be directly related to the epilepsy itself. There are now standardized experimental tasks which tend to objectively evaluate problems such as set-shifting, processing speed and double tasks, and which can help to explain why an apparently normally intelligent child with epilepsy fails in school, or give early indices of future difficulties (Schouten et al 2001).

13.6.5 Rapid, Short, Screening Neuropsychological Tests (BREV)

The availability of a reliable baseline rapid, sensitive neuropsychological battery screening several aspects of cognitive functioning is an important potential advance, particularly in epilepsy because of its very nature and frequency. A group of French paediatric neurologists has developed such a battery, called BREV, in normal children (500 children aged 4 to 8 years) and has validated this tool in children with epilepsy (Billard et al 2002a, 2002b).

The BREV, as opposed to other 'mini-mental state' examinations (Ouvrier et al 1999), has been standardized for each cognitive function, allowing the detection of specific disorders, which is especially relevant to many instances of childhood epilepsy. In their study of 202 children aged 4 to 8 years with various epilepsy syndromes, the results obtained with the BREV were compared with results obtained with the WISC and with other more specific subtests from existing classic batteries (MacCarthy, Kaufman). The authors found that every function evaluated with the BREV was significantly correlated with the items of the reference battery testing a similar function. Specificity and sensitivity of the BREV verbal and non-verbal scores were correlated with those of the Wechsler scale in more than 75 per cent of the cases.

The BREV has been devised as a screening test that can be administered by physicians. It does not provide a diagnosis, nor does it replace clinical judgement, but it can help to identify areas of delay or dysfunction necessitating more detailed neuropsychological assessment. As long as this is recognized, as well as the wide range of normal scores found in some tests, especially in the younger age group, it may become a very useful adjunct to clinical evaluation of children with epilepsy in whom a full neuropsychological evaluation is not warranted or not possible and also difficult to repeat frequently.

It will be important to evaluate whether data obtained with the BREV in an early phase of epilepsy in a child who subsequently stagnates, regresses or has highly fluctuating cognitive performance will allow the diagnosis of significant changes directly related to the epilepsy, which would never have been picked up otherwise.

13.6.6 Documentation of Temporary Cognitive or Behavioural Problems Linked to Epileptic Activity (Cognitive Seizures)

There are children with epilepsy in whom, from the history, one may suspect fluctuations in a particular cognitive task, such as reading or writing, and in whom one would like to try to document this, ideally while the child is having an EEG recorded. If the examiner happens to be present when the EEG is done, he or she may be able to document the suspected disturbance, provided that adequate material is at hand. This may be created *ad hoc* or taken from existing tests (text to read, paper and pencil, objects to show or words to say for recall, or tests for a given language function, e.g. naming or verbal comprehension). These fleeting opportunities occur rarely, but may provide important information. If a transient deficit can be documented, one has in fact recorded a 'cognitive seizure'. One can occasionally plan such investigations in a child with frequent non-convulsive status epilepticus, especially when this can be triggered by hyperventilation (see case K.C. with ring chromosome 20, in Chapter 8, section 8.7).

Despite convincing descriptions by parents and observations by clinicians that the unusual behaviours and/or cognitive difficulties they had seen had disappeared with appropriate therapy, the conditions necessary to document these cognitive manifestations of epilepsy are not easily met and this explains the rarity of published observations.

13.7 Computerized tests

In some situations, computerized tests can offer complementary information to that obtained by conventional clinical testing. These tests have the advantage of allowing a quantifiable assessment of some basic neuropsychological parameters, such as reaction time or short-term memory, and some features of attention, such as sustained attention in visual, verbal or spatial modality. They can be coupled with videoEEG monitoring when very short-term changes are looked for (Alpherts and Aldenkamp 1995; and see also Chapter 4, section 4.3.2 on transient cognitive impairment).

In clinical neuropsychology, such tests have been developed mainly for the testing of children with attention deficit disorders and those with epilepsy, and to monitor central side-effects of drugs (Alpherts and Aldenkamp 1990, Conner's Continuous performance test 1995). Assessment of multiple domains with the FEPSY, in a child with, for example, frequent lapses in vigilance or other 'online' epilepsy-related dysfunctions, can show precisely quantitative changes in speed, accuracy, etc., in all or specific tasks during the prolonged (hour or more) testing period. These tests, however, cannot replace the richness and completeness of the usual clinical neuropsychological testing. For research purposes, computerized tests can be an important tool to address a specific neuropsychological question – for instance, evaluation of attention with different distractors on the screen, with responses that can be precisely measured and compared in different populations.

13.8 Questionnaires

Questionnaires have inherent problems of bias and subjectivity. Marked differences can be found in responses from different people (parents, teachers) close to the child, especially when the questions deal with abnormal behaviours and their severity. However, when they are completed repeatedly by the same individuals in the course of the disease, this can give a useful indication of the changes.

Sometimes, questionnaires can be used as a diagnostic tool, but more often they are used to document a wide range of behaviours that may disappear or worsen in the course of the epilepsy and are not always observed in consultation. There are general standardized questionnaires on child behaviour (Achenbach 1991), and others focused on more specific domains: autistic behaviours (CARS), executive functions (BRIEF) and language development.

We have developed a questionnaire that we use for epilepsies with a severe cognitive-behavioural impact, which covers a wide range of behaviours (including sleep, food habits, etc.). The questionnaire is particularly helpful as a baseline in a situation where one cannot predict what problems are likely to show up or disappear, and in evaluating the effect of therapy or of a spontaneous change in the evolution of the epileptic disease (Roulet-Perez et al 1993). A selection of the most abnormal or significant behaviours (aberrant or new), as perceived by the family ('target items'), can be used in a semiquantitative way for follow-up. The items chosen come from the existing questionnaire or from the parents' own observations. The important point is to document a limited number of behaviours which are relevant, easily observed and pertinent to the family, especially those which are new or most disturbing.

The rapidity of the behavioural improvement and its correlation with changes in cognitive abilities or communication may be significant for determining what was the most affected domain. For instance, a child with improving auditory agnosia who becomes able to recognize and give meaning to sounds may rapidly change their attitude towards the sound environment and communication in general.

In many countries, early stimulation and support programmes are provided during preschool years, by special education teachers, sometimes in the child's own house, for children at risk and those with recognized developmental delay. These teachers can be usefully involved in helping to make specific regular written and ad hoc comments on pre-established questionnaires, or in writing down informal but sometimes crucial observations.

13.9 Evaluation of children (especially very young children) with behaviour-communication disorders

Standardized developmental or more elaborate cognitive-communicative, language or domain-specific evaluations may be very difficult to perform in young children with epilepsy and primarily behaviour-communication disorders. However, it is important to gather as many objective and comparable data as possible if one suspects that the observed deficit may change significantly and possibly rapidly. A baseline evaluation, including present level in all fields of development (and not only the one which seems most affected), must rely on different approaches, including spontaneous behaviour recorded on video in a natural setting, documentation of the communicative level (for instance, with the ESCS communication scale), and behaviour in different structured play situations (Lowe and Costello 1982), together with specific questionnaires (for example, the CARS or MacArthur scale of language development). The cognitive and behavioural phenotype can then be compared with those observed in the classically recognized developmental disorders, such as specific language impairment, autistic spectrum disorders, developmental coordination disorder, etc. The underlying premise should be that unusual patterns of development or neuropsychological profiles are more likely to be found in cases where epileptic dysfunction is playing a role than in the usual developmental disorders.

13.10 Integrating the results of the neuropsychological evaluation with epilepsy data (Table 13.2)

In epilepsy, more than in other childhood brain disorders, it is essential that the neuropsychological data are discussed with the clinician and put in the context of the often changing neurological situation – a difficult issue when evaluations are done outside the clinical setting. The conclusion that a significant cognitive or behavioural change can be attributed to the epilepsy itself is sometimes only possible when data obtained with different methods,

TABLE 13.2
Conclusions from neuropsychological evaluation and other data: direct relationship with epilepsy?

This table summarizes the main sources of information on which one has to rely in evaluating the direct role of epilepsy in situations where no rapid, direct and simple clinical–EEG correlation can be made.

- Results of serial neuropsychological tests and behavioural questionnaires
- Observations from caregivers (educational team, teachers)
- Videorecording of specific behaviours (e.g. language, motricity)
- Evaluation of EEG changes and correlations with clinical data
- Overall clinical impression and family judgement of changes

from different sources and at different times are combined. It is useful to have a checklist of all possible sources of information to see if important data are still missing, especially when a therapeutic or other decision has to be made (see Table 13.1).

In addition to the neuropsychological evaluation, the clinical impression during consultations, the behaviour at home and in school, the results of questionnaires and school progress, as well as video observations, can all be important components of the final judgement, in correlation with the EEG changes and other indices of epilepsy control (better sleep, decrease of the seizures or of fluctuations in behaviour or cognition). When all data are concordant, and rapid changes in a specific domain are seen, the impression is reinforced. When this is not the case, the reasons for the discrepancies have to be analysed specifically before therapeutic decisions are taken. If they remain unexplained, one may have to wait and compare the present findings with the next evaluation, for which a clear timing and objective should be defined.

14
PRACTICAL CLINICAL ISSUES IN DIAGNOSIS AND ANTIEPILEPTIC DRUG THERAPY

14.1 Evaluation of a possible direct role of epilepsy on cognition and behaviour

The circumstances in which the question of a possible direct effect of epilepsy on cognition and behaviour is raised in an individual child are extremely variable. It is not always easy to draw a clear line between dismissing the possibility of a direct role of epilepsy and leaving some doubt about it, especially with the parents. This book would be doing a disservice, if it left the impression that epilepsy itself is the main or even a frequent cause of cognitive and behavioural problems in the majority of otherwise normal children with epilepsy, which it is not. However, this possibility is often in the parent's mind at one moment or another of the evolution, even in benign cases, and has to be frequently considered. Here are some typical clinical situations in which these questions are raised.

14.1.1 Children with Known Epilepsy Currently with or without Therapy

During clinical follow-up, there are several types of complaints that parents express concerning their child's behaviour or school performance which can suggest temporary dysfunctions directly due to epilepsy. Not infrequently, parents or children express in very telling simple or metaphorical language the rapid and temporary changes in brain function intuitively understood or easily interpretable as an epileptic dysfunction. For example: 'it is like a blackboard that has been erased'; 'like a computer suddenly unplugged'; 'sudden bout of fatigue, there is no fuel any more'. Sudden mood changes are referred to: 'Good child/bad child' or 'Jekyll and Hyde'.

Difficulty in waking

Parents of children with epilepsy can often tell from the way the child wakes up if he/she has had seizures during sleep, even after this has happened only once. So, difficulty in waking in a child who fails in school may be due to unrecognized nocturnal seizures (see Chapter 5, section 5.4).

See-saw school results

Very uneven school performances may be due to unrecognized seizures. For example, parents may report: 'He can do the best and the worst' or 'She can have very good and very bad marks'.

Temporary abnormal behaviours or cognitive changes resembling a known pre- or postictal state

Parents may recognize a similarity between present behavioural disorders and what they have observed (even if only once) before or after the first seizure, although they do not always spontaneously make the connection.

Increasing cognitive difficulties in a specific domain

This may suggest a focal dysfunction of epileptic origin. It may only be a worsening in a domain which was weak to start with and is fragile for many possible reasons, but it may be an indication of the site of origin of this epilepsy.

14.1.2 Children with Cognitive, Learning or Behavioural Problems in Whom the Question of Epilepsy is Raised

Some of the reasons why this possibility is considered are discussed above. It is inadvisable to consider epilepsy and obtain routine EEGs just because of school failure, unless a true cognitive regression, stagnation and unexplained fluctuations are documented or suspected clinically. In children with an isolated attention deficit (for instance, if they have the criteria for ADHD), a routine EEG is not necessary. The prevalence of paroxysmal EEG abnormalities may be slightly higher in this population than in control groups, but this has no clear diagnostic and therapeutic implications, and their presence is not a contraindication to methylphenidate (Richer et al 2002, Holtmann et al 2003). If inattention is clearly a new problem and if there are other possible hints for epilepsy, the situation is of course different, and an EEG (waking and sleep) can be useful.

The decision to perform an EEG is a serious one for different reasons. First of all, the EEG must include a sleep period, because in some cognitive epilepsies the EEG 'epileptic' abnormalities are seen only during sleep. A normal waking and sleep EEG probably does rule out epilepsy as playing a major role at that moment, but it does not rule out the possibility that it did in the past and it should not rule it out for ever. There are many examples of children whose epileptic disorder was recognized very late, because the first EEG was normal.

If the EEG shows epileptiform abnormalities, it is still not proof that these are causally related to the clinical problem. These abnormalities can occur in otherwise normal children as a familial trait, or they can be a marker of brain dysfunction in children with developmental disorders, and in both situations they have no special significance. The clinical context can usually help in deciding if the finding is possibly relevant to the problem. If discharges are frequent enough (but not continuous) and if the child is cooperative, videoEEG monitoring during cognitive tasks could be carried out, looking for transient cognitive impairment. It must be said that this is not an easy procedure and it is not done routinely in most centres treating children with epilepsy. The decision to try an antiepileptic drug in these situations is discussed later (section 14.2).

14.1.3 Young Children with a Developmental Disorder and Epilepsy and/or Paroxysmal EEG Abnormalities

The question of a possible direct role of epilepsy and/or paroxysmal EEG discharges on development and cognitive functions in a young child may arise in different clinical circumstances.

Child with developmental delay without history of regression or clinical epilepsy

This is the situation of a child with developmental delay whose etiological diagnostic work-up reveals paroxysmal EEG epileptic abnormalities. Some special EEG patterns can be useful markers in the identification of a known syndrome (e.g. fragile X syndrome, Angelman syndrome, 15q11–q13 duplication syndromes, cortical malformations), but do not explain or play the main role in the cognitive or behavioural problems. When no specific diagnosis can be made and if the EEG shows sustained diffuse epileptic activity, or if this abnormality is localized in particular areas (frontal or temporal), the search for subtle unrecognized clinical seizures and other indices of epileptic activity in the cognitive-behavioural domain (such as marked variability in mood, vigilance, performance) is particularly warranted and may justify a trial of antiepileptic medication, after a period of careful baseline observation.

Developmental delay with regression/fluctuations, but no 'evident' epilepsy

Rare neurometabolic-degenerative disorders of early onset have to be ruled out first (e.g. Rett syndrome, see Chapter 11). The possibility of 'hidden' epilepsy to explain regression or fluctuation must be seriously considered, and unusual 'epileptic' behaviours such as stereotypies or abnormal laughter (gelastic seizures) should be especially looked for. In such situations, the first EEG is not always revealing, because the child is still very young or because epileptic discharges can start from areas (mesiofrontal, limbic) too far from the brain surface to show on a scalp EEG.

Developmental delay with clinical epilepsy

Epilepsy here is often the presenting symptom of an underlying encephalopathy, the cause of which needs to be investigated. It is important to have good documentation of behaviour and cognitive level before prophylactic antiepileptic therapy, because, occasionally, rapid and surprising developmental progress is seen, suggesting that a long-standing unrecognized epilepsy has played a direct additional negative role in that particular case (see below).

Epilepsy and behaviour may also be directly improved in rare metabolic situations in which a specific therapy is possible (e.g. ketogenic diet in glucose-transported deficiency (GT1) or vitamin B6 dependency, see Chapter 11, section 11.5).

14.2 Antiepileptic drug therapy

> Many physicians in attempting to extinguish seizures only succeed in drowning the finer intellectual processes of their patients. . . . The intelligent and individualistic use of antiepileptic drugs should not and does not impair the patient's mind.
>
> (Lennox 1960)

14.2.1 General Considerations and Choice of Antiepileptic Drugs

The admirable wish of Lennox is unfortunately not easy to accomplish, especially when one is dealing with epilepsies with a direct cognitive impact. Antiepileptic therapy can improve, impair or make no change to the patient's overall cognitive and affective functioning, depending on many factors which have been analysed elsewhere. It is obvious, but not always fully realized, that when an epilepsy which has no cognitive impact occurs in a very bright child, even minor cognitive side-effects of drugs will be noticeable. On the other hand, when epilepsy directly impairs cognitive functioning and if the drug is effective, the overall improvement will far outweigh any possible side-effects (see Chapter 5, section 5.2).

One must also keep in mind that antiepileptic drugs can have powerful effects on the central nervous system, independently of their specific antiepileptic effects.

Choice of antiepileptic drugs

When the risk of recurrence of seizures and other particular characteristics of the case favour the use of prophylactic antiepileptic drugs, the same kind of thinking as used in the different childhood epilepsies should be applied. This will not be discussed further as it is covered in several recent epilepsy textbooks.

However, when there is a suspicion that this particular epilepsy has a direct cognitive impact (in addition to the seizures) or if it manifests mainly as such ('cognitive epilepsies'), special consideration should be given to the potential positive or negative cognitive side-effects of some antiepileptic drugs. These are summarized in Table 14.1.

Evaluation of cognitive effects of antiepileptic drugs, especially in newly diagnosed and treated epilepsy

When a child with newly diagnosed epilepsy is started on antiepileptic drugs and the seizures are under control, three typical situations can be encountered:

1. Behaviour and cognitive capacities are unchanged: the therapy has no side-effects. This is usually the best one hopes for.
2. The epilepsy is controlled, but the child's behaviour is altered, or learning capacities or cognitive performance are affected. There are several possible reasons. Probably the most frequent is that this is a side-effect of the medication. This is usually rapidly evident to the family and sometimes to the child, unless the dose is slowly increased over a long period. The possibility of an insidious and progressive drug intoxication or

TABLE 14.1
Antiepileptic drugs: special features relevant to cognitive aspects of epilepsy

This table lists the usual indications for the main antiepileptic drugs and some of their characteristic effects which may be relevant to the cognitive dimension of the disorder. It is not intended to give all the potential behavioural or cognitive problems but to highlight some of their positive or negative features which are typical or that we have found particularly relevant.

Drug	Usual indications	Comments on epileptic effect: important features	Comments on cognitive/behavioural aspects
Phenobarbital	Febrile seizures (complex), various epilepsies in neonates and children <18 months	Simple metabolism, few general side-effects	Cognitive slowing at high (moderate?) doses – irritability in one-third of children
Carbamazepine	Partial epilepsies (lesional)	May be efficacious even at low doses	Possible language/cognitive regression in partial epilepsies with focal sharp waves (↑ of EEG discharges) – rarely agitation and irritability
Diphenylhydantoin	Partial epilepsies (lesional)	May be efficacious even at low doses, risk of progressive intoxication (in slow metabolizers)	Cognitive slowing from gradual intoxication
Valproate	Primary generalized epilepsy or mixed (cf. lamotrigine)	Broad spectrum, tremor frequent	Cases of valproate dementia reported (reversible, insidious) – rarely irritability
Ethosuximide	Absence epilepsy, partial epilepsies with CSWS, rolandic epilepsies with 'negative myoclonus'	May act when other drugs have failed	Fatigue, irritability, sleep disturbances
Diazepines (clobazam, nitrazepam)	Infantile spasms (2nd or 3rd choice), some lesional partial epilepsies, partial epilepsies with CSWS	Rapid result visible in good responders, frequent 'escape' phenomenon	Cognitive improvement in some partial epilepsies with CSWS, irritability, hyperactivity frequent in young children
Vigabatrin	Infantile spasms	Effective, rapid response – good tolerance, fewer side-effects than steroids, long-term visual field defects	Improvement in infant behaviour and development, progress may be easily seen, sedation – irritability at high doses
Lamotrigine	Atypical absences, mixed epilepsies (general and focal)	May suppress 'subclinical' EEG discharges	Possible psychotropic effect, positive or negative (irritability)
Topiramate	Partial epilepsies	May control seizures when other antiepileptic drugs have failed – frequent decrease of appetite	Cognitive slowing frequent – specific(?) word-finding difficulties in adults

TABLE 14.1 *continued*
Antiepileptic drugs: special features relevant to cognitive aspects of epilepsy

Drug	**Usual indications**	**Comments on epileptic effect: important features**	**Comments on cognitive/behavioural aspects**
Sulthiame	Partial epilepsies with 'focal sharp waves' (rolandic epilepsies)	Rapid suppression of focal sharp waves on EEG, sometimes only temporary – well tolerated	No, or very rare cognitive/behavioural side-effects
Corticosteroids (orACTH)	Infantile spasms (if failure on vigabatrin), acquired epileptic aphasia and CSWS	Often very effective on both clinical seizures and EEG discharges – side-effects of steroids (↓ on alternate dosage) relapse on withdrawal	Cognitive improvement may be masked by physical and behavioural side-effects, behavioural effects very variable, negative (irritability) or positive (mood)

the rare direct negative idiosyncratic effects of the drug on cognition, as can be seen with any antiepileptic drug, including the most recent and effective ones (valproate, topiramate), has to be considered. It may sometimes be very difficult to decide if apathy, inattention, slow or inadequate thinking or even depression is due to a direct drug effect or to other factors, mainly psychological, and only drug withdrawal may answer the question. A psychological reaction to the diagnosis of epilepsy and to its personal and family consequences is always a possibility to keep in mind, which is probably underestimated, and not always considered.

One should try to clarify this issue of tolerance early on, because the natural tendency (especially of teachers and caregivers) to blame medication will often occur at one point or another in the course of the disease.

3 Epilepsy is not only controlled, but behaviour and learning are much improved. This situation occurs not infrequently and suggests a direct effect of epilepsy on higher cognitive functions. If cognitive and/or behavioural deterioration had occurred prior to the recognition of epilepsy and improves clearly with antiepileptic drugs, this is an even clearer argument for thinking that this particular epilepsy indeed had an impact in this domain. The positive change noted by the parents makes them clearly aware that the visible seizure element was not the only effect of the epilepsy, but that it altered their child's mental or psychological well-being in a much more profound way. These parents usually do not question the benefit of treatment and are even reluctant when a withdrawal is proposed after a certain period. The improvement may come from the suppression of the focal epileptic discharges in areas important for cognitive functions, or because frequent EEG epileptic discharges causing transient cognitive impairment (see Chapter 4, section 4.3.2) disappear, or through control of nocturnal epileptic activity. A direct psychotropic drug effect is also a possibility, especially when anxiety or a mood disturbance were in the forefront, but this is unlikely when the change is sudden and improves a specific cognitive function, vigilance or speed of processing.

The special issue of forced normalization

The term 'forced normalization' has been used to describe the sudden occurrence of severe behavioural problems of psychotic type coinciding with abrupt seizure cessation and normalization of the EEG by drugs. It is a well-described special clinical situation in adults, mainly with temporal lobe epilepsy (Trimble and Schmidt 2002). It has been reported in a few children with severe epilepsy by Amir and Gross-Tsur (1994). We have not encountered this situation or, if we have, we have not called it forced normalization. It occasionally happens that a drug which is effective in controlling clinical seizures and causes the suppression of the EEG discharges is accompanied by acute and very abnormal behaviours. These disappear on withdrawal of the drug. Only if other antiepileptic drugs had the same effect on the same child could a special mechanism be invoked, directly related to the suppression of the epileptic activity. This did not occur in Amir's study. The psychotic behaviour might be due to a change in neurotransmitter balance, but also to the experience of a new psychological state made possible by the control of the epileptic process. The rarity of the phenomenon of forced normalization in children, as opposed to adults, is still unexplained, but may be related to the duration of the epileptic disorder.

Severe and new behavioural problems are sometimes seen immediately after successful epilepsy surgery, although this appears exceptional (Anderman et al 1999, Holthausen, personal communication). This seems to occur when a child discovers new capacities and is capable of an independence and choices which were not available before, but this issue needs to be clarified. Epilepsy surgery cases should be a particularly interesting group for a systematic study of these phenomena.

14.2.2 Special Clinical Situations Where the Effect of Antiepileptic Drugs on Cognitive Functions is the Main Goal

Transient cognitive impairment associated with epileptic EEG discharges in children without seizures

> TCI [transient cognitive impairment] confronts the clinical electroencephalographer with an intriguing paradox. Having learned to avoid overinterpretation of the EEG, and having persuaded colleagues that spikes are not diagnostic of epilepsy nor closely related to its severity or prognosis, one has to adopt the seemingly inconsistent position of stressing the practical importance of subclinical discharges.
>
> (Binnie and Marston 1992)

The role of epileptic EEG discharges as a contributing or causal factor in children with cognitive problems but without other evidence of epilepsy, or after a first or rare seizure such as in BPERS, is an extremely delicate issue with a great risk of overdiagnosis and inappropriate treatment. Excessive enthusiasm in this domain has been publicly criticized, particularly in the UK (White 2001).

As discussed (see Chapter 4, section 4.3.2 on transient cognitive impairment), it is not easy to demonstrate, even with videoEEG monitoring, the role of these discharges on cognitive functions. If in doubt, one may first decide to monitor the situation without treatment, after precise documentation of the child's cognitive abilities (including attention and memory) using standardized tests and after discussion with teachers or other professionals involved. A repeat clinical evaluation after a few months may be reassuring about continuing acquisitions, or, on the contrary, show a stagnation or regression which would justify an attempt at drug treatment.

A therapeutic trial may be considered for a limited period of time and stopped if there is no clear clinical benefit and if the EEG is unchanged, but failure with one drug does not mean that others will not be useful. Spike-waves or other epileptic features on the EEG can be due to very different epilepsies with different sensitivity to drugs. This usually cannot be predicted. Sometimes the EEG is improved before clinical improvement is noted and a further period of treatment may be justified.

This approach to trying antiepileptic drugs and evaluating the child on and off therapy on certain precise and repeatable psychological measures (the child being their own control) is quite difficult. Unsurprisingly, studies on this problem are very rare.

Marston et al (1993) studied 10 children and showed improved psychosocial functioning in correlation with reduced amount of EEG discharges (due to added valproate). The authors could not rule out the role of confounding variables, the main one being that treatment decreased the clinical seizure frequency in 9/10. These positive results have not been replicated in any large study since.

Ronen et al (2000) conducted a randomized, double-blind, single cross-over trial also using valproate or placebo in eight children with different learning and behaviour problems and electroencephalographic epileptiform discharges but without clinical seizures. Neuropsychological testing and behavioural questionnaires were carried out in each treatment phase. None of the children improved clinically or in formal test results while on valproate. It should be noted that 4/8 children had either an increased (one child) or an unchanged amount of EEG discharges while on valproate, and the whole group was heterogeneous in terms of age, type of cognitive problem and type of epileptic EEG abnormalities. One can only conclude from this study that valproate was not effective in suppressing the EEG discharges in 1/2 of the children and had possible negative cognitive side-effects in the whole group. It does not mean that another drug would not have been beneficial.

This detailed and careful study illustrates the complexity of the issue and the need for further and more individualized drug trials. Group results from heterogeneous cases with variable response to a given medication may hide significant individual responses. For instance, an epileptic focus in a crucial area for cognition and with rapid generalization can manifest on the EEG as generalized spike-waves without other signs of epilepsy besides cognitive and behavioural problems.

A drug trial in which the child is their own control and in which an attempt is made to correlate the amount of epileptiform abnormalities with cognitive performance on and off therapy, at successive times, remains a valid research approach. When a positive change is found and if repeated on/off drug trials show the same results, this can be accepted as scientific evidence of the drug effect, and also in this case of its mechanism (suppression

TABLE 14.2
Practical approach in a child with paroxysmal discharges on the waking EEG and no clinical seizures

This table shows the practical approach one may follow in a child who has no clinical evidence of epilepsy at the time he/she is found to have many paroxysmal epileptiform EEG abnormalities, especially when behaviour or learning is a problem.

No apparent dysfunction: clinical follow-up without treatment
If associated with present or past cognitive dysfunction or history of cognitive/behavioural fluctuations:

- Document precisely present level, looking for specific dysfunctional areas
- Carry out close follow-up looking for stagnation, regression or new problems
- If poor learning, behavioural problems (new) or documented cognitive stagnation/regression are documented: consider antiepileptic drug therapy with EEG before and on therapy

or decrease of EEG discharges (Gordon et al 1996)). Obviously, this on/off method, which is often applied and diagnostically useful in children with attention deficit disorders treated with methylphenydate or in children with tics treated with neuroleptics, may be difficult to justify in children with epilepsy, especially when there is a clinical impression of progressive cognitive improvement.

At the very least, careful clinical documentation of relevant neuropsychological functions before and after therapy should be carried out to avoid prolonged and useless trials.

Specific cognitive epileptic syndromes with or without seizures (Landau–Kleffner syndrome and partial epilepsy with CSWS)

In children with language or cognitive deterioration and focal sharp waves on EEG (Landau–Kleffner and related syndromes, partial epilepsy with CSWS), suppression of EEG discharges is of paramount importance.

No controlled therapeutic studies have been done in these syndromes, despite frequent insistence on the need for this for more than two decades by various experts including Professor Landau himself (Landau and Kleffner 2001). One can speculate whether this is just laziness or lack of scientific rigour on the part of clinicians, or a practical impossibility given the number of variables, or just not the right approach for this type of disorder. Important data, however, are available.

Numerous single case studies or small series of cases, especially those followed longitudinally, have demonstrated several generally accepted facts (Marescaux et al 1990). Paroxysmal EEG abnormalities are uninfluenced or can be aggravated by classic antiepileptic drugs (phenobarbital, diphenylhydantoins, carbamazepine), but can be suppressed, often temporarily, by benzodiazepines (clobazam).

Corticosteroids are definitely useful (but not always). This is based on several lines of evidence:

1 The rapid disappearance or marked decrease of paroxysmal EEG abnormalities, with concomitant, sometimes delayed, clinical improvement.

2 Recurrence of the symptoms (clinical and EEG) on withdrawal of corticosteroids.
3 Positive responses on repeat courses of treatment during relapses.

The possible benefit is sometimes obscured by intolerable side-effects and too rapid withdrawal. There are some limited data on immunoglobulins which have been tried with success in a few cases. A particularly indicative, well-documented case was published by Lagae: this child with acquired epileptic aphasia who initially responded to steroids was later, on several occasions, given repeated courses of immunoglobulins, with corresponding clinical and EEG improvement (Lagae et al 1998).

There are several isolated reports in the literature of either positive response or aggravation (or even appearance of cognitive symptoms, e.g. aphasia) with the newer antiepileptic drugs (vigabatrin, lamotrigine, topiramate) (Battaglia et al 2001). This indicates that important and unpredictable differences between cases with an apparently similar syndrome do exist. This should dictate an open and empirical attitude towards the use of the new antiepileptic drugs, without prejudice.

Given all the uncertainties, it is not possible to give precise guidelines for treatment of these syndromes. A reasonable attitude would be to try diazepines (clobazam) first and, if unsuccessful, sulthiame and/or ethosuximide. This may help gain some time before deciding on a course of steroids, which there may be some reluctance to do. The problem with this approach is that a long time may elapse before these clinical trials are completed. The decision to start rapidly or delay corticosteroids will depend on the severity and duration of the symptoms, and the presence of already observed spontaneous fluctuation at the time the child is first diagnosed, indicating that the course will possibly be short-lived.

As acquired epileptic aphasia and the idiopathic cases of epilepsy with CSWS share a probable common physiopathology with the 'benign partial epilepsies of childhood', one should also capitalize on the new knowledge which has become available in the treatment of these more frequent conditions (Rating et al 2000, Bast et al 2003, Engler et al 2003).

A few children with severe persistent acquired epileptic aphasia resistant to antiepileptic drugs and corticosteroids have been treated surgically with multiple subpial transection, by Morrell in Chicago, and subsequently in other centres in the USA and in Europe (Morrell et al 1995, Irwin et al 2001), with apparently good results. Clearly, the multiple subpial transection abolished the epileptic discharges on the EEG and the CSWS, but in most cases language improvement did not occur rapidly. However, in cases with severe additional behavioural problems, these improved rapidly and spectacularly (Irwin et al 2001). A follow-up study of the initial cases operated on by Morrell was reported several years later (Grote et al 1999). All children continued to show improvement in the years after surgery but had persistent sequelae. Whether their final outcome would have been different if treated medically is a difficult question to answer.

Contrary to earlier reports suggesting minimal or no progress in cases with severe aphasia unresponsive to medical therapy in the first years after onset of aphasia, several recent reports have shown surprising late and progressive recovery after years of complete auditory agnosia and mutism (Roulet-Perez et al 2001). We still do not know enough about the natural history of the disease and its great variability in severity to assess the value and superiority of multiple subpial transection over medical therapies in the long run. Multiple subpial transection must still be considered experimental in this context.

Developmental disorders with cognitive-behavioural problems of suspected epileptic origin (paroxysmal EEG discharges)

In developmental disorders with cognitive-behavioural problems of suspected epileptic origin (because of paroxysmal EEG discharges) the relationship between the clinical disorder and epilepsy is most often uncertain, and the evidence of a direct link can be proven only with a positive drug trial. This option should be pursued only with the greatest care, making sure that the family has understood the problem and that a psychologist will be able to evaluate the child extensively and repeatedly. If it is decided to go ahead, the baseline EEG and neuropsychological evaluation should be done at the same period. Often too much time has elapsed between the initial diagnostic work-up, the judgement of a possible role of the epilepsy and the treatment proposal to make a correlation meaningful. The parameters of improvement, namely a measurable and rapid progress in a given cognitive task together with decrease of EEG epileptic activity, may be difficult to obtain, particularly in young disturbed children. Considering the very nature of the basic symptoms (cognitive and behavioural), a limited tolerance to the negative cognitive-behavioural effects of the drug is more likely to occur than in other epileptic situations. The tendency to judge the therapeutic effect as negative if not striking and rapid is understandable, and it may be difficult to persuade the family and caregivers to pursue treatment with other drugs. Finally, the result may be a mixed blessing. The child's cognitive functions may improve but his/her behaviour become worse, for many possible reasons.

All these factors explain why most drug trials reported in these situations are either negative and not reported or if positive are usually not reported either, because no convincing hard clinical data can be produced. In the published series with more than a few cases, indices of improvement are either lacking in detail or occur over a long time frame, during which many other factors could have played a role, besides a direct role of antiepileptic treatment (Nass et al 1998, Lewine et al 1999). If the results are convincing, they may not be accepted as scientific evidence, because there is no control group, a condition which is almost impossible to obtain in such situations.

15
PSYCHOLOGICAL AND EDUCATIONAL ASPECTS: SPECIAL IMPLICATIONS FOR EPILEPSIES WITH COGNITIVE MANIFESTATIONS

In most child psychiatry textbooks, there is surprisingly little place given to epilepsy and its psychological consequences, especially considering the general existential dimension of the problem. In most countries, children with epilepsy are usually treated by paediatricians or neurologists. Child psychiatrists, with few exceptions, rarely have direct access and are not involved in their care, especially at the crucial moments of diagnosis. They are not in a position to influence the general management of these children, despite the fact that so much preventive work in the psychological domain is necessary (Deonna 2003, 2005). They tend to be involved in severe cases where the disease has major familial consequences, in complex epilepsies with major behavioural problems, or rare syndromes with cognitive-behavioural manifestations, all of which are the exception in the general population of children with epilepsy.

Taylor is one of the exceptions. His initial medical contribution was in the neuropathology of epilepsy (Taylor and Falconer 1971) and he described what is now recognized as the first example of cortical dysplasia, one of the main causes of intractable epilepsy in children. He spent his career as a child psychiatrist working with children with epilepsy, in the latter part of it as a consultant in one of the first major childhood epilepsy surgery centres in the world (Great Ormond Street Hospital for Children, London). He has written extensively on this unique experience. He tried to identify and explain which behaviours could be the direct consequence of the epileptic condition or that of the brain disease which caused it. In parallel he analysed all the consequences of 'living with epilepsy', with its social consequences, both in the child's own perception of him/herself and in the perceptions that close relatives and society at large have about epilepsy (Taylor and Lochery 1991).

Soulayrol worked in close association with the Centre St-Paul for children with epilepsy in Marseille, and has written about his experience in this position (Soulayrol 1999), with a psychoanalytical frame of reference. He did not specifically study the direct cognitive and psychiatric manifestations of epilepsy and how they can influence the child's emotional development and learning abilities. The types of family psychodynamics resulting from the presence of a child with epilepsy have also been the subject of systematic study (Beauchesne 1980).

It is a common clinical experience that emotional well-being and, on the contrary, emotional crises or unusual stressful situations can sometimes contribute either to seizure freedom or to recurrence of epilepsy. Whether or not it is true in a given situation, parents invariably ask the question or have made up their own mind about it, and this should be acknowledged. Some child psychoanalysts, however, have gone too far, constructing theories to explain epilepsy and/or its circumstances of occurrence as being the direct result of psychological conflicts or crisis (Bouchard et al 1975), rather than this being only one of the possible factors.

15.1 General psychological factors linked to epilepsy

The potentially important sources of psychological problems in children with epilepsy are now well recognized and some can be prevented. They should be in the clinician's mind when trying to analyse what components of the child's emotional-behavioural problems are a direct consequence of the epileptic disorder or of its underlying cause and what are due to reactive psychological phenomena. These factors are briefly reviewed below. Note that these can affect the child directly but also result from the family's attitude and reactions to the disease.

1. General psychological consequences of having a chronic disease.
2. Current myths about epilepsy and their influence on the family and child (Deonna 2003).
3. Specificity of the epileptic symptom: unpredictability, shameful visibility, absence of control, variability of cognitive functioning, anxiety about attacks (Matthews et al 1982, Taylor and Lochery 1991).

   The child with epilepsy depends upon an unreliable and transiently non-functioning cognitive system. A lack of confidence in their own abilities, so typical of children with specific learning disabilities, takes on another dimension here. The same type of task may be difficult for the child to solve at one moment, but not at another: 'Sometimes it is very easy, sometimes I don't understand or don't know what to do.' The child with epilepsy may feel that there is no good strategy that will help them to learn. They may lose any confidence that they have control over their own faculties and that they can trust them.
4. Family reaction to the disease: overprotection, overindulgence. Changed familial interactions (Lerman 1977, Beauchesne 1980, Berg et al 1993, Ziegler et al 1994).
5. Psychological and psychiatric consequences of brain dysfunction.

   Children with brain dysfunction of whatever cause have an increased frequency of psychopathology (Rutter 1981). Mental retardation, when accompanied by epilepsy, is more often associated with significant psychopathology (Caplan and Austin 2000).

15.2 Psychopathological syndromes in childhood epilepsies

The typologies used in the past to describe the 'epileptic personality' appear from our modern perspective very primitive, the more so when applied to children. Having a chronic disease and the unique characteristics of the epileptic symptoms can induce common behavioural reactions, but this does not imply any specific personality. Given the variety of childhood epilepsy types, the severity of associated cognitive dysfunction and underlying brain disorders, one should not expect any typical psychological profiles. However, the site of onset of epilepsy and the propagation of epileptic discharges in particular brain regions can be of special significance, as in the temporal lobe epilepsies (Caplan et al 1992b). This is not very surprising considering the role of the structures involved, and their connections (limbic system), in emotional life.

Children with temporal lobe epilepsies have long been recognized as having frequent and often severe behavioural problems, more so than those with generalized epilepsies and epilepsies in other locations (Dixon and Glaser 1956, Ounsted 1969, Lindsay et al 1979). Some adults with temporal lobe epilepsy develop a so-called interictal psychosis ('schizophrenia-like'). In children with temporal lobe epilepsy, a full-blown psychosis, as seen in adults, appears exceptional. There has been very limited systematic research on this aspect.

The question arises whether milder forms of psychosis might be unrecognized because the child does not manifest obvious 'externalizing behaviours' (Caplan et al 1991), and whether early epilepsy affecting specific maturing brain systems could affect their structural or chemical organization (neurotransmitters) in a way similar to that implicated in chronic psychiatric disorders of genetic or other causes. Caplan et al (1997) have looked specifically for a 'formal thought disorder' and other psychopathology, using structured interviews comparing children with complex partial, generalized seizures and normal controls. They found that illogical thinking, associated with 'schizophrenia-like symptoms', might be a feature of 'complex partial seizures'.

Like other cross-sectional studies on cognitive problems in childhood epilepsy, one cannot know the exact role of epilepsy as opposed to that of the focal brain disorder, and whether these deficits constitute a mild form or are the precursors of a more severe schizophrenia-like psychosis which will develop in adolescence or early adulthood. Interestingly, children with intractable temporal epilepsy, and particularly those with hippocampal sclerosis which is the most frequent cause, do not seem to be those who will develop adult-onset interictal psychosis (Umbricht et al 1995).

A severe early onset obsessive-compulsive disorder in a young girl with intractable anterior cingulate epilepsy was reported by Levine and Duchowny (1991). Anterior cingulectomy stopped clinical seizures and led to a marked improvement of the behavioural disorder. Whether the obsessive-compulsive disorder was the direct manifestation of epilepsy in relevant circuits or an epiphenomenon of a dysfunctional circuitry that also generated the epilepsy remains an open question, but such observations open a very interesting and new link between some epilepsies and psychiatric disorders. A remarkable recent personal case with similarities to the one reported by Levine and Duchowny raises exactly the same questions. The rapid improvement of behaviour together with the cessation of seizures with antiepileptic drug treatment suggests a very close relationship between the two disorders.

Case D.V.

A girl aged 5 years 3 months was seen for suspected epilepsy. In fact, she had had early onset unrecognized seizures (diurnal 'absences' and frontal nocturnal seizures) since infancy, and had been treated and even hospitalized several times in a psychiatric unit because of a severe behaviour disorder, with anxieties, phobias, panic attacks and tantrums provoked when 'things were not done as neatly as she wants', and because 'things need to be perfect'. In the last few months she had developed an eating disorder, with refusal of any foods other than smooth ones, and a fear of eating crumbs. The girl was otherwise very intelligent and even advanced for her age in some skills. The EEG showed predominant right-sided bifrontal paroxysmal activity (no generalized spike-waves) and the brain MRI was normal. Carbamazepine was immediately effective, with disappearance of all paroxysmal phenomena and abnormal behaviours. More prolonged follow-up is not available.

15.3 Special psychological implications in epilepsies with cognitive and behavioural manifestations

The psychological consequences of the epileptic disease for the child and their family are sometimes more important in children with mainly cognitive-behavioural manifestations of epilepsy, in whom seizures themselves are usually rare and not the main concern. In these situations, psychological reactions to the disease must be differentiated from quite similar symptoms that can be understood and explained as a direct effect of epilepsy.

There are many conflicts and pitfalls of interpretation of the various abnormal behaviours and learning difficulties, depending on one's explanatory model (psychological or neurophysiological), but also because the apparently same behaviours may have a different explanation at different periods of the epileptic disease. For instance, a child may be unable to concentrate or learn when epilepsy and/or drugs affect these abilities, but later on, when this is no longer a problem, the child may be depressed, angry or not motivated when they become able to recognize their failures. The absence of good scientific data and clinical experience of these puzzling clinical pictures, for instance in children with frontal epileptic syndromes, poses a problem. Some behaviours are hard to understand, accept or even conceptualize by non-medical specialists as possible epileptic manifestations.

Behavioural or emotional disturbances of suspected epileptic origin must be documented, if possible quantitatively, if the aim is to correlate such disturbances with the epileptic condition. However, the description of the disturbances or the use of questionnaires by neurologists is not equivalent to understanding the emotional-affective dimension of the problem. This is a major but under-recognized source of misunderstanding between neurobiologically and psychodynamically trained colleagues. The level of the child's emotional development, the emotional changes induced by the epilepsy itself and the child's reactions to the epileptic disease are not captured by formal neuropsychological tests or questionnaires. The 'epileptic experience' and its emotional consequences can be understood only in a subject-oriented psychological approach, which is often difficult or unrealistic or not considered a priority in the acute or fluctuating phases of the child's epilepsy.

The medical management of the cognitive-behavioural manifestations of epilepsy means a need for frequent EEGs and cognitive assessments, and this can have negative psychological consequences. The child may receive the message that all their problems are due to the epilepsy. They may feel that they are not responsible and not in control of their own emotions or actions. This is comparable to what can occur in children with ADHD treated with methylphenidate, when an exclusive pharmacological approach is taken, and when the need for methylphenidate is compared to the need for insulin in diabetes. The child is also reminded that their brain is not functioning well and needs frequent 'looking at' by an EEG. This may be an additional reason for anxiety and confusion about the adequacy of their cognitive function, which can be underestimated. This is especially true when the child does not have clinical seizures and does not consider him/herself as sick. Telling a child that he/she has a medical problem when the child has never had personal experience of its physical reality is a very particular situation.

In the school, it is not always easy for teachers or school authorities to accept the idea that a child who presently functions at a very deficient level because of an active epilepsy has a different problem – and potential for improvement, if given time – from that of a child with congenital mental retardation.

15.4 The role of the psychiatrist in a childhood epilepsy team

The evaluation and management of the psychological dimension of epilepsy require knowledge of psychiatric models of family functioning and of the development of the child's personality in such complex circumstances (which are the same as those of any chronic disease, but with the addition of the unique brain symptoms). This knowledge is all typically within the expertise of the child psychiatrist.

The child psychiatrist may see their role mainly as helping to understand and cope with the psychological consequences of the disease for the child and their family, and giving their expertise in the diagnosis and therapy of an associated psychiatric disorder (comorbidity), so frequent in epilepsy. The psychiatrist should also be asked to participate in the evaluation of what the neuropaediatrician believes to be direct psychiatric manifestations of epilepsy.

The acute psychiatric symptoms of epileptic origin, and their sometimes dramatic improvement when control of epilepsy (medical or surgical) is achieved, could be better described and possibly handled if the child psychiatrist was part of the neuropaediatric team treating such children on a regular basis. This is particularly true in very young children with severe lesional epilepsies and behavioural regression. At the moment, the child psychiatrist's involvement in this aspect of epilepsy is not actively sought by neuropaediatricians, despite claims to the contrary.

The observations of behavioural improvements after successful medical or surgical therapy of most epilepsies accompanied by psychiatric problems, which are regularly made (and probably justifiably so) by neuropaediatricians or neurosurgeons, could be better substantiated by an independent professional observer in an area where good follow-up data are badly needed. Also, the behavioural changes which can follow abrupt cessation of seizures, sometimes attributed to the phenomenon of 'forced normalization' (see Chapter 14, section 14.2.1), could be better understood and dealt with.

Finally, these epilepsies offer a remarkable and unique opportunity to study brain–behaviour relationships in a developing brain, and their consequences, from a combined neurobiological and psychological perspective, which is the definition of what modern child neuropsychiatry should be about (Bax 2002).

16
ADULT OUTCOME OF CHILDHOOD EPILEPSIES WITH 'COGNITIVE' EPILEPTIC MANIFESTATIONS: UNEXPECTED LESSONS FROM FOLLOW-UP STUDIES

16.1 The importance of long-term follow-up

We have now entered an important period in the history of modern epilepsy in which precisely defined groups of children with epilepsy diagnosed according to modern classifications and followed by the same surviving clinicians are reported in adulthood with regard to psychosocial outcome (Kokkonen et al 1997, Sillanpää et al 1998, Sillanpää 2000). These studies stress the importance of 'non-biological factors' and the difficulty of predicting outcome in childhood. The social disabilities in adulthood have been found to correlate more with the psychological and cognitive impairments than with the variables related to the epileptic disease itself, such as still being on medication or quality of seizure control (Camfield et al 1993, Kokkenen et al 1997). Since learning disabilities and psychiatric disabilities are generally considered as 'non-biological' factors, the possible contribution of the underlying brain dysfunction and that of the direct effects of epilepsy to these problems cannot be isolated (Camfield et al 1993).

Childhood epilepsies which directly and durably impinge on cognitive development but which finally remit before adulthood constitute a special neurophysiological situation. The long-term consequences must be expected to be different from those seen in other static childhood brain diseases, and this is still largely unknown territory.

Epileptic syndromes such as acquired epileptic aphasia and partial epilepsy with continuous spike-waves during sleep, which typically remit before adolescence, are examples in point. In these situations the deficit observed in adulthood (or its disappearance) is mainly the result of the damage the epilepsy did to the affected part of the developing brain during the active period of the disease and of the brain's capacity for compensation. Clinical data in this area are still rare (Mantovani and Landau 1980, Deonna et al 1989, Baynes et al 1998, Praline et al 2003). To reach valid conclusions, it is important that the initial deficit and its direct relationship to epilepsy have been clearly defined, and that progress in the affected domain is monitored for a long period. Global IQ data and psychosocial adaptation, although very important to document, cannot indicate whether and to what extent a given cognitive capacity can recover.

TABLE 16.1
Follow-up of childhood cognitive epilepsies: open questions

This table lists new questions about the possible original influence of chronic epileptic brain dysfunction on adult cognitive outcome and brain reorganization that can be tackled by long-term follow-up studies of some childhood 'cognitive' epilepsies.

	Opportunity for study	Example chosen (source)
1 Dynamics of dysfunction	close and distant follow-up	graphomotor study (see case S.C.)
2 Compensation for deficit (adaptive strategies)	opportunity to learn new strategies	sign language proficiency in auditory agnosia (Roulet-Perez et al 2001)
3 Relocation/maintenance of function in affected areas	• cortical stimulation	cortical stimulation (preop. 26 years: Roulet-Perez et al 1998)
	• hemispherectomy	see text
	• functional imaging	Hertz-Pannier et al 2002 (see Fig. 10.1)
4 Time limit for recovery	follow-up throughout life	acquired aphasia (see case M.R. 5–37 years)
5 Selective vulnerability of certain brain areas and influence on sequelae	compare focal epileptic lesion in different locations at long follow-up	insufficient data

Individual long-term follow-up of children with either acquired aphasia or dementia occasionally shows surprising continuous improvement in the affected domains during late childhood, adolescence and beyond: for example, recovery of verbal language after years of almost total absence of comprehension and productive speech (Roulet-Perez et al 2001). This suggests that a unique reorganization of functions may take place in these pathologies, which needs further study, clinically, with functional imaging and newer electrophysiological techniques (evoked potentials).

Table 16.1 shows some of the data obtained by systematic long-term follow-up study of children whose epilepsy had a major cognitive impact, and the questions that these data raise.

16.2 Dynamics of the epileptic dysfunction and its recovery

The rapidity and mode of the recovery are sometimes obvious clinically and do not seem to need detailed evaluation, but they can occur over a more subtle, prolonged and also variable time period. The same child may lose function over a few days or even abruptly, then recover or regress again at very different tempos in the course of time. It is likely that different mechanisms are responsible for these modes of recovery and relapse. The child with acquired dysgraphia described in Chapter 8 (see p. 91) illustrates this point in relation to a very specific developing ability, graphomotricity.

Each developmental domain has its own innate critical period of development. The exercise and explicit teaching needed for the function to develop is variable. From the evolutionary point of view, one may think that functions which are not taught and are 'automatically' acquired have a stronger, more determined, innate programme that unfolds 'by itself', whereas the trained, late acquired (school-taught) competences, such as writing, have a wider more plastic programme. Epilepsy may interfere at different moments in these organizational processes and for differing periods of duration. Whether the child recovers by relearning a lost competence, or capitalizes on previously unavailable 'hidden' knowledge, is unknown, and is probably different according to each particular developmental 'biography' of the involved domain. At this state of knowledge, follow-ups need to be frequent and detailed during the active phase of the disease, and later need to be continued for long periods, possibly into adulthood, in order to document, without any preconceived ideas, how fast and for how long recovery can still occur.

16.3 Compensation for deficits in cases with prolonged course, and development of adaptive strategies

A striking example of this is the use of sign language in children with prolonged auditory agnosia in Landau–Kleffner syndrome (Roulet-Perez et al 2001). A level of competence in sign language comparable to that of a congenitally deaf child, in whom sign language was the natural language, was documented in a 13-year-old child with Landau–Kleffner syndrome. Of course, this may not be attained in all cases, but our study showed that it is possible, provided that the brain dysfunction is limited to central auditory dysfunction and that the child has early exposure to and opportunity to use sign language within their family or at school. Very importantly also, the child described above, who recovered excellent oral language, illustrates that the learning of sign language did not hinder, but on the contrary may have facilitated, the re-emergence of oral language, when the brain areas which subserve this modality again became available. Written language acquired initially without using the normal phonological route was an important learning and communicative tool for the child, and later, when sound and phonemic decoding abilities recovered, was a support in the (re)learning of phonological representations of words. These prolonged but potentially reversible epileptic deficits can thus be very interesting models for the study of important questions in developmental neuropsychology.

16.4 Relocation or maintenance of function in affected areas: importance of follow-up studies

Children with congenital or early acquired focal brain lesions in the dominant hemisphere, particularly in the perisylvian region, may or may not shift their language representation to the other hemisphere. There are different conditions for this to occur. Older invasive studies of brain dominance using the Wada test and the results of hemispherectomy for intractable epilepsy, and more recently the use of functional imaging, have shown that this shift occurs with large ischemic lesions around the sylvian fissure. In smaller lesions, in those outside the sylvian region and in focal brain pathologies which are not destructive but developmental in nature (focal dysplasias), there may be no change in dominance for language. Epilepsy, arising in any of these lesions, may by itself create an additional structural pathology.

The organization and stabilization of the networks in the region affected by epilepsy (which acts during intermittent but usually prolonged periods of childhood) is a unique situation referred to as a 'functional lesion'. The final organization of the brain for language and, for that matter, for any developing function in children with an early focal pathology, is thus determined by many different constraints. The severity, location, duration and mode of spread of the epilepsy and the nature of the epileptic process (structural static or progressive pathology or only a focal hyperexcitability without structural disease) can all have an original influence (see Chapter 9, section 9.1.1 on focal cortical dysplasias).

The situation is quite different in children with functional epilepsies, such as acquired epileptic aphasia and partial epilepsies with CSWS, compared with that in those with epilepsy due to a progressive focal pathology such as Rasmussen's encephalitis or Sturge–Weber syndrome. In the child with refractory epilepsy due to Sturge–Weber syndrome treated by hemispherectomy (discussed in Chapter 10), functional imaging of language functions before and after surgery showed a shift from left to right hemisphere, suggesting that epilepsy and the increasingly damaged dominant hemisphere had 'prepared' the right hemisphere to sustain language (Hertz-Pannier et al 2002). In idiopathic partial epilepsies with cognitive deficits, functional imaging carried out after long follow-up and final remission of the epileptic disease will be most informative, but data are only just emerging (Majerus et al 2003).

The brain representation for language in epilepsy has been studied by direct focal brain stimulation in cases with severe epilepsy prior to epilepsy surgery. This is a biased sample, but can be quite informative as to what happens in these situations, especially since in most of these patients the epilepsy started in early childhood. The data obtained have shown a great variability between patients in the extent of the zone in which stimulation of the dominant hemisphere interfered with speech (Ojeman 1983, Devinsky et al 2000). It appears that language representation in the brain of persons with early focal epilepsies is quite different from that in those with a normal brain or with lesions which are not epileptogenic. Whether this applies to other functions is unknown but probable.

16.5 Duration of possible recovery: time-limited or lifelong?

Studies of the long-term outcome in children with a prolonged epileptic cognitive dysfunction, precisely documented from early childhood with parallel electroencephalographic data, are understandably very rare. We want to illustrate what can be learned from such studies, and the questions that these types of study can answer or the new questions that they are raising.

Case A.O.

This boy has been followed from the age of 3 years when he developed hard-to-control, frequent seizures of various types (mainly atypical absences, epileptic falls, peribuccal myoclonias), with frequent polymorphic generalized EEG discharges, increased during sleep (but no CSWS), with some frontal predominance. Repeat MRI showed a small left frontal parasagittal arachnoid cyst, which has remained unchanged. He was considered to have frontal seizures with rapid generalization. Several antiepileptic drugs were tried, with some effects but little change in the EEG abnormalities (see Fig. 16.1). His IQ, which was initially normal, gradually decreased over the years, and he was in the retarded range at 13 years (IQ 48). This drop in IQ was related to the total stagnation in raw scores on successive testings and not true loss of skills.

At 13 years, his epilepsy subsided, his EEG normalized, and he improved markedly, and is still progressing and learning at 18 years (total IQ 71). The lower verbal IQ was due to poor results on the 'information' and 'comprehension' items of the WAIS and not to any aphasic difficulty. The careful longitudinal evaluation

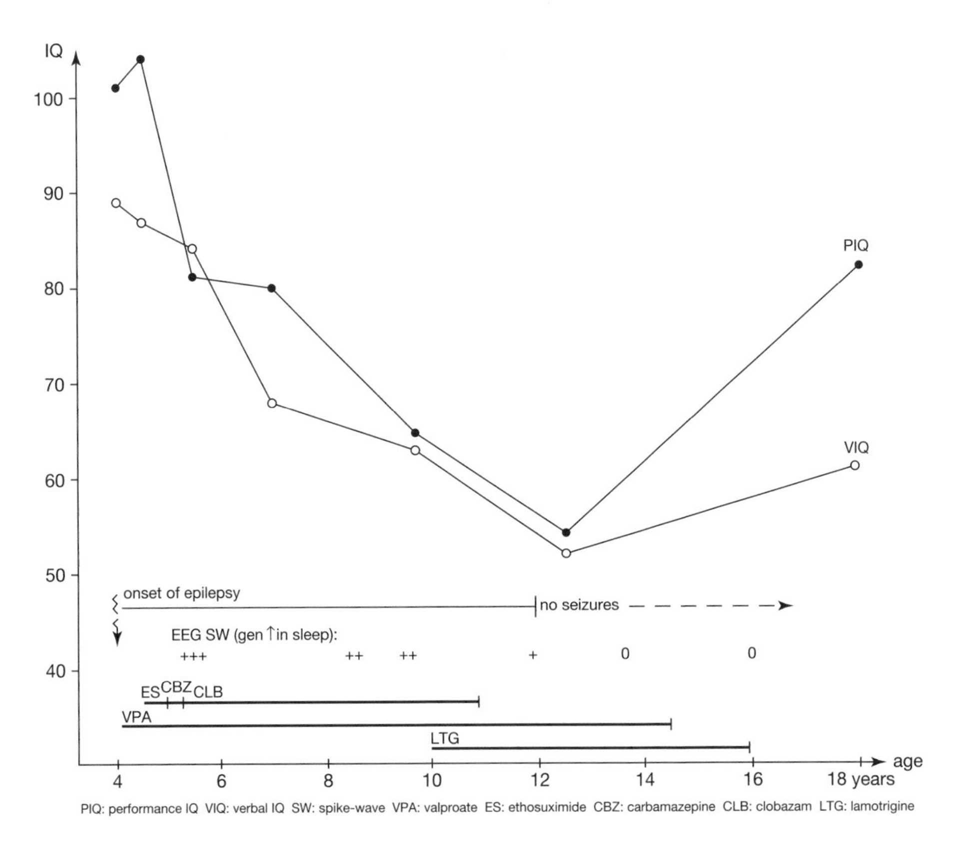

Fig. 16.1 Case A.O., boy: mixed epilepsy with left prefrontal parasagittal cyst. Clinical evolution from 3 to 18 years.

Prolonged cognitive arrest with delayed recovery associated with severe mixed epilepsy with left prefrontal parasagittal cyst (see description).

of cognitive functions, the monitoring of possible drug side-effects and epileptic activity (clinical and EEG) from an early age had led us to conclude that he had a prolonged learning arrest directly related to his epilepsy.

The delayed and marked continuous improvement after adolescence was also observable in other areas of his life. He now has total social independence, he has undertaken a successful apprenticeship, he has achieved excellent sport results and he has obtained his driving licence. Neither he nor his family had anticipated these possibilities.

The following very long-term study (from 5 years to 37 years) of a child with acquired epileptic aphasia (Landau–Kleffner syndrome) is rather exceptional for several reasons. This boy was studied in detail and published as a child and again in a follow-up study of acquired epileptic aphasia as a young adult (Deonna et al 1977, 1989). When seen again a few years later for administrative reasons (invalidity claim), we were surprised at his continuing progress and this prompted us to see him again 10 years later.

Case R.M.

This boy lost all verbal comprehension and expression and also became demented within a few weeks at the age of 5 years. He recovered his cognitive capacities and language comprehension during the next three years but had no expressive language. He was unable to say more than a few words and short sentences until 11 years. From the history and clinical contacts, there continued to be significant progress in expressive language after adolescence, and this surprised us when we saw him at 20 and 29 years. We had comparative videotaped recordings of his spontaneous speech and conversation at 29 years and 37 years. The comparison showed that there was a definite increase in speech fluency (speed, rhythm), naming, and content (grammatical complexity, vocabulary, length of sentences), and a decrease of phonemic paraphasias.

In contrast to his improved expressive abilities, his non-linguistic oromotor functions had not significantly improved (moderate oromotor apraxia). He started to learn to read very late (11 years), because he was not considered really capable, and now continues to study as an adult. We could also document an improvement in written text comprehension over the years. His reading level is limited but functional for simple matters (he works as a mechanic and drives a lot for his firm).

It is difficult to know how much the speech improvement is due to practice rather than a continuing 'true' reorganization of his linguistic system, because other abilities such as oromotor functions did not improve. It may be that the cortical areas dedicated to oromotor control, which were the earliest and most severely affected by the epileptic process, were more permanently damaged, while the areas for speech programming were involved later and less severely, allowing the possibility of continued improvement of the latter function. Also, the cerebral plasticity for these different functions may be different.

These two cases show what can be learned from follow-up studies in these cognitive childhood epilepsies, and the necessity of keeping an open mind in the prognosis of these situations. A.O.'s case showed a late improvement in global cognitive functioning, starting in adolescence and continuing into early adulthood, after many years of total stagnation and inability to learn. R.M. taught us that the language impairment in acquired epileptic aphasia, and the extent of the associated problems, is quite variable and may be mostly expressive,

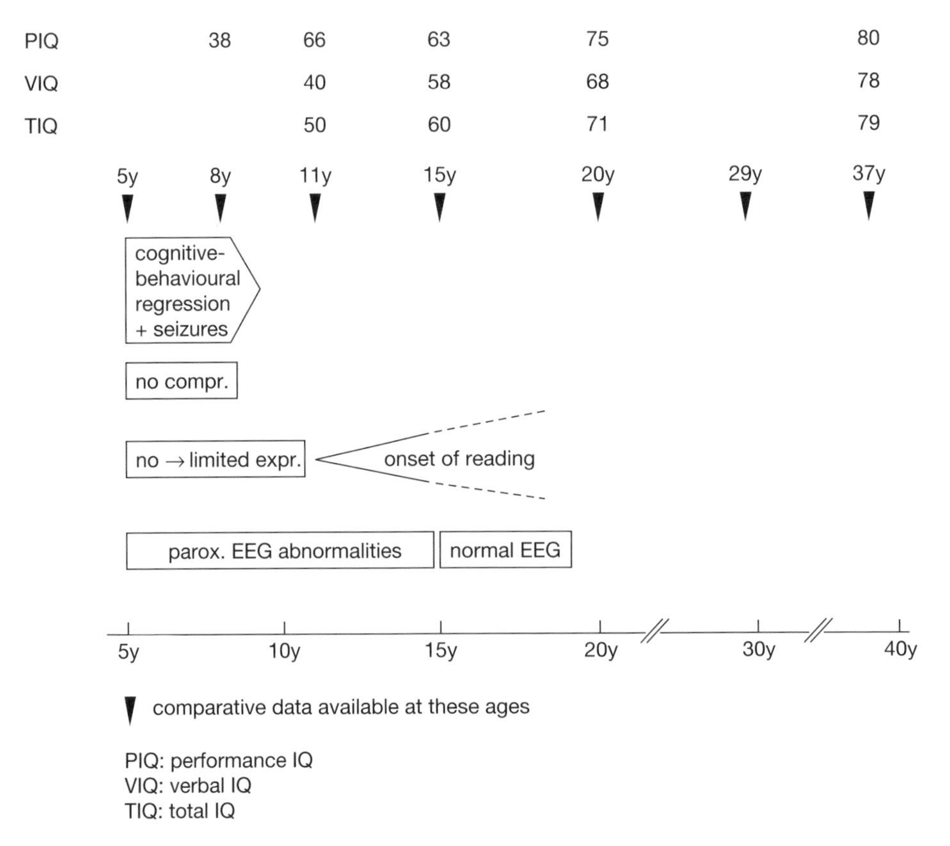

Fig. 16.2 Case R.M., boy: acquired epileptic aphasia (expressive, prolonged).

Summary of evolution and regular observations from the age of 5 to 37 years.

and that continuing progress in language expression can occur beyond the adolescent period through early adulthood and into middle age. Also the acquisition of some functional written language can start late and progress in adulthood. This evolution, which is a continuing and encouraging surprise, tells us how little we still know about these disorders. It is likely that there are many more surprises to come as more and better-treated children with such syndromes become adults, if they are re-examined long after their epilepsy has subsided. This should be done regardless of how well or how poorly they seem to have recovered.

16.6 Cerebral plasticity in the context of epilepsy

Functional imaging and clinical studies are increasingly showing that brain reorganization can occur with injuries sustained well beyond early childhood and adolescent years, and probably across the whole life span (Stiles 2000). Most of the clinical and experimental data on the reorganization of functions in an injured brain concern acute destructive brain pathologies which occurred in a single location in the brain and at a unique moment in its developmental history. As discussed before (see Chapter 3), epilepsy is a different situation because it may affect brain function over prolonged periods, rather than at a single point in time. Also, it may have consequences not only in its region of origin but also at a distance in functionally connected areas.

Epilepsy may be symptomatic of brain lesions of various types and locations – that is, in brain regions which mature at different tempos and have their own selective vulnerability at different ages and to different types of pathology, including the epileptic damage. One has to distinguish plasticity changes which occur after a lesion from those due to epilepsy itself. Removal of brain tissue in epilepsy surgery may still trigger another kind of plasticity (Chugani and Muller 1999). Long-term follow-ups of larger groups of children with cognitive epilepsies will hopefully help in finding out whether the kind of brain changes induced by epilepsy are really unique in terms of their late consequences, as compared to other types of brain damage or dysfunction.

Plasticity for memory functions is a special and important aspect of plasticity in the context of childhood epilepsy and has been discussed in Chapter 7, sections 7.3.2 and 7.3.3 on memory.

17 CONCLUSIONS

This book has been an attempt to give a view on childhood epilepsies which is centred, as opposed to most clinical texts, not on the seizure disorder itself, but on the consequences of the epileptic dysfunction for cognition and behaviour, particularly those of a chronic nature. It is increasingly recognized that these are often more important for the final prognosis than the remission of seizures, and are not limited to severe epilepsies in the classic sense. In fact, in some epileptic situations with predominant cognitive effects, the seizures may be rare, easy to treat or even absent.

The different types of childhood epilepsies have a variable impact on cognitive functions and behaviour, from none to severe, and of course no generalizations can be made. Even in the most frequent and 'benign' epilepsies, e.g. benign partial epilepsy with rolandic spikes, cognitive consequences can occur. The direct role of epilepsy has to be considered at some point or another in many different epilepsies of childhood.

Some clinical situations have been particularly important for the recognition and study of the direct but often elusive consequences of epilepsy for behaviour and cognition, and are discussed in more detail. These are:

1 The ictal-postictal, sometimes prolonged deficits.
2 The brief transitory cognitive impairment measurable during some EEG epileptic discharges in the absence of 'visible' clinical seizures.
3 Epileptic syndromes with loss of cognitive function as the main or only manifestation of epilepsy, e.g. acquired epileptic aphasia and partial epilepsies with continuous spike-waves during sleep.
4 Epilepsy surgery cases where suppression of seizures may occasionally allow evaluation of the direct role of epilepsy.
5 Newly diagnosed epilepsies in which reversible cognitive or behavioural changes preceded the first recognized seizures and diagnosis of epilepsy.

The various types of epileptic brain lesions or developmental brain disorders, now better defined anatomically, and the increasing number of genetically determined epileptic syndromes may each have a special and different relevance for the study of epilepsy-related cognitive and behaviour dysfunction, and can be a source of important information, which has been amply utilized in this book.

There are many ways and mechanisms by which the different epilepsies can interfere with cognitive functions and behaviour in an acute, subacute, chronic, reversible, persistent or even permanent manner. The clinical consequences can range from absence of or aberrant development, to stagnation of acquisitions or loss of fully mastered capacities and behaviours. Childhood epilepsies, besides their typical seizure manifestations, can be seen as a unique form of brain disorder in which any isolated or several developing functions may be temporarily or constantly interrupted. The affected child needs to adapt to frequently changing inner conditions, at different periods of his/her life, level of brain organization and experience. Epileptic activity itself, especially when early and long-standing or when involving particular developing areas, can lead to original (re)organizations or cause permanent or even progressive structural brain changes, the mechanisms and long-term consequences of which are still largely unknown.

These considerations forced us to challenge several traditional notions. The first was the distinction between paroxysmal and non-paroxysmal (persistent) symptoms, only the former being usually considered as typical of epilepsy. The second was the distinction between cognitive deficits due to a pre-existing or acquired brain pathology and those which are due to the epilepsy itself. In reality, there is a frequent interplay between these factors, with either one or the other or both being important during the whole duration of the disease or at different periods of its evolution. Finally, emotional-behavioural symptoms, as opposed to cognitive ones, should not be seen only as reactive to the disease and its consequences; they can also be direct manifestations of focal epilepsy arising in areas such as prefrontal or mesiotemporal regions, both highly epileptogenic zones belonging to the complex limbic circuits, and this often from a very early age.

It should be emphasized that the clinical importance of these cognitive-behavioural effects of epilepsy is not limited to otherwise normal (or at least initially normal) children with epilepsy, but extends also to already learning disabled or mentally retarded children in whom these constitute an additional disability.

The clinical evaluation of the direct effects of epilepsy on cognition and behaviour and the benefit of antiepileptic therapy requires very different methods from those traditionally used in epileptology which mainly rely on seizure counts. An individually tailored approach is necessary, using comparative standardized neuropsychological tests, questionnaires, videos and learning curves. These are not always available in young children, and they are time-consuming, often difficult to interpret and hardly applicable to large numbers of patients. Neuropsychological expertise, which is not yet available in many centres, and cooperation with the many professionals caring for developmentally or learning disabled children are also needed.

These difficulties present great limitations to progress in the study of the cognitive effects of epilepsy, in which hard data are difficult to obtain. Most of the experience discussed in this book is based on longitudinal single case studies, often considered 'anecdotal' and with scepticism. However, large group studies with controls are easy to aspire to, but often present their own pitfalls, when it comes to evaluating complex developing functions, with major individual variations, at least in our present state of knowledge. The numerous case reports reported in this book illustrate the value and limits of our approach; and the frequent and often long follow-ups offer some reassurance that the initial arguments and hypotheses were not contradicted by the passage of time.

One should also bear in mind that the outcome of children now, who are diagnosed early and treated aggressively with drugs or surgery and active rehabilitative measures, is likely to be different from those diagnosed 30 or 40 years ago and untreated, even though in many cases the epilepsy remains very difficult to treat or even resistant to all available drugs. There is still a wide gap between our current awareness of and ability to recognize and study these important aspects of epilepsy, and our therapeutic possibilities. We think, however, that accurate diagnosis of these problems, as always in medicine, is a necessary first step.

Finally, the authors fully acknowledge that the psychological and social consequences of 'being epileptic' can have a major impact on the so-called 'quality of life', and sometimes be the main cause of learning and behaviour disorders – a topic on which there has been important recent systematic work. However, it should also be accepted that the abilities of a child to adapt to these adverse circumstances are strongly dependent upon the child's cognitive and emotional resources and that these can be directly affected by the epileptic process itself, a recurring theme of this book.

17.1 Practical implications for the clinician

When cognitive and behavioural problems arise in a child with epilepsy, the possible direct causal or contributing role of the epileptic activity will almost always be thought of by parents, even if not entertained openly, and it needs to be approached directly.

The syndromic or etiological classification of the epilepsy may give a general hint as to what can be expected at the cognitive and behavioural level statistically. However, except for a few known constantly severe forms, there are major individual differences in cognitive impact even in medically well-defined situations.

For these reasons, each situation has to be examined as a unique one from the cognitive and behavioural point of view. A clinical approach has been proposed which is meant to help the clinician, either at the first encounter with the child and his family or during follow-up, or even when the possibility of epilepsy is suspected and no diagnosis has yet been made. Very often, only a hypothesis can be formulated on the importance of the epileptic activity *per se*, which will be confirmed or abandoned by observing the natural course of events and/or monitoring the effects of therapy, providing that the initial state has been well documented. The situation has to be reviewed regularly, at times over a prolonged period, keeping an open mind for what is probably the most complex form of chronic childhood neurological disorder that can interfere with learning and behaviour.

APPENDIX 1
BIBLIOGRAPHIC REFERENCES FOR NEUROPSYCHOLOGICAL TESTS AND OTHER TOOLS

BELEC Batterie d'évaluation du langage écrit et de ses troubles
Mousty P, Leybaert J, Alegria J, Content A, Morais J. (1994) Laboratoire de Psychologie Expérimentale, Université Libre de Bruxelles.

BELSKY Belsky J, Most RK. (1981) From exploration to play: a cross-sectional study of infant free play behaviour. *Dev Psychol* 17: 630–639.

BEM Batterie d'efficience mnésique
Signoret JL. (1991) Paris: Elsevier.

BEPL Batterie d'évaluation psycholinguistique
Chevrie-Muller C, Simon AM, Le Normand MT, Fournier S. (1988) Paris: Les Editions du Centre de Psychologie Appliquée.

BORB Birmingham object recognition battery
Riddoch MJ, Humphreys GW. (1993) Hove, UK: Lawrence Erlbaum Associates.

BREV Batterie rapide d'évaluation
Billard C, Livet MO, Motte J, Vallee L, Gillet P. (2002) The BREV neuropsychological test. Part I. Results for 500 normally developing children. *Dev Med Child Neurol* 44(6): 391–397.

BRIEF Behavior rating inventory of executive functions
Gioia GA, Isquith PK, Guy SC, Kenworthy L. (2000) Odessa, FL: PAR.

BSID Bayley scale of infant development
The Pyschological Corporation. (1993) 2nd edition. San Antonio, TX: Harcourt Brace.

CARS Childhood autism rating scale
Schopler E, Reichler RJ, De Vellis RF, Daly K. (1980) Toward objective classification of childhood autism. *J Autism Dev Disord* 10(1): 91–103.

CBCL Child behaviour checklist
Achenbach TM, Edelbrock CS. (1983) Manual for the child behaviour checklist and revised child behaviour profile. Burlington, VT: University of Vermont. Department of Psychiatry.
French adaptation: Fombonne E, Chedhan F, Carradec AM, Achard S,

	Navarro N, Reis S. (1988) Le Child Behaviour Checklist: un instrument pour la recherche en psychiatrie de l'enfant. *Psychiatr Psychobiol* 3: 409–418.
CBTT	Corsi-block tapping test French adaptation: Van Der Linden M, Closset A. Examen neuropsychologique de l'enfant, Liège, Belgium.
CCC	Children's communication checklist Bishop DVM. (1998) Development of the children's communication checklist: a method for assessing qualitative aspects of communicative impairment in children. *J Child Psychol Psychiatr* 39(6): 879–891.
CELF-3	Semel E, Wiig EH, Secord WH. (1995) *Clinical Evaluation of Language Fundamentals*. 3rd edition. San Antonio, TX: Psychological Corporation.
CMS	Children memory scale French translation: Cohen MJ. Echelle de mémoire pour enfants (2001) Paris: ECPA.
CORKUM	Corkum V, Byrne JM, Ellsworth C. (1995) Clinical assessment of sustained attention in preschoolers. *Child Neuropsychol* 1(1): 3–18.
CPRS-R	Revised Conners parent rating scale Conners CK, Sitarenios G, Parker JD, Epstein JN. (1998) The revised Conners parent rating scale (CPRS-R). *J Abnormal Child Psychol* 26(4): 257–268.
CPT	Conners' continuous performance test (1995) Toronto: Multi-Health Systems Inc.
CVLT	California verbal learning test French adaptation: Van Der Linden M, Closset A. Examen neuropsychologique de l'enfant, Liège, Belgium.
D2	Test D2 d'attention concentrée French adaptation: (1966) Editest.
DIGIT SPAN	From WISC-III
ECOSSE	Epreuve de compréhension syntaxique-sémantique Lecocq P. (1996) Lille: Presses Universitaires du Septentrion. English equivalent: TROG (Bishop)
EEL	Epreuves pour l'examen du langage Chevrie-Muller C, Simon AM, Decante P. (1981) Paris: Les Editions du Centre de Psychologie Appliquée.
ERC-N	Evaluation résumée du comportement – nourrisson (1984) LXXXIIe Session du Congrès de Psychiatrie et de Neurologie de Langue Française, Masson, pp 189–193.
ESCS	Early social communication scale Seibert JM, Hogan AE, Mundy P. (1982) Assessing interactional competencies: the early social communication scale. *Inf Mental Hlth J* 3: 244–258.

EVIP	Echelle de vocabulaire en images Peabody Dunn LD, Thériault-Wahlen CM, Dunn LM. (1993) Toronto: Psycan. English equivalent: Peabody picture vocabulary test.
FEPSY	Alphert WCJ, Aldenkamp AP. (1995) *FEPSY: The Iron Psyche.* Heemsteede, The Netherlands: Instituut voor Epilepsiebestrijding.
HANOI TOWER	Adapted by Sevino O. (1998) Les fonctions exécutives chez l'enfant: développement, structure et évaluation. Dissertation, Geneva.
HOOPER	The Hooper visual organization test Hooper HE. (1985) Los Angeles: Western Psychological Services.
K-ABC	Kaufmann assessment battery for children Kaufmann A, Kaufmann N. (1983) Circle Pines, MN: American Guidance Service. French adaptation: Kaufmann AS, Kaufmann NL. (1993) Batterie pour l'examen psychologique de l'enfant. Paris: Les Editions du Centre de Psychologie Appliquée.
L2MA	Langage oral, langage écrit, mémoire, attention Chevrie-Muller C, Simon AM, Fournier S. (1997) Paris: ECPA.
LOBROT	Batterie d'épreuves pour mesurer la lecture et l'orthographe Lobrot M. (1967) Bureau d'études et de recherches de Beaumont-sur-Oise.
LOWE & COSTELLO	Lowe M, Costello AJ. (1982) *The Manual for the Symbolic Play Test.* Berkshire: NFER-Nelson.
MACCARTHY	MacCarthy scales of children's abilities MacCarthy D. (1972) New York: Psychological Corporation.
MAZES	From WISC-III
NEEL	Nouvelles épreuves pour l'examen du langage Chevrie-Muller C, Plaza M. (2001) Paris: ECPA.
O-52	Epreuve d'évaluation des stratégies de compréhension en situation orale Khomsi A. (1987) Paris: Les Editions du Centre de Psychologie Appliquée.
PEABODY	Peabody picture vocabulary test – revised Dunn LM. (1981) Circle Pines, MN: American Guidance Service.

PMS	Raven's progressive matrices French adaptation: (1981) Issy-Les-Moulineaux: Editions Scientifiques et Psychologiques.
PRESCHOOL LANGUAGE SCALE – 3	Zimmerman IL, Steiner V, Pond R. (1992) San Antonio, TX: Psychological Corporation.
PURDUE	Purdue Pegboard. French adaptation: (1961) Paris: Centre de Psychologie Appliquée.
RAVLT	Rey's auditory verbal learning test Rey A. (1964) L'examen clinique en psychologie. Paris: Presses Universitaires de France.
RBMT	Rivermead behavioural memory test, for children aged 5 to 10 years Wilson BA, Ivani-Chaliam R, Aldrich F. (1991) Suffolk: The Thames Valley Test Company.
RCFT	Rey complex figure test Rey A. (1959) Paris: Editions du Centre de Psychologie Appliquée.
RENFREW LANGUAGE SCALES	Renfrew CE. (1988) Bicester: Winslow Press.
REY'S VISUAL DESIGN LEARNING TEST	Rey A. (1968) Epreuves mnésiques et d'apprentissage Neuchâtel, Switzerland: Delachaux & Niestlé.
STROOP	Stroop JR. (1935) Studies of interference in serial verbal reactions. *J Exp Psychol* 18: 643–662.
TEST OF LANGUAGE DEVELOPMENT: PRIMARY	Newcomer P, Hammill DD. (1997) 3rd edition. Austin, TX: Pro-Ed.
TLP	Test de langage parlé Caracosta H, Piterman Scoatarian S, van Waeyenberghe M, Zivy J. (1975) Test de langage pour enfants de 5 à 10 ans. Issy-les-Moulineaux: Etablissements scientifiques et Psychotechniques.
TMT	Trail-making test. Adapted by Sevino O. (1998) Les fonctions exécutives chez l'enfant: développement, structure et évaluation. Dissertation, Geneva.
TROG	Test for the reception of grammar Bishop D. (1989) Cambridge: Medical Research Council/ Chapel Press.

TVPS	Test of visual-perceptual skills Gardner MF, Burlingame CA. (1982) Psychological and Educational Publications.
VERBAL AND FIGURAL FLUENCY TEST	Adapted by Sevino O. (1998) Les fonctions exécutives chez l'enfant: développement, structure et évaluation. Dissertation, Geneva.
WISC-III	Wechsler intelligence scale for children Wechsler D. (1974) Wechsler intelligence scale for children – revised manual. New York: Psychological Corp. French adaptation: (1996) version III. Paris: Les Editions du Centre de Psychologie Appliquée.
WISCONSIN	Wisconsin card sorting test Chelune G, Baer R. (1986) Developmental norms for the Wisconsin card sorting test. *J Clin Exp Neuropsychol* 8: 219–228.
WPPSI-R	Wechsler preschool and primary scale of intelligence French adaptation: (1995) Paris: Les Editions du Centre de Psychologie Appliquée.
Z2B	Test des 2 barrages Zazzo R. (1992) Issy-les-Moulineaux: Editions scientifiques et psychologiques.

REFERENCES

Aarts JPH, Binnie CD, Smit AM, Wilkins J. (1984) Selective cognitive impairment during focal and generalized epileptiform EEG activity. *Brain* 107: 293–308.

Acharya JN, Wyllie E, Luders HO, Kotagal P, Lancman M, Coelho M. (1997) Seizures symptomatology in infants with localization-related epilepsy. *Neurology* 48: 189–196.

Achenbach TM. (1991) *Manual for the Child Behaviour Checklist and Revised Child Behaviour Profile.* Burlington, VT: Department of Psychiatry, University of Vermont.

Adrien JL, Lenoir P, Martineau J, Perrot A, Hameury L, Larmande C, Sauvage D. (1993) Blind ratings of early symptoms of autism based upon family home movies. *J Am Acad Child Adolesc Psychiatry* 32: 617–626.

Aicardi J. (1994) *Epilepsy in Children*, 2nd edition. New York: Raven Press, pp 130–164.

Aicardi J. (1999) Epilepsy: the hidden part of the iceberg. *Eur J Pediatr Neurol* 3: 197–200.

Aicardi J, Chevrie JJ. (1982) Atypical benign partial epilepsy of childhood. *Dev Med Child Neurol* 24: 281–292.

Alajouanine T. (1963) Dostoiewsky's epilepsy. *Brain* 31(2): 181–188.

Aldenkamp AP, Alperts WCJ, De Bruïne-Seeder D, Dekker MJA. (1990) Test-retest variability in children with epilepsy. A comparison of WISC-R profiles. *Epilepsy Res* 7: 165–172.

Aldenkamp AP, Alpherts WC, Blennow G, Elmqvist D, Heijbel J, Nilsson HL, Sandstedt P, Tonnby B, Wahlander L, Wosse E. (1993) Withdrawal of antiepileptic medication in children – effects on cognitive function: the Multicenter Holmfrid Study. *Neurology* 43(1): 41–50.

Alpherts WC, Aldenkamp AP. (1990) Computerized neuropsychological assessment of cognitive functioning in children with epilepsy. *Epilepsia* 31 Suppl 4: S35–S40.

Alpherts WC, Aldenkamp AP. (1995) *FEPSY: The Iron Psyche.* Heemsteede, The Netherlands: Instituut voor Epilepsiebestrijding.

Alvarez N, Besag F, Iivanainen M. (1998) Use of antiepileptic drugs in the treatment of epilepsy in people with intellectual disability. *J Intellect Disabil Res* 42 Suppl 1: 1–15.

American Psychiatric Association. (1994) *Diagnostic and Statistical Manual of Mental Disorders (DSM IV),* 4th edition. Washington, DC: APA.

Amir N, Gross-Tsur V. (1994) Paradoxical normalization in childhood epilepsy. *Epilepsia* 35(5): 1060–1064.

Andermann F, Robb JP. (1972) Absence status: a reappraisal following review of 38 patients. *Epilepsia* 13: 177–187.

Andermann LF, Savard G, Meenke HJ, McLachlan R, Moshe S, Andermann F. (1999) Psychosis after resection of ganglioglioma or DNET. *Epilepsia* 40(1): 83–87.

Annett M. (1992) Five tests of handskill. *Cortex* 28(4): 583–600.

Arroyo S, Lesser RP, Gordon B, Uematsu S, Hart J, Schwerdt P, Andreasson K, Fisher RS. (1993) Mirth, laughter and gelastic seizures. *Brain* 116: 757–780.

Arzimanoglou A, Guerrini R, Aicardi J, editors. (2004) *Aicardi's Epilepsy in Children.* Philadelphia: Lippincott Williams and Wilkins.

Astur RS, Taylor LB, Mamelak AN, Philpott L, Sutherland RJ. (2002) Humans with hippocampus damage display severe spatial memory impairments in a virtual Morris water task. *Behav Brain Res* 132(1): 77–84.

Augustijn PB, Parra J, Wouters CH, Joosten P, Lindhout D, van Emde Boas W. (2001) Ring chromosome 20, epilepsy syndrome in children: electroclinical features. *Neurology* 57(6): 1108–1111.

Austin JK, Dunn DW. (2002) Progressive behavioral changes in children with epilepsy. In: Sutula T, and Pitkainen A, editors. *Progress in Brain Research* 135. Amsterdam: Elsevier, pp 419–427.

Austin JK, Smith MS, Risinger MW, McNelis AM. (1994) Childhood epilepsy and asthma: comparison of quality of life. *Epilepsia* 35(3): 608–615.
Austin JK, Huberty TJ, Huster GA, Dunn DW. (1999) Does academic achievement in children with epilepsy change over time? *Dev Med Child Neurol* 41: 473–479.
Austin JK, Harezlak J, Dunn DW, Huster GA, Rose DF, Ambrosius WT. (2001) Behavior problems in children before first recognized seizures. *Pediatrics* 107: 115–122.
Austin JK, Dunn DW, Caffrey HM, Perkins SM, Harezlak J, Rose DF. (2002) Recurrent seizures and behavior problems in children with first recognized seizures: a prospective study. *Epilepsia* 43: 1564–1573.
Avanzini G. (2001) Functional organization of the limbic system. In: Avanzini G, Beaumanoir A, Mira L, editors. *Limbic Seizures in Children*. London: John Libbey, pp 21–31.
Badinand H, Bastuji H, De Bellecize J, Cortinovis P, Kocher L, Rousselle C, Revol M. (1995) Three unpublished new cases of continuous spikes and waves during slow sleep. In: Beaumanoir A, Bureau A, Deonna T, Mira C, Tassinari CA, editors. *Continuous Spikes and Waves during Slow Sleep. Electrical Status Epilepticus during Slow Sleep*. Mariani Foundation Neurology Series: 3. London: John Libbey, pp 186–187.
Baglietto MG, Battaglia FM, Nobili L, Tortorelli S, De Negri E, Calevo MG, Veneselli E, De Negri M. (2001) Neuropsychological disorders related to interictal epileptic discharges during sleep in benign epilepsy of childhood with centrotemporal or rolandic spikes. *Dev Med Child Neurol* 43: 407–412.
Bailet LL, Turk WR. (2000) The impact of childhood epilepsy on neurocognitive and behavioral performance: a prospective longitudinal study. *Epilepsia* 41(4): 426–431.
Baird G, Robinson R. (2000) Sleep EEGs in children under 48 months with autism but without epilepsy. *Dev Med Child Neurol* 85(42 Suppl 1): 12. (Abstract.)
Ballaban-Gil K, Tuchman R. (2000) Epilepsy and epileptiform EEG: association with autism and language disorders. *Ment Retard Dev Disabil Res Rev* 6(4): 300–308.
Baram TZ. (2003) Longterm plasticity and functional consequence of simple versus recurrent early-life seizures. *Ann Neurol* 54(6): 701–705.
Barkovich AJ, Kuzniecky RI, Dobyns WB, Jackson GD, Becker LE, Evrard P. (1996) A classification scheme for malformations of cortical development. *Neuropediatrics* 27: 59–63.
Bast T, Volp A, Wolf C, Rating D, Sulthiame Study Group. (2003) The influence of sulthiame on EEG in children with benign childhood epilepsy with centrotemporal spikes. *Epilepsia* 44(2): 215–220.
Bates E, Thal D, Janowsky JJ. (1992) Early language development and its neural correlates. In: Segalowitz JJ, Rapin I, editors. *Handbook of Neuropsychology,* Vol 7. New York: Elsevier, pp 69–110.
Battaglia D, Iuvone L, Stefanini MC, Acquafondata C, Lettori D, Chiricozzi F, Pane M, Mittica A, Guzzetta F. (2001) Reversible aphasic disorder induced by lamotrigine in atypic benign childhood epilepsy. *Epileptic Disorders* 3(4): 217–222.
Battaglia D, Dravet C, Veredice C, Donvito V, Pane M, Lettori D. (2003) Early thalamic injury in epileptic children and continuous spike wave during slow sleep (CSWC): causal or casual link? *Eur J Paediatr Neurol* 7(5): 319.
Battros AM. (2000) *Half a Brain is Enough: The History of Nico*. Cambridge: Cambridge University Press.
Baumbach HD, Chow KL. (1981) Visuocortical epileptiform discharges in rabbits: differential effects on neuronal development in the lateral geniculate nucleus and superior colliculus. *Brain Res* 209(1): 61–76.
Bax MCO. (2002) Neurology or psychiatry? *Dev Med Child Neurol* 44: 291.
Baxter P. (1999) Epidemiology of pyridoxine-dependent and pyridoxine-responsive seizures in the UK. *Arch Dis Child* 81(5): 431–433.
Bayley N. (1993) *Manual for the Bayley Scales for Infant Development*, 2nd edition. San Antonio: Psychological Corporation/Harcourt Brace & Co.
Baynes K, Kegl JA, Brentari D, Kussmaul C, Poizner H. (1998) Chronic auditory agnosia following Landau–Kleffner syndrome: a 23 year outcome study. *Brain and Language* 63: 381–425.
Beauchesne H. (1980) *L'épileptique*. Paris: Bordas.
Beaumanoir A, Andermann F, Mira L, Zifkin B, editors. (2003) *Frontal Lobe Seizures and Epilepsies in Children.* Montrouge: John Libbey.
Beaussart M. (1972) Benign epilepsy in children with rolandic (centro-temporal) paroxysmal foci. *Epilepsia* 13: 795–811.
Bebek N, Gurse C, Gokyigit A, Baykan B, Ozkara C, Dervent A. (2001) Hot water epilepsy: clinical and electrophysiologic findings based on 21 cases. *Epilepsia* 42(9): 1180–1184.
Beckung E, Uvebrant P. (1997) Hidden dysfunction in childhood epilepsy. *Dev Med Child Neurol* 39: 72–79.

Bednarek N, Motte J, Soufflet C, Plouin P, Dulac O. (1998) Evidence for late infantile spasms. *Epilepsia* 39: 55.

Berg I, Butler A, Ellis M, Foster J. (1993) Psychiatric aspects of epilepsy in childhood treated with carbamazepine, phenitoin or sodium valproate: a random trial. *Dev Med Child Neurol* 35(2): 149–157.

Bergin PS, Thompson PJ, Fish DR, Shorvon SD. (1995) The effect of seizures on memory for recently learned material. *Neurology* 45(2): 236–240.

Berkovic SF. (2003) Hypothalamic hamartoma and seizures. A treatable epileptic encephalopathy. *Epilepsia* 44: 969–973.

Berkovic SF, Kuzniecky RI, Andermann F. (1997) Human epileptogenesis and hypothalamic hamartomas: new lessons from an experiment of nature. *Epilepsia* 38(1): 1–3.

Berroya AG, Melntyre J, Webster R, Lah S, Sabaz M, Lawson J. (2004) Speech and language deterioration in benign rolandic epilepsy. *J Child Neurol* 19(1): 53–58.

Berry-Kravis E. (2002) Epilepsy in fragile X-syndrome. *Dev Med Child Neurol* 44(11): 724–728.

Besag FMC. (1987) Cognitive deterioration in children with epilepsy. In: Trimble MR, Reynolds EH, editors. *Epilepsy, Behavior and Cognitive Function*. Chichester: John Wiley, pp 113–127.

Bever TG. (1982) *Regression in Mental Development: Basic Phenomena and Theories*. Hillsdale, NJ: Erlbaum.

Billard C, Livet MO, Motte J, Vallee L, Gillet P. (2002a) The BREV neuropsychological test. Part I. Results for 500 normally developing children. *Dev Med Child Neurol* 44(6): 391–397.

Billard C, Motte J, Farmer M, Livet MO, Vallee L, Gillet P, Vol S. (2002b) The BREV neuropsychological test. Part II. Results of validation in children with epilepsy. *Dev Med Child Neurol* 44(6): 398–404.

Binnie CD. (1991) Behavioral correlates of interictal spikes. *Adv Neurol* 55: 113–126.

Binnie CD, Marston D. (1992) Cognitive correlates of interictal discharges. *Epilepsia* 33 Suppl 6: S11–S17.

Binnie CD, Kasteleijn-Nolst Trenité DGA, Smit AM, Wilkins AJ. (1987) Interactions of epileptiform EEG discharges and cognition. *Epilepsy Res* 1: 239–245.

Binnie CD, De Silva M, Hurst A. (1992) Rolandic spikes and cognitive function. *Epilepsy Res* Suppl 6: S71–S73.

Biraben A, Taussig D, Thomas P, Even C, Vignal JP, Scarabin JM, Chauvel P. (2001) Fear as the main feature of epileptic seizures. *J Neurol Neurosurg Psychiatry* 70(2): 186–191.

Bishop D. (1997) *Uncommon Understanding: Development and Disorders of Language Comprehension in Children*. Hove: Psychology Press.

Bishop D. (2000) Pragmatic language impairment: a correlate of SLI, a distinct subgroup, or part of the autistic continuum? In: Bishop DVM, Leonard LB, editors. *Speech and Language Impairments in Children: Causes, Characteristics, Intervention and Outcome*. Hove: Psychology Press, pp 99–113.

Bishop D, Mogford K. (1988) *Language Development in Exceptional Circumstances*. Edinburgh: Churchill Livingstone.

Blake RV, Wroe SJ, Breen EK, McCarthy RA. (2000) Accelerated forgetting in patients with epilepsy. Evidence for an impairment in memory consolidation. *Brain* 123 Pt 3: 472–483.

Boatman D, Freeman J, Vining E, Pulsifer M, Miglioretti D, Minahan R, Carson B, Brandt J, McKhann G. (1999) Language recovery after left hemispherectomy in children with late-onset seizures. *Ann Neurol* 46: 579–586.

Boel M, Casaer P. (1989) Continuous spikes and waves during slow wave sleep: a 30 month follow-up study of neuropsychological recovery and EEG findings. *Neuropediatrics* 20(3): 176–180.

Bolton PF, Park RJ, Higgins JN, Griffiths PD, Pickles A. (2002) Neuro-epileptic determinants of autism spectrum disorders in tuberous sclerosis complex. *Brain* 125 Pt 6: 1247–1255.

Boniface SJ, Kennett RP, Oxbury SM. (1994) Changes in focal interictal epileptiform activity during and after the performance of verbal and visuospatial tasks in a patient with intractable partial seizures. *J Neurol Neurosurg Psychiatry* 57: 227–228.

Boone KB, Miller BL, Rosenberg l, Durazo A, Mclntyre H, Weil M. (1988) Neuropsychological and behavioral abnormalities in an adolescent with frontal lobe seizures. *Neurology* 38: 583–586.

Bornstein M, Coddon D, Song S. (1956) Prolonged alterations in behavior associated with a continuous electroencephalographic (spike and dome) abnormality. *Neurology* 6: 444–448.

Bouchard A, Lorilloux J, Guedeney C, Kipman DS. (1975) *Childhood Epilepsy. A Pediatric-Psychiatric Approach*. New York: International University Press.

Boulloche J, Husson A, Le Luyer B, Le Roux P. (1990) Dysphagie, troubles de la parole et pointes-ondes centrotemporales. *Arch Fr Pediatr* 47: 115–117.

Bourgeois BF. (1998) Antiepileptic drugs, learning and behavior in childhood epilepsy. A review. *Epilepsia* 39(9): 13–21.

Bourgeois BF, Prensky AL, Palkes HS, Talent BK, Bush SG. (1983) Intelligence in epilepsy: a prospective study in children. *Ann Neurol* 14: 438–444.
Boyd, SG, Rivera-Gaxiola M, Towel AD, Harkness W, Neville BGR. (1996) Discrimination of speech sounds in a boy with Landau–Kleffner syndrome: an intraoperative event-related potential study. *Neuropediatrics* 27(4): 211–215.
Camfield C, Camfield P, Smith B, Gordon K, Dooley J. (1993) Biological factors as predictors of social outcome of epilepsy in intellectually normal children. A population based study. *J Pediatr* 122: 869–875.
Campbell BG, Ostrach LH, Crabtree JW, Chow KL. (1984) Characterization of penicillin- and bicuculline-induced epileptiform discharges during development of striate cortex in rabbits. *Dev Brain Res* 15: 125–128.
Caplan R, Austin JK. (2000) Behavioral aspects of epilepsy in children with mental retardation. *Ment Retard Dev Disabil Res Rev* 6(4): 293–299.
Caplan R, Shields D, Mori L, Yudovin S. (1991) Middle childhood onset of interictal psychosis. *J Am Acad Child Adolesc Psychiatry* 30(6): 893–896.
Caplan R, Guthrie D, Mundy P, Sigman M, Shields D, Sherman T, Peacock W. (1992a) Nonverbal communication skills of surgically treated children with infantile spasms. *Dev Med Child Neurol* 34: 499–506.
Caplan R, Comain Y, Shewmon DA, Jackson L, Chugani HT, Peacock W. (1992b) Intractable seizures, compulsions, and coprolalia: a pediatric case study. *J Neuropsychiatry Clin Neurosci* 4(3): 315–319.
Caplan R, Arbelle S, Guthrie D, Komo S, Shields WD, Hansen R, Chayasirisobhon S. (1997) Formal thought disorder and psychopathology in pediatric primary generalized and complex partial epilepsy. *J Am Acad Child Adolesc Psychiatry* 36(9): 1286–1294.
Caraballo R, Cersosimo R, Fejerman N. (1999) A particular type of epilepsy in children with congenital hemiparesis associated with unilateral polymicrogyria. *Epilepsia* 40: 865–871.
Cassé-Perrot C, Wolf M, Dravet C. (2001) Neuropsychology of severe myoclonic epilepsy in infancy. In: Jambaqué I, Lassonde M, Dulac O, editors. *Neuropsychology of Childhood Epilepsy*. New York: Kluwer Academic/Plenum Press, pp 131–140.
Catalano R. (1998) *When Autism Strikes. Families Cope with Childhood Disintegrative Disorder*. New York: Plenum Press.
Caviness VS, Hatten ME, McConnel II SK, Takahashi T. (1995) Developmental neuropathology and childhood epilepsies. In: Schwartzkroin PA, Moshé SL, Noebels JL, Swan JW, editors. *Brain Development and Epilepsy*. New York and Oxford: Oxford University Press, pp 94–121.
CCPT. (1995) *Conner's Continuous Performance Test*. Toronto: Multihealth System Inc.
Cendes F, Andermann F, Gloor P, Gambardella A, Lopes-Cendes I, Watson C, Evans A, Carpenter S, Olivier A. (1994) Relationship between atrophy of the amygdala and ictal fear in temporal lobe epilepsy. *Brain* 117: 739–746.
Chang BS, Lowenstein DH. (2003) Mechanisms of disease. Epilepsy. *New Engl J Med* 349: 1257–1266.
Chaudhry MR, Pond DA. (1961) Mental deterioration in epileptic children. *J Neurol Neurosurg Psychiatry* 24: 213–219.
Chen YJ, Chow JC, Lee IC. (2001) Comparison of the cognitive effect of antiepileptic drugs in seizure-free children with epilepsy before and after drug withdrawal. *Epilepsy Res* 44(1): 65–70.
Chevalier H, Metz-Lutz MN, Segalowitz SJ. (2000) Impulsivity and control of inhibition in benign focal childhood epilepsy. *Brain and Cognition* 43 (1–3): 86–90.
Chilosi AM, Cipriani P, Bertuccelli B, Pfanner PL, Cioni PG. (2001) Early cognitive and communication development in children with focal brain lesions. *J Child Neurol* 16(5): 309–316.
Chiron C, Jambaqué I, Nabbout R, Lounes R, Syrota A, Dulac O. (1997) The right brain hemisphere is dominant in human infants. *Brain* 120 Pt 6: 1057–1065.
Chival G, Thibault de Beauregard A. (2000) Evaluation du langage oral dans ses aspects structurels et fonctionnels chez six enfants atteints d'épilepsie avec POCS (pointes-ondes continues de sommeil). Dissertation, Université Claude-Bernard Lyon I.
Chugani HT, Muller RA. (1999) Plasticity associated with cerebral resections. *Adv Neurol* 81: 241–250.
Chugani HT, Da Silva E, Chugani DC. (1996) Infantile spasms: III. Prognostic implications of bitemporal hypometabolism on positron emission tomography. *Ann Neurol* 39(5): 643–649.
Colamaria V, Sgro V, Caraballo R, Simeone M, Zullini E, Fontana E, Zanetti R, Grimau-Merino R, Dalla Bernardina B. (1991) Status epilepticus in benign rolandic epilepsy manifesting as anterior operculum syndrome. *Epilepsia* 32: 329–334.

Croona C, Kihlgren M, Lundberg S, Eeg-Olofson D, Edebon-Eeg-Olofson K. (1999) Neuropsychological findings in children with benign childhood epilepsy with centrotemporal spikes. *Dev Med Child Neurol* 41: 813–818.

Culhane-Shelburne K, Chapieski L, Hiscock M, Glaze D. (2002) Executive functions in children with frontal and temporal lobe epilepsy. *J Int Neuropsychol Soc* 8: 623–632.

Curatolo P, editor. (2003) *Tuberous Sclerosis Complex: From Basic Science to Clinical Phenotypes,* International Review of Child Neurology Series. London: Mac Keith Press.

D'Alessandro P, Piccirilli M, Tiacci C, Ibba A, Maiotti M, Sciarma T, Testa A. (1990) Neuropsychological features of benign partial epilepsy in children. *Ital J Neurol* 11: 265–269.

D'Alessandro P, Piccirilli M, Sciarma T, Tiaci C. (1995) Cognition in childhood epilepsy: a longitudinal study. *Abstract Epilepsia* 36 Suppl 3: S124.

Dalla Bernardina B, Fontana E, Zullini E, Avesani E, Zoccante L, Perez Jimenez A, Giardina L. (1994) Unusual partial complex status with autisticlike behavior in infancy. *Abstract Epilepsia* 35 Suppl 7: S43.

Dall'Oglio AM, Bates E, Volterra V, Di Capua M, Pezzini G. (1994) Early cognition, communication and language in children with focal brain injury. *Dev Med Child Neurol* 36(12): 1076–1098.

Damasio A. (1999) *The Feeling of What Happens: Body and Emotion in the Making of Consciousness.* London: William Heinemann, p 101.

Daniel RT, Villemure KM, Roulet E, Villemure JG. (2004) Surgical treatment of temporoparietooccipital cortical dysplasia in infants: report of two cases. *Epilepsia* 45(7): 1–5.

Deas D, Gerding L, Hazy J. (2000) Marijuana and panic disorder. *J Am Acad Child Adolesc Psychiatry* 39: 1466–1467.

De Grauw TJ, Salomons GS, Cecil KM, Chuck G, Newmeyer A, Schapiro MB, Jakobs C. (2002) Congenital creatine transporter deficiency. *Neuropediatrics* 33(5): 232–238.

Delgado Escueta AV, Mattson RH, King L, Goldensohn ES, Spiegel H, Madsen J, Crandall P, Dreifuss F, Porter RJ. (1981) Special report. The nature of aggression during epileptic seizures. *New Engl J Med* 305(12): 711–716.

DeLong GR, Heinz ER. (1997) The clinical syndrome of early life bilateral hippocampal sclerosis. *Ann Neurol* 42(1): 11–17.

Deonna T. (1991) Acquired epileptiform aphasia in children (Landau–Kleffner syndrome). *J Clin Neurophysiol* 8(3): 288–298.

Deonna T. (1993) Annotation: Cognitive and behavioural correlates of epileptic activity in children. *J Child Psychol Psychiatry* 34(5): 611–620.

Deonna T. (1995) Cognitive and behavioral disturbances as epileptic manifestations in children: an overview. *Semin Pediatr Neurol* 2: 254–260.

Deonna T. (1996) Epilepsies with cognitive symptomatology. In: Wallace S, editor. *Epilepsies in Childhood.* London: Chapman and Hall, pp 315–322.

Deonna T. (1999) Developmental consequences of epilepsies in infancy. In: Nehling A, Motte J, Moshé SL, Plouin P, editors. *Childhood Epilepsies and Brain Development.* London: John Libbey, pp 113–122.

Deonna T. (2000a) Rolandic epilepsy (RE) – neuropsychology of the active epilepsy phase. *Epileptic Disord* 2 Suppl 1: S59–S61.

Deonna T. (2000b) Acquired epileptic aphasia (AEA) or Landau–Kleffner syndrome: from childhood to adulthood. In: Bishop DVM, Leonard LB, editors. *Speech and Language Impairments in Children. Causes, Characteristics, Intervention and Outcome.* Hove: Psychology Press, pp 261–272.

Deonna T. (2003) Childhood epilepsy: secondary prevention is crucial. *Dev Med Child Neurol* 45 Suppl 95: 38–41.

Deonna T. (2004) Cognitive and behavioral manifestations of epilepsy in children. In: Wallace SJ, Farrell K, editors. *Epilepsy in Children*, 2nd edition. London: Arnold, pp 250–256.

Deonna T. (2005) Management of epilepsy. Can quality of care be improved? *Arch Dis Child* 90(1): 5–10.

Deonna T, Roulet E. (1995) Acquired epileptic aphasia (AEA): definition of the syndrome and current problems. In: Beaumanoir A, Bureau M, Deonna T, Mira L, Tassinari CA, editors. *Continuous Spikes and Waves during Slow Sleep. Electrical Status Epilepticus during Slow Sleep.* Mariani Foundation Neurology Series: 3. Paris: John Libbey, pp 37–45.

Deonna T, Ziegler AL. (2000) Hypothalamic hamartoma, precocious puberty and gelastic seizures: a special model of 'epileptic' developmental disorder. *Epileptic Disord* 2: 33–37.

Deonna T, Beaumanoir A, Gaillard F, Assal G. (1977) Acquired aphasia in childhood with seizure disorder: a heterogeneous syndrome. *Neuropädiatrie* 8: 265–273.

Deonna T, Fletcher P, Voumard C. (1982) Temporary regression during language acquisition: a linguistic analysis of a 2-year-old child. *Dev Med Child Neurol* 24: 156–163.
Deonna T, Chevrie C, Hornung E. (1987) Childhood epileptic speech disorder: prolonged, isolated deficit of prosodic features. *Dev Med Child Neurol* 29: 100–105.
Deonna T, Peter C, Ziegler AL. (1989) Adult follow-up of the acquired aphasia-epilepsy syndrome in childhood. Report of 7 cases. *Neuropediatrics* 20: 132–138.
Deonna T, Roulet E, Fontan D, Marcoz JP. (1993a) Speech and oromotor deficits of epileptic origin in benign partial epilepsy of childhood with rolandic spikes (BPERS). Relationship to the acquired aphasia-epilepsy syndrome. *Neuropediatrics* 24: 83–87.
Deonna T, Ziegler AL, Moura-Serra J, Innocenti G. (1993b) Autistic regression in relation to limbic pathology and epilepsy: report of two cases. *Dev Med Child Neurol* 35: 166–176.
Deonna T, Davidoff V, Roulet E. (1993c) Isolated disturbance of written language acquisition as an initial symptom of epileptic aphasia in a 7-year-old child: a 3-year follow-up study. *Aphasiology* 7(5): 441–450.
Deonna T, Ziegler AL, Maeder IM, Ansermet F, Roulet E. (1995) Reversible behavioural autistic-like regression: a manifestation of a special (new?) epileptic syndrome in a 28-month-old child. A 2-year longitudinal study. *Neurocase* 1: 91–99.
Deonna T, Davidoff V, Ingvar-Maeder M, Zesiger P, Marcoz JP. (1997) The spectrum of cognitive disturbances in children with partial epilepsy and continuous spike waves during sleep. A 4-year follow-up case study with prolonged reversible learning arrest and dysfluency. *Eur J Child Neurol* 1: 19–29.
Deonna T, Zesiger P, Davidoff V, Maeder M, Mayor C, Roulet E. (2000) Benign partial epilepsy of childhood: a neuropsychological and EEG study of cognitive function. *Dev Med Child Neurol* 42: 595–603.
Deonna T, Fohlen M, Jalin C, Delalande O, Ziegler AL. (2002) Epileptic stereotypies in children. In: Guerrini R, Aicardi J, Andermann F, Hallett M, editors. *Epilepsy and Movement Disorders.* Cambridge: Cambridge University Press, pp 319–332.
Deonna T, Ziegler AL, Roulet-Perez E. (2003) Acquired epileptic frontal syndrome in children. In: Beaumanoir A, Andermann F, Chauvel P, Mira L, Zifkin B, editors. *Frontal Lobe Seizures and Epilepsies in Children.* Montrouge: John Libbey, pp 133–146.
de Saint-Martin A, Petiau C, Massa R, Maquet P, Marescaux C, Hirsch E, Metz-Lutz MN. (1999) Idiopathic rolandic epilepsy with 'interictal' facial myoclonia and oromotor deficit: a longitudinal EEG and PET study. *Epilepsia* 40(5): 614–620.
de Saint-Martin AD, Carcangiu R, Arzimanoglou A, Massa R, Thomas P, Motte J, Marescaux C, Metz-Lutz MN, Hirsch E. (2001) Semiology of typical and atypical rolandic epilepsy: a video-EEG analysis. *Epileptic Disord* 3(4): 173–182.
Devinsky O, Gershengorn J, Brown E, Perrine K, Vazquez B, Luciano D. (1997) Frontal functions in juvenile myoclonic epilepsy. *Neuropsychiatr Neuropsychol Behav Neurol* 10(4) 243–246.
Devinsky O, Perrine K, Hirsch J, McCullen W, Paacia S, Doyle W. (2000) Relation of cortical language distribution and cognitive function in surgical epilepsy patients. *Epilepsia* 41(4): 400–404.
Devlin AM, Cross JH, Harkness W, Chong WK, Harding B, Vargha-Khadem F, Neville BG. (2003) Clinical outcomes of hemispherectomy for epilepsy in childhood and adolescence. *Brain* 126: 556–566.
Di Martino A, Tuchman R. (2001) Antiepileptic drugs: affective use in autism spectrum disorders. *Pediatr Neurol* 25(3): 199–207.
Dixon MS, Glaser GH. (1956) Psychomotor seizures in childhood. A clinical study. *Neurology* 6(9): 646–655.
Dlugos DJ, Moss EM, Duhaime AC, Brooks-Kayal AR. (1999) Language-related cognitive declines after left temporal lobectomy in children. *Pediatr Neurol* 21(1): 444–449.
Doose H, Völzke E. (1979) Petit mal status in early childhood and dementia. *Neuropädiatrie* 10(1): 10–14.
Doose H, Bayer WK, Ernst JP, Tuxhorn I, Völzke E. (1988) Benign partial epilepsy. Treatment with sulthiame. *Dev Med Child Neurol* 30: 683–684.
Doose H, Neubauer B, Carlsson G. (1996) Children with benign focal sharp waves in the EEG – developmental disorders and epilepsy. *Neuropediatrics* 27: 227–241.
Dreifuss FE. (1983) *Pediatric Pileptology. Classification and Management of Seizures in the Child.* Boston, MA: John Wright PSG.
Drinkenburg WHIM, Schuurmans MLEJ, Coenen AML, Vossen JMH, van Luijtelaar ELJM. (2003) Ictal stimulus processing during spike-wave discharges in genetic epileptic rats. *Behav Brain Res* 14: 141–146.
Duchowny M, Jayacar P, Harvey AS, Resnick T, Alvarez L, Dean P, Levin B. (1996) Language cortex representation: effects of developmental versus acuired pathology. *Ann Neurol* 40(1): 31–38.
Dulac O. (2001) Epileptic encephalopathy. *Epilepsia* 42 Suppl 3: S23–S26.

Dulac O, Billard C, Arthuis M. (1983) Aspects electrocliniques et évolutifs de l'épilepsie dans le syndrome aphasie-épilepsie. *Arch Fr Pediatr* 40: 299–308.
Dusser A. (1992) Analyse des troubles du comportement associés aux crises gélastiques: à propos d'une observation d'un enfant porteur d'un hamartome hypothalamique. *ANAE* 1: 22–25.
Duvelleroy-Hommel C, Billard C, Lucas P, Gillet M, Barthez A, Santini JJ, Degiovanni E, Henry F, De Toffel B, Autret A. (1995) Sleep EEG and developmental dysphasia: lack of a consistent relationship with paroxysmal EEG activity during sleep. *Neuropediatrics* 26(1): 14–18.
Echenne B, Cheminal R, Rivier F, Negre C, Touchon J, Billiard M. (1992) Epileptic encephalopathic abnormalities and developmental dysphasias: a study of 32 patients. *Brain Dev* 14: 216–225.
Efron R. (1961) Post-epileptic paralysis: theoretical critique and report of a case. *Brain* 84: 281–294.
Ellenberg JH, Hirtz DG, Nelson KB. (1986) Do seizures in children cause intellectual deterioration? *New Engl J Med* 14: 216–225.
Engel J, Lufwig BI, Fetell M. (1986) Prolonged partial complex status epilepticus: EEG and behavioral observations. *Neurology* 28: 863–869.
Engler F, Maeder-Ingvar M, Roulet E, Deonna T. (2003) Treatment with Sulthiame (Ospolot®) in benign partial epilepsy of childhood and related syndromes: an open clinical and EEG study. *Neuropediatrics* 34: 105–109.
Eriksson K, Kylliainen A, Hirvonen K, Nieminen P, Koivikko M. (2003) Visual agnosia in a child with non-lesional occipito-temporal CSWS. *Brain Dev* 25(4): 262–267.
Evans-Jones LG, Rosenbloom L. (1978) Disintegrative psychosis in childhood. *Dev Med Child Neurol* 20: 462–470.
Fejerman N. (1987) Status epilepticus of benign partial epilepsies in children: report of two cases. *Epilepsia* 28: 351–355.
Fejerman N, Caraballo R, Tenembaum SN. (2000) Atypical evolutions of benign localization-related epilepsies in children: are they predictable? *Epilepsia* 41(4): 380–390.
Fenwick PBC. (1992) The relationship between mind, brain and seizures. *Epilepsia* 33 Suppl 6: S1–S6.
Ford FE. (1952) *Diseases of the Nervous System in Infancy, Childhood and Adolescence*, 3rd edition. Springfield, IL: Charles C. Thomas.
Frattali CM, Liow K, Craig GH, Korenman LM, Makhlouf F, Sato S, Biesecker LG, Theodore WH. (2001) Cognitive deficits in children with gelastic seizures and hypothalamic hamartoma. *Neurology* 57(1): 43–46.
Freeman JL, Coleman LT, Smith LJ, Shield LK. (2002) Hemiconvulsion-hemiplegia-epilepsy syndrome: characteristic early magnetic resonance imaging findings. *J Child Neurol* 17(1): 10–16.
Fröscher W, Vassella F. (1993) *Die Epilepsien, Grundlagen. Klinik, Behandlung*. Berlin: De Gruyter.
Gaily E, Appelqvist K, Kantola-Sorsa E, Liukkonen E, Kyyrönen P, Sarpola M, Huttunen H, Valanne L, Granström ML. (1999) Cognitive deficits after cryptogenic infantile spasms with benign seizure evolution. *Dev Med Child Neurol* 41: 660–664.
Gateaux-Mennecier J (1989) *Bourneville et l'enfance altérée. L'humanisation du déficient mental au XIXe siècle.* Paris: Edition Centurion.
Gayatri NA, Hughes MI, Clarke MA, Martland TR. (2002) Epilepsy with reversible bulbar dysfunction. *Dev Med Child Neurol* 44: 770–772.
Geschwind N. (1982) Disorders of attention: a frontier in neuropsychology. *Trans Roy Soc London* Ser B 298: 173–185.
Gillberg C, Coleman M. (2000) *The Biology of the Autistic Syndromes*, 3rd edition. Clinics in Developmental Medicine. London: Mac Keith Press.
Gillberg C, Schaumann H. (1983) Epilepsy presenting as infantile autism? Two case studies. *Neuropediatrics* 14: 206–212.
Gillberg C, Uvebrant P, Carlsson G, Heditorström A, Silfvenius H. (1996) Autism and epilepsy (and tuberous sclerosis?) in two pre-adolescent boys: neuropsychiatric aspects before and after epilepsy surgery. *J Intellect Disabil Res* 40: 75–81.
Gioia GA, Isquith PK, Guy SC, Kenworthy L. (1996) *Behavior Rating Inventory of Executive Function (BRIEF).* Odessa, FL: Psychological Assessment Resources.
Gleissner U, Sassen R, Lendt M, Clusmann H, Elger CE, Helmstaedter C. (2002) Pre- and postoperative verbal memory in pediatric patients with temporal lobe epilepsy. *Epilepsy Res* 51(3): 287–296.
Gloor P. (1986) Consciousness as a neurological concept in epileptology: a critical review. *Epilepsia* 27 Suppl 2: S14–S26.

Gloor P. (1991) Neurobiological substrates of ictal behavioral changes. In: Smith D, Treiman D, Trimble M, editors. *Advances in Neurology*: 55. New York: Raven Press, pp 1–34.
Gloor P, Olivier A, Quesney LF, Andermann F, Horowitz S. (1982) The role of the limbic system in experiential phenomena of temporal lobe epilepsy. *Ann Neurol* 12: 129–144.
Goldensohn ES, Gold AP. (1960) Prolonged behavioral disturbances as ictal phenomena. *Neurology* 10(1): 1–9.
Gordon K, Badwen H, Camfield P, Mann S, Orlik P. (1996) Valproic acid treatment of learning disorder and severely epileptiform EEG without clinical seizures. *J Child Neurol* 11: 41–43.
Gordon N. (1999) Episodic dyscontrol syndrome. *Dev Med Child Neurol* 41(11): 786–788.
Green JB. (1961) Association of behavior disorder with an electroencephalographic focus in children without seizures. *Neurology* 11: 337–344.
Grigonis AM, Murphy EH. (1994) The effects of epileptic cortical activity on the development of callosal projections. *Dev Brain Res* 77: 251–255.
Gross-Tsur V, Manor O, van der Meere J, Joseph A, Shalev RS. (1997) Epilepsy and attention deficit hyperactivity disorder: is methylphenidate safe and effective? *J Pediatr* 130(1): 40–44.
Grote CL, Van Slike P, Hoeppner JA. (1999) Language outcome following multiple subpial transection for Landau–Kleffner syndrome. *Brain* 122 Pt 3: 561–566.
Gucuyener K, Erdemoglu AK, Senol S, Serdaroglu A, Soysal S, Koch AI. (2003) Use of methylphenidate for attention-deficit hyperactivity disorder in patients with epilepsy or electroencephalographic abnormalities. *J Child Neurol* 18(2): 109–112.
Guerreiro MM, Andermann F, Andermann E, Palmini A, Hwang P, Hoffman HJ, Otsubo H, Bastos A, Dubeau F, Snipes GJ, Olivier A. (1998) Surgical treatment of epilepsy in tuberous sclerosis: strategies and results in 18 patients. *Neurology* 51(5): 1263–1269.
Guerrini R, Aicardi J. (2003) Epileptic encephalopathies with myoclonic seizures in infants and children (severe myoclonic epilepsy and myoclonic-astatic epilepsy). *J Clin Neurophysiol* 20(6): 449–461.
Guerrini R, Belmonte A, Genton P. (1998) Antiepileptic drug-induced worsening of seizures in children. *Epilepsia* 39 Suppl 3: S2–S10.
Gülgonen S, Demirbilek V, Korkmaz B, Dervent A, Townes BD. (2000) Neuropsychological functions in idiopathic occipital lobe epilepsy. *Epilepsia* 41(4): 405–411.
Gurrieri F, Battaglia A, Torrisi L, Tancredi R, Cavallaro C, Sangiorgi E, Neri G. (1999) Pervasive developmental disorder and epilepsy due to maternal derived duplication of 15q11–q13. *Neurology* 52(8): 1694–1697.
Guyatt G, Sackett D, Taylor DW, Chong J, Roberts A, Pugsley S. (1992) Determining optimal therapy. Randomized trials in individual patients. *New Engl J Med* 314: 889.
Guzzetta F, Crisafulli A, Isaya Crine M. (1993) Cognitive assessment of infants with West syndrome. How useful in diagnosis and prognosis? *Dev Med Child Neurol* 35: 379–387.
Guzzetta F, Frisone MF, Ricci D, Randò T, Guzzetta A. (2002) Development of visual attention in West syndrome. *Epilepsia* 43: 757–763.
Hahn A, Pistohl J, Neubauer BA, Stephani U. (2001) Atypical 'benign' partial epilepsy or pseudo-Lennox-syndrome – clinical symptomatology and long-term prognosis. *Neuropediatrics* 32(1): 9–13.
Harvey AS, Jayakar P, Duchowny M, Resnick T, Prats A, Altman N, Renfroc JB. (1996) Hemifacial seizures and cerebellar ganglioglioma: an epilepsy syndrome of infancy with seizures of cerebellar origin. *Ann Neurol* 40(1): 91–98.
Hashimoto T, Sasaki M, Sugai K, Hanakoa S, Fukumizu M, Kato T. (2001) Paroxysmal discharges on EEG in young autistic patients are frequent in frontal regions. *J Med Invest* 48: 175–180.
Heijbel J, Bohman M. (1975) Benign epilepsy of childhood with centrotemporal EEG foci: intelligence, behavior and school adjustement. *Epilepsia* 16: 679–687.
Heller T. (1930) Über dementia infantilis. *Zeitschrift für Kinderforschung* 37: 661–667.
Helmstaedter C, Kurthen M, Lux S, Reuber M, Elger CE. (2003) Chronic epilepsy and cognition: a longitudinal study in temporal lobe epilepsy. *Ann Neurol* 54(4): 425–432.
Hemmer SA, Pasternak JF, Zecker SG, Trommer BL. (2001) Stimulant therapy and seizure risk in children with ADHD. *Pediatr Neurol* 24(2): 99–102.
Henin N. (1980) Développement des praxies orofaciales chez l'enfant normal de 3 à 12 ans. Dissertation, Université de Marseille, France.
Hermann BP, Seidenberg M, Wyler AR, Davies KG, Foley KT, Dohan Jr FC. (1997) Memory outcome following anterior temporal lobectomy and its relationship to the neuropathological status of the mesial temporal lobe. In: Tuxhorn I, Holthausen H, Boenigk H, editors. *Paediatric Epilepsy Syndromes and their Surgical Treatment*. London: John Libbey, pp 291–310.

Hernandez MT, Sauerwein HC, Jambaqué I, de Guise E, Lussier F, Lortie A, Dulac O, Lassonde M. (2003) Attention, memory, and behavioral adjustment in children with frontal lobe epilepsy. *Epilepsy Behav* 4(5): 522–536.

Hershey T, Craft S, Glauser TA, Hale S. (1998) Short-term and long-term memory in early temporal lobe dysfunction. *Neuropsychology* 12(1): 52–64.

Hertz-Pannier L, Chiron C, Jambaqué I, Renaux-Kieffer V, van de Moortele PF, Delalande O, Fohlen M, Brunelle F, Le Bihan D. (2002) Late plasticity for language in a child's non-dominant hemisphere. *Brain* 125: 361–372.

Hill AE, Rosenbloom L. (1986) Disintegrative psychosis of childhood: teenage follow-up. *Dev Med Child Neurol* 28(1): 34–40.

Hirsch E, Marescaux C, Maquet P, Metz-Lutz MN, Kiesmann M, Salmon E, Frank G, Kurtz D. (1990) Landau–Kleffner syndrome: a clinical and EEG study of 5 cases. *Epilepsia* 31: 768–777.

Hobson JA, Pace-Schott EF. (2002) The cognitive neuroscience of sleep: neuronal systems, consciousness and learning. *Neuroscience* 3(9): 679–693.

Hobson P. (1995) *Autism and the Development of Mind.* Hove: Lawrence Erlbaum.

Holmes GL. (1997) Epilepsy in the developing brain: lessons from the laboratory and clinic. *Epilepsia* 38: 12–30.

Holmes GL, Ben-Ari Y. (2001) The neurobiology and consequences of epilepsy in the developing brain. *Pediatr Res* 49: 320–325.

Holtmann M, Becker K, Kentner-Figura B, Schmidt MH. (2003) Increased frequency of rolandic spikes in ADHD children. *Epilepsia* 44(9): 1241–1244.

Hommet C, Billard C, Barthez MA, Gillet P, Perrier D, Lucas B, de Toffol B, Autret A. (2000) Continuous spikes and waves during slow sleep (CSWS): outcome in adulthood. *Epileptic Disord* 2(2): 107–112.

Hoon AH, Reiss AL. (1992) The mesial-temporal lobe and autism: case report and review. *Dev Med Child Neurol* 34: 252–259.

Huttenlocher PR, Hapke RJ. (1990) A follow-up study of intractable seizures in childhood. *Ann Neurol* 28(5): 699–705.

ICD-10 (1992) *Classification of Mental and Behavioral Disorders: Clinical Descriptions and Guidelines.* Geneva: WHO.

Illingworth RS. (1955) Sudden mental deterioration with convulsions in infancy. *Arch Dis Child* 30: 529–537.

Inoue Y, Fujiwara T, Matsuda K, Kubota H, Tanaka M, Yagi K, Yamamori K, Takahashi Y. (1997) Ring chromosome 20 and nonconvulsive status epilepticus. A new epileptic syndrome. *Brain* 120: 939–953.

Irwin K, Birch V, Lees J, Polkey C, Alarcon G, Binnie C, Smedley M, Baird G, Robinson RO. (2001) Multiple subpial transection in Landau–Kleffner syndrome. *Dev Med Child Neurol* 43: 248–252.

Jacobs R, Anderson V, Harvey AS. (2001) Neuropsychological profile of a 9-year-old child with subcortical band heterotopia or 'double cortex'. *Dev Med Child Neurol* 43: 628–633.

Jambaqué I, Dulac O. (1989) Syndrome frontal réversible et épilepsie chez un enfant de 8 ans. *Arch Fr Pediatr* 46: 525–529.

Jambaqué I, Dellatolas G, Dulac O, Ponsot G, Signoret JL. (1993a) Verbal and visual memory impairment in children with epilepsy. *Neuropsychologia* 31(12): 1321–1337.

Jambaqué I, Chiron C, Dulac O, Raynaud C, Syrota P. (1993b) Visual inattention in West syndrome: a neuropsychological and neurofunctional imaging study. *Epilepsia* 34: 692–700.

Jambaqué I, Chiron C, Kaminska A, Plouin P, Dulac O. (1998) Transient motor aphasia and recurrent partial seizures in a child: language upon seizure control. *J Child Neurol* 13(6): 296–300.

Jambaqué I, Mottron L, Chiron C. (2001) Neuropsychological outcome in children with West syndrome: a 'human model' for autism. In: Jambaqué I, Lassonde M, Dulac O, editors. *Neuropsychology of Childhood Epilepsy*. New York: Kluwer Academic/Plenum Press, pp 175–184.

Kallay C. (2005) Reversible frontal syndrome after hemispherectomy in a child with congenital hemiplegia and epilepsy with CSWS, due to a prenatal middle central artery infarction. Dissertation, Faculty of Medicine, University of Lausanne, Switzerland. In preparation.

Kanner AM. (2000) Commentary: the treatment of seizure disorders and EEG abnormalities in children with autistic spectrum disorders: are we getting ahead of ourselves? *J Autism Dev Disord* 30(5): 491–495.

Karmiloff-Smith A, Thomas M. (2003) What can developmental disorders tell us about the neurocomputational constraints that shape development? The case of the Williams syndrome. *Dev Psychopathol* 15(4): 969–990.

Kasteleijn-Nolst Trenité DGA, Smith AM, Velis DN, Van Emde Boas W. (1990a) On-line detection of transient neuropsychological disturbances during EEG discharges in children with epilepsy. *Dev Med Child Neurol* 32: 46–50.

Kasteleijn-Nolst Trenité DGA, Siebelink BM, Berends SCG, Van Strien JW, Meinardi H. (1990b) Lateralized effects of subclinical epileptiform EEG discharges on scholastic performance in children. *Epilepsia* 31(6): 740–745.

Kasteleijn-Nolst Trenité DGA, de Saint-Martin A. (2004) Cognitive aspects. In: Wallace SJ, Farrel K, editors. *Epilepsy in Children*, 2nd edn. London: Arnold, pp 433–446.

Kaufman AS, Kaufman NL. (1993) *K-ABC: Batterie pour l'examen psychologique de l'enfant.* Paris: Editions du Centre de Psychologie Appliquée.

Kelemen A, Halasz P, Barsi P, Sarac J, Gyorsok Z, Szücs A. (2003) Mediodorsal perinatal thalamic lesion and electrical status epilepticus in slow wave sleep – report of 2 cases. *Eur J Paediatr Neurol* 7(5): 328.

Kiper DC, Zesiger P, Maeder P, Deonna T, Innocenti GM. (2002) Vision after early-onset lesions of the occipital cortex: I. Neuropsychological and psychophysical studies. *Neural Plast* 9(1): 1–25.

Klepper J. (2004) Impaired glucose transport into the brain: the expanding spectrum of glucose transporter type 1 deficiency syndrome. *Curr Opin Neurol* 17(2): 193–196.

Knyaseva MG, Maeder P, Kiper DC, Deonna T, Innocenti GM. (2002) Vision after early-onset lesions of the occipital cortex: II. Physiological studies. *Neural Plast* 9(1): 27–40.

Kokkonen J, Kokkonen ER, Saukkonen AL, Pennanen P. (1997) Psychological outcome of young adults with epilepsy in childhood. *J Neurol Neurosurg Psychiatry* 62: 265–268.

Koo B, Hwang P. (1996) Localization of focal cortical lesions influences age of onset of infantile spasms. *Epilepsia* 37(11): 1068–1071.

Korkman M, Granström ML, Appelqvist K, Liukkonen E. (1998) Neuropsychological characteristics of five children with the Landau–Kleffner syndrome: dissociation of auditory and phonological discrimination. *J Int Neuropsychol Soc* 4: 566–575.

Kramer U, Ben-Zeev B, Harel S, Kivity S. (2001) Transient oromotor deficits in children with benign childhood epilepsy with central temporal spikes. *Epilepsia* 42(5): 616–620.

Kurita H. (1985) Infantile autism with speech loss before the age of thirty months. *J Am Acad Child Psychiatry* 24: 191–196.

Kuzniecky R, Guthrie B, Mountz J, Bebin M, Faught E, Gillam F, Liu HG. (1997) Intrinsic epileptogenesis of hypothalamic hamartomas in gelastic epilepsy. *Ann Neurol* 42: 60–67.

Kyllerman M, Nyden A, Prauin N, Rasmussen P, Wetterquist AK, Heditorström A. (1996) Transient psychosis in a girl with epilepsy and continuous spikes and waves during slow sleep (CSWS). *Eur Child Adolesc Psychiatry* 5(4): 216–221.

Laan LA, Renier WO, Aarts WF, Buntinx IM, Burgt IJ, Stroink H, Beuten J, Zwinderman KH, van Dijk JG, Brouwer OF. (1997) Evolution of epilepsy and EEG findings in Angelman syndrome. *Epilepsia* 38(2): 195–199.

Lagae LG, Silberstein J, Gillis PL, Casaer PJ. (1998) Successful use of intravenous immunoglobulins in Landau–Kleffner syndrome. *Pediatr Neurol* 18(2): 165–168.

Landau WM, Kleffner FR. (1957) Syndrome of acquired aphasia with convulsive disorder in children. *Neurology* 7: 523–530.

Landau WM, Kleffner FR. (2001) Syndrome of acquired aphasia with convulsive disorder in children 1956. *Neurology* 57(11) Suppl 4: S29–S36.

Laporte N, Sebire G, Gillerot Y, Guerrini R, Ghariani S. (2002) Cognitive epilepsy: ADHD related to focal EEG discharges. *Pediatr Neurol* 27(4): 307–311.

Lelord G, Barthelemy C. (1989) *Echelle d'évaluation des comportements autistiques ECA*. Paris: Editions EAP.

Lenard HG. (1999) Dacrystic seizures reconsidered. *Neuropediatrics* 30(2): 107–108.

Lendt H, Helmstaedter C, Elger CE. (1999) Pre- and postoperative neuropsychological profiles in children and adolescents with temporal lobe epilepsy. *Epilepsia* 40(11): 1543–1550.

Lendt M, Helmstaedter C, Kuczaty S, Schramm J, Elge CE. (2000) Behavioural disorders in children with epilepsy: early improvement after surgery. *J Neurol Neurosurg Psychiatry* 69(6): 739–744.

Lennox WG. (1960) *Epilepsy and Related Disorders*. Boston, MA: Little, Brown & Co.

Le Normand MT, Cohen H. (1997) L'acquisition du langage chez l'enfant épileptique: retard de compréhension et déficit de production. In: Lambert J, Nespoulous, JL, editors. *Perception auditive et compréhension du langage*. Marseille: Solal.

Lerman P. (1977) The concept of preventive rehabilitation in childhood epilepsy: a plea against over protection and over indulgence. In: *Epilepsy, the Eighth International Symposium.* New York: Raven Press, pp 265–268.

Lesser R, Gordon B, Uematsu S. (1994) Electrical stimulation and language. Review. *J Clin Neurophysiol* 11(2): 191–204.

Levine B, Duchowny M. (1991) Childhood obsessive-compulsive disorder and cingulate epilepsy. *Biol Psychiatry* 30: 1049–1055.

Lewine JD, Andrews R, Chez M, Patil AA, Devinsky O, Smith M, Kanner A, Davis JT, Funke M, Jones G, Chong B, Provencal S. Weisend M, Lee RR, Orrison Jr WW. (1999) Magnetoencephalographic patterns of epileptiform activity in children with regressive autism spectrum disorders. *Pediatrics* 104(3) Pt 1: 405–418.

Lindsay J, Ounsted C, Richards P. (1979) Long-term outcome in children with temporal lobe seizures III: Psychiatric aspects in childhood and adult life. *Dev Med Child Neurol* 21(5): 630–636.

Lindsay J, Ounsted C, Richards P. (1980) Long-term outcome in children with temporal lobe seizures IV: Genetic factors, febrile convulsions and the remission of seizures. *Dev Med Child Neurol* 22(4): 429–439.

Loiseau P, Cohadon F, Mortureux Y. (1967) A propos d'une forme singulière d'épilepsie de l'enfant. *Rev Neurol* 116(3): 244–248.

Loiseau P, Pestre M, Dartigues JF, Commenges D, Berbeyer-Gateau C, Cohadon S. (1983) Long-term prognosis in two forms of childhood epilepsy: typical absence seizures and epilepsy with rolandic (centrotemporal) EEG foci. *Ann Neurol* 13: 642–648.

Lowe M, Costello AJ. (1982) *The Manual for the Symbolic Play Test.* Berkshire: NFER-Nelson.

Luscher C, Nicoll RA, Maleuka RC, Muller D. (2000) Synoptic plasticity and dynamic modulation of the postsynaptic membrane. *Nat Neurosci* 3(6): 545–546.

Mabbott DJ, Smith ML. (2003) Memory in children with temporal or extra-temporal excisions. *Neuropsychologia* 41: 995–1007.

Maccario M, Hefferen SJ, Keblusek SJ, Lipinski KA. (1982) Developmental dysphasia and electroencephalographic abnormalities. *Dev Med Child Neurol* 24(2): 141–155.

Majerus S, Laureys S, Collette F, Del Fiore G, Degueldre C, Luxen A, Van der Linden M, Maquet P, Metz-Lutz MN. (2003) Phonological short-term memory networks following recovery from Landau–Kleffner syndrome. *Hum Brain Mapp* 19(3): 133–144.

Manford M, Cvejic H, Minde K, Andermann F, Taylor L, Savard G. (1998) Case study: neurological brain waves causing serious behavioral brainstorms. *J Am Acad Child Adolesc Psychiatry* 37(10): 1085–1090.

Manning DJ, Rosenbloom L. (1987) Non-convulsive status epilepticus. *Arch Dis Child* 62: 37–40.

Mantovani JF. (2000) Autisic regression and Landau–Kleffner syndrome: progress or confusion? *Dev Med Child Neurol* 42(5): 349–353.

Mantovani JF, Landau WM. (1980) Acquired aphasia with convulsive disorder: course and prognosis. *Neurology* 30: 524–529.

Maquet P, Hirsch E, Metz-Lutz MN, Motte J, Dive D, Marescaux C, Franck G. (1995) Regional cerebral glucose metabolism in children with deterioration of one or more cognitive functions and continuous spike-and-wave discharges during sleep. *Brain* 118: 1497–1520.

Marescaux C, Hirsch E, Finck S. (1990) Landau–Kleffner syndrome: a pharmacological study of 5 cases. *Epilepsia* 31: 768–777.

Marston D, Besag F, Binnie CD, Fowler M. (1993) Effects of transitory cognitive impairment on psychosocial functioning of children. *Dev Med Child Neurol* 35(7): 574–581.

Massa R, de Saint-Martin A, Carcangiu R, Rudolf G, Seegmuller C, Kleitz C, Metz-Lutz MN, Hirsch E, Marescaux C. (2001) EEG criteria predictive of complicated evolution in idiopathic rolandic epilepsy. *Neurology* 57(6): 1071–1079.

Mathern GW. (1997) Hippocampal pathology in children with severe epilepsy. In: Tuxhorn I, Holthausen H, Boenigk H, editors. *Paediatric Epilepsy Syndromes and their Surgical Treatment.* London: John Libbey, pp 236–241.

Matsuoka H, Okuma T, Ueno T, Saito H. (1986) Impairment of parietal cortical functions associated with episodic prolonged spike-and-wave discharges. *Epilepsia* 27(4): 432–436.

Matsuoka H, Takahashi T, Sasaki M, Matsumoto K, Yoshida S, Numachi Y, Saito H, Ueno T, Sato M. (2000) Neuropsychological EEG activation in patients with epilepsy. *Brain* 123 Pt 2: 318–330.

Matthews WS, Barabas G, Ferrari M. (1982) Emotional concomitants of childhood epilepsy. *Epilepsia* 23: 671–681.

Mayor C, Zesiger P, Roulet-Perez E, Maeder-Ingvar M, Deonna T. (2003) Acquired epileptic dysgraphia: a longitudinal study. *Dev Med Child Neurol* 45: 807–812.
Mayor-Dubois C, Gianella D, Chaves-Vischer V, Haenggeli CA, Deonna T, Roulet-Perez E. (2004) Speech delay due to a prelinguistic regression of epileptic origin. *Neuropediatrics* 35: 50–53.
Menkes JH. (1985) *Textbook of Child Neurology*, 3rd edition. Philadelphia and London: Lea and Febiger.
Menkes JH. (1990) *Textbook of Child Neurology*, 4th edition. Philadelphia and London: Lea and Febiger.
Metz-Lutz MN, Kleitz C, De Saint-Martin A, Massa R, Hirsch E, Marescaux C. (1999) Cognitive development in benign focal epilepsies of childhood. *Dev Neurosci* 21(3–5): 182–190.
Metz-Lutz MN, Maquet P, de Saint-Martin A, Rudolf G, Wioland N, Hirsch E, Marescaux C. (2001) Pathophysiological aspects of Landau–Kleffner syndrome: from the active epileptic phase to recovery. *Int Rev Neurobiol* 45: 505–526.
Mintzer S, Lopez F. (2002) Comorbidity of ictal fear and panic disorder. *Epilepsy Behav* 3(4): 330–337.
Mitchell WG, Chavez JM, Lee H, Guzman BL. (1991) Academic underachievement in children with epilepsy. *J Child Neurol* 6: 65–72.
Mitchell WG, Scheier LM, Baker SA. (1994) Psychosocial, behavioral and medical outcomes in children with epilepsy: a developmental risk factor model using longitudinal data. *Pediatrics* 94: 471–477.
Monteiro JP, Roulet-Perez E, Davidoff V, Deonna T. (2001) Primary neonatal thalamic haemorrhage and epilepsy with continuous spike-wave during sleep: a longitudinal follow-up of a possible significant relation. *Eur J Paediatr Neurol* 5: 41–47.
Morrell F, Whisler WW, Smith MC, Hoeppner TJ, de Toledo-Morrell L, Pierre-Louis SJC, Kanner AM, Buelow JM, Ristanovic R, Bergen D, Chez M, Hasegawa H. (1995) Landau–Kleffner syndrome: treatment with subpial intracortical transection. *Brain* 118: 1529–1546.
Mouridsen SE, Rich B, Isager T. (1999) Epilepsy in disintegrative disorder and infantile autism: a long-term validation study. *Dev Med Child Neurol* 41(2): 110–114.
Nass R, Devinsky O. (1999) Autistic regression with rolandic spikes. *Neuropsychiatr Neuropsychol Behav Neurol* 12(3): 193–197.
Nass R, Gross A, Devinsky O. (1998) Autism and autistic epileptiform regression with occipital spikes. *Dev Med Child Neurol* 40: 453–458.
Nass R, Gross A, Wisoff J, Devinsky O. (1999) Outcome of multiple subpial transections for autistic epileptiform regression. *Pediatr Neurol* 21(1): 464–470.
Nehlig A, Motte J, Moshé SL, Plouin P, editors. (1999) *Childhood Epilepsies and Brain Development*. London: John Libbey.
Neville BGR, Nicol HG, Barss A, Forster KL, Garrett MF. (1991) Syntactically based sentence processing classes: evidence from event-related brain potentials. *J Cognitive Neurosci* 3: 151–163.
Neville BGR, Harkness WFJ, Cross JH, Cass HC, Burch VC, Lees JA, Taylor DC. (1997) Surgical treatment of severe autistic regression in childhood epilepsy. *Pediatr Neurol* 16: 137–140.
Neville BGR, Burch V, Cass H, Lees J. (2000) Behavioural aspects of Landau–Kleffner syndrome. *Clin Dev Med* 149: 56–63.
Neville BGR, Spratt HC, Birtwistle J. (2001) Early onset epileptic auditory and visual agnosia with spontaneous recovery associated with Tourette's syndrome. *J Neurol Neurosurg Psychiatry* 71(4): 560–561.
Niedermeyer E, Naidu SB. (1990) Further EEG observations with the Rett syndrome. *Brain Dev* 12(1): 53–54.
O'Donohue NV. (1981) *Epilepsies of Childhood*, 2nd edition. London: Butterworths.
Oguni H, Hayashi K, Osawa M. (1996) Long-term prognosis of Lennox–Gastaut syndrome. *Epilepsia* 37 Suppl 3: S44–S47.
Ojeman GO. (1983) Brain organization for language from the perspective of electrical stimulation mapping. *Behav Brain Sci* 6: 189–230.
Olsson I, Steffenburg S, Gillberg C. (1988) Epilepsy in autism and autisticlike conditions. A population-based study. *Arch Neurol* 45: 666–668.
O'Regan ME, Brown JK, Goodwin GM, Clarke M. (1998) Epileptic aphasia: a consequence of regional hypometabolic encephalopathy. *Dev Med Child Neurol* 40: 508–516.
Otsubo H, Chitoku S, Ochi A, Jay V, Rutka JT, Smith ML, Elliott IM, Snead OC. (2001) Malignant rolandic-sylvian epilepsy in children. Diagnosis, treatment, and outcomes. *Neurology* 57: 590–596.
Ounsted C. (1964) Some relationships between bio-electric paroxysms and performance in epileptic children. *Proc Roy Soc Med* 57: 1177–1178.
Ounsted C. (1969) Aggression and epilepsy rage in children with temporal lobe epilepsy. *J Psychosom Res* 13(3): 237–242.

Ouvrier RA, Goldsmith RF, Ouvrier S, Williams IC. (1993) The value of the Mini Mental State examination in childhood: a preliminary study. *J Child Neurol* 8: 145–148.
Ouvrier R, Hendy J, Bornohlt L, Black FH. (1999) SYSTEMS: school years screening test for the evaluation of mental status. *J Child Neurol* 14: 772–780.
Oxbury S, Oxbury J, Renowden S, Squier W, Carpenter K. (1997) Severe amnesia: an unusual late complication after temporal lobectomy. *Neuropsychologia* 35(7): 975–988.
Paetau R. (1994) Sounds trigger spikes in the Landau–Kleffner syndrome. *J Clin Neurophysiol* 11(2): 231–234.
Palmini A, Andermann F, Dubeau F, Gloor P, Olivier A, Quesney LF, Salanova V. (1992) Pure amnesic seizures in temporal lobe epilepsy. Definition, clinical symptomatology and functional anatomical considerations. *Brain* 115: 749–769.
Pan A, Luders HO. (2000) Epileptiform discharges in benign focal epilepsy of childhood. *Epileptic Disord* 2 Suppl 1: S29–S36.
Panayotopoulos CP. (1999) *Benign Childhood Partial Seizures and Related Epileptic Syndromes.* London: John Libbey.
Parkinson GM. (2002) High incidence of language disorder in children with focal epilepsies. *Dev Med Child Neurol* 44: 533–537.
Parry-Fielder B, Nolan TM, Collins KJ, Stojcevski Z. (1997) Developmental language disorders and epilepsy. *J Paediatr Child Health* 33(4): 277–280.
Patry G, Lyagoubi S, Tassinari A. (1971) Subclinical 'electrical status epilepticus' induced by sleep in children. *Arch Neurol* 24: 242–252.
Pavao Martins I, Lobo Antunes N, Levy Gomes A. (1993) Acquired visual agnosia in a child: a neuropsychological study. *Approche Neuropsychologique des Apprentissages chez l'Enfant* 5: 70–75.
Pavone P, Bianchini R, Trifiletti RR, Incorpora G, Pavone A, Parano E. (2001) Neuropsychological assessment in children with absence epilepsy. *Neurology* 56: 1047–1051.
Pellock JM, Dodson WE, Bourgeois BF. (2001) *Pediatric Epilepsy*, 2nd edition. New York: Demos Medical Publishing Inc.
Penfield W, Jasper H. (1954) *Epilepsy and the Functional Anatomy of the Human Brain.* Boston, MA: Little, Brown, pp 515–520.
Perez-Jimenez A, Villarejo FJ, Fournier del Castillo MC, Garcia-Perez JJ, Carreno M. (2003) Continuous giggling and autistic disorder associated with hypothalamic hamartoma. *Epileptic Disord* 5(1): 31–37.
Perucca E, Gram L, Avanzini G, Dulac O. (1998) Antiepileptic drugs as a cause of worsening seizures. *Epilepsia* 39: 5–17.
Picard A, Cheliout Heraut F, Bouskraoui M, Lacert P. (1998) Sleep EEG and developmental dysphasia. *Dev Med Child Neurol* 40(9): 595–599.
Piccirilli M, D'Alessandro P, Tiacci C, Ferroni A. (1988) Language lateralization in children with benign partial epilepsy. *Epilepsia* 29(1): 19–25.
Piccirilli M, D'Alessandro P, Sciarma T, Cantoni C, Dioguardi MS, Giulietti M, Ibba A, Tiacci C. (1994) Attention problems in epilepsy: possible significance of the epileptogenic focus. *Epilepsia* 35: 1091–1096.
Pineau-Valencienne V. (2000) *Une cicatrice dans la tête. Un témoignage sur l'épilepsie.* Paris: Plon.
Plioplys AV. (1994) Autism: electroencephalogram abnormalities and clinical improvement with valproic acid. *Arch Pediatr Adolesc Med* 148: 220–222.
Poblano A, Ibarra J, Muniz A, Garza S. (2001) Absence seizures effects on reading revealed by video-electroencephalography. *Rev Invest Clin* 53(2): 136–140.
Posner MI. (1994) Attention: the mechanisms of consciousness. *Proc Natl Acad Sci USA* 91(16): 7398–7403.
Praline J, Hommet C, Barthez MA, Brault F, Perrier D, Passage GD, Lucas B, Bonnard J, Billard C, Toffol BD, Autret A. (2003) Outcome at adulthood of the continuous spike-waves during sleep and Landau–Kleffner syndromes. *Epilepsia* 44(11): 1434–1440.
Prats JM, Garaizar C, Garcia-Nieto ML, Madoz P. (1998) Antiepileptic drugs and atypical evolution of idiopathic partial epilepsy. *Pediatr Neurol* 18(5): 402–406.
Prats JM, Garaizar C, Garcia-Nieto ML, Madoz P. (1999) Opercular epileptic syndrome: an unusual form of benign partial epilepsy in childhood. *Rev Neurol* 29(4): 375–380.
Pressler RM. (1997) *Entwicklung eines computerisierten EEG-getriggerten Testsystem zur Erkennung kognitiver Leistungsstörungen während subklinischen epileptiformen Enladungen im Kindesalter.* Munich: These.

Pressler RM, Brandl U. (1995) Transitory cognitive impairment during very brief subclinical EEG discharges in children. *Epilepsia* 36 Suppl 3: A93. (Abstract.)

Putnam (1941) Dullness as an epileptic equivalent. *Arch Neuro Psychiatr* 45: 797.

Rapin I. (1965) Dementia infantilis (Heller's disease). In: Carter CH, editor. *Medical Aspects of Mental Retardation*. Springfield, IL: CC Thomas, pp 760–767.

Rapin I. (1982) *Children with Brain Dysfunction. Neurology, Cognition, Language, and Behavior.* New York: Raven Press.

Rapin I. (1991) Autistic children: diagnosis and clinical features. *Pediatrics* 87: 751–760.

Rapin I. (1995) Autistic regression and disintegrative disorder: how important is the role of epilepsy? Review. *Semin Pediatr Neurol* 2: 278–285.

Rapin I, Allen DA. (1988) Syndromes in developmental and adult aphasia. *Res Publ Assoc Res Nerv Ment Dis* 66: 57–75.

Rapin I, Dunn M. (2003) Update on the language disorders of individuals on the autistic spectrum. *Brain Dev* 25: 166–172.

Rapin I, Mattis S, Rowan AJ, Golden GG. (1977) Verbal auditory agnosia in children. *Dev Med Child Neurol* 19: 192–207.

Rating D, Wolf C, Bast T. (2000) Sulthiame as monotherapy in children with benign childhood epilepsy with centrotemporal spikes: a 6-month randomized, double-blind, placebo-controlled study. Sulthiame study group. *Epilepsia* 41(10): 1284–1288.

Regard M, Cook ND, Wieser HG, Landis T. (1994) The dynamics of cerebral dominance during unilateral limbic seizures. *Brain* 117: 91.

Rey A. (1959) *Test de copie d'une figure complexe.* Paris: Editions du Centre de Psychologie Appliquée.

Richer LP, Shevell MI, Rosenblatt BR. (2002) Epileptiform abnormalities in children with attention-deficit-hyperactivity disorder. *Pediatr Neurol* 26(2): 125–129.

Riva D, Pantaleoni C, Milani N, Giorgi C. (1993) Hemispheric specialization in children with unilateral epileptic focus, with and without computed tomography-demonstrated lesion. *Epilepsia* 34(1): 69–73.

Robinson RJ. (1991) Causes and associations of severe and persistent specific speech and language disorders in children. *Dev Med Child Neurol* 9: 943–962.

Robinson RO, Baird G, Robinson G, Simonoff E. (2001) Landau–Kleffner syndrome: course and correlates with outcome. *Dev Med Child Neurol* 43: 243–247.

Ronen GM, Richards JE, Cunningham C, Secord M, Rosenbloom D. (2000) Can sodium valproate improve learning in children with epileptiform bursts but without clinical seizures? *Dev Med Child Neurol* 42: 751–755.

Rosenbaum DH, Siegel M, Barr WB, Rowan AJ. (1986) Epileptic aphasia. *Neurology* 36: 822–825.

Rosenblatt B, Vernet O, Montes JL, Andermann F, Schwartz S, Taylor LB, Villemure JG, Farmet JP. (1998) Continuous unilateral epileptiform discharge and language delay: effect of functional hemispherectomy on language acquisition. *Epilepsia* 39(7): 787–792.

Rossi PG, Parmeggiani A, Posar A, Scaduto MC, Chiodo S, Vatti G. (1999) Landau–Kleffner syndrome (LKS): long-term follow-up and links with electrical status epilepticus during sleep (ESES). *Brain Dev* 21: 90–98.

Roubertie A, Petit J, Genton P. (2000) Ring chromosome 20: an identifiable epileptic syndrome. *Rev Neurol* (Paris) 156(2): 149–153.

Roubertie A, Humbertclaude V, Rivier F, Cheminal R, Echenne B. (2003) Interictal paroxysmal epileptic discharges during sleep in childhood: phenotypic variability in a family. *Epilepsia* 44(6): 864–869.

Roulet E, Deonna T, Despland PA. (1989) Prolonged intermittent drooling and oromotor dyspraxia in benign childhood epilepsy with centrotemporal spikes. *Epilepsia* 30(5): 564–568.

Roulet E, Deonna T, Gaillard F. Peter-Favre C, Despland PA. (1991) Acquired aphasia, dementia and behavior disorder with epilepsy and continuous spike and waves during sleep in a child. *Epilepsia* 32(4): 495–503.

Roulet-Perez E. (1995) Syndromes of acquired apileptic aphasia and epilepsy with continuous spike-wave discharges during sleep. Model of prolonged cognitive impairment of epileptic origin. *Semin Pediatr Neurol* 2: 269–277.

Roulet-Perez E, Davidoff V, Despland PA, Deonna T. (1993) Mental and behavioural deterioration of children with epilepsy and CSWS: acquired epileptic frontal syndrome. *Dev Med Child Neurol* 35: 661–674.

Roulet-Perez E, Seek M, Mayer E, Despland PA, De Tribolet N, Deonna T. (1998) Childhood epilepsy with neuropsychological regression and continuous spike waves during sleep: epilepsy surgery in a young adult. *Eur J Paediatr Neurol* 2: 303–311.

Roulet-Perez E, Maeder P, Villemure KM, Chaves Vischer V, Villemure JG. (2000) Acquired hippocampal damage after temporal lobe seizures in 2 infants. *Ann Neurol* 48: 384–387.

Roulet-Perez E, Davidoff V, Prélaz AC, Morel B, Rickli F, Metz-Lutz MN, Boyes Braem P, Deonna T. (2001) Sign language in childhood epileptic aphasia (Landau–Kleffner syndrome). *Dev Med Child Neurol* 43(11): 739–744.

Roulet-Perez E, Mayor C, Davidoff V, Seek M, Maeder-Ingvar M, Gubser-Mercati D, Haenggeli CA, Villemure JG, Deonna T. (2003) Dynamics of development before and after early epilepsy surgery: sorting out the direct effects of epilepsy. *Eur J Paediatr Neurol* 7(5): 345–346. (Abstract.)

Rousselle C, Revol M. (1995) Relations between cognitive functions and continuous spikes and waves during slow sleep. In: Beaumanoir A, Bureau M, Deonna T, Mira L, Tassinari CA, editors. *Continuous Spikes and Waves during Slow Sleep. Electrical Status Epilepticus during Slow Sleep.* Mariani Foundation Neurology Series: 3. London: John Libbey.

Rutter M. (1981) Psychological sequelae of brain damage in children. *Am J Psychiatry* 138(12): 1533–1544.

Sato S, Dreifuss SE, Penry JK, Kirby DD, Palesch Y. (1983) Long-term follow-up of absence seizures. *Neurology* 33: 1590–1595.

Sauvage D. (1988) *Autisme du nourrisson et du jeune enfant (0–3 ans). Signes précoces et diagnostic.* Paris: Masson Ed.

Scheffer IE, Berkovic SF. (1997) Generalized epilepsy with febrile seizures plus. A genetic disorder with heterogeneous clinical phenotypes. *Brain* 120: 479–490.

Scheffer IE, Jones L, Pozzebon M, Howel A, Saling M, Berkoovic SF. (1995) Autosomal dominant rolandic epilepsy and speech dyspraxia: a new syndrome with anticipation. *Ann Neurol* 38: 633–664.

Schinzel A, Niedrist D. (2001) Chromosome imbalance associated with epilepsy. *Am J Med Genet* 106(2): 119–124.

Schopler E, Reichler RJ. (1985) *The Childhood Autism Rating Scale (CARS*). New York: Irvington.

Schouten A. (2000) Set-shifting in healthy children with idiopathic or cryptogenic epilepsy. *Dev Med Child Neurol* 42(6): 392–397.

Schouten A, Oostrom K, Jennekens-Schinkel A, Peters ACB. (2001) School career of children is at risk before diagnosis of epilepsy only. *Dev Med Child Neurol* 43: 575–576.

Schouten A, Oostrom KJ, Pestman WR, Peters AC, Jennekens-Schinkel A. (2002) Dutch study group of epilepsy in childhood. Learning and memory of school children with epilepsy: a prospective controlled longitudinal study. *Dev Med Child Neurol* 44(12): 803–811.

Schwartzkroin PA, Moshé SL, Noebels JL, Swan JW, editors. (1995) *Brain Development and Epilepsy.* New York and Oxford: Oxford University Press.

Seibert JM, Hogan AE, Mundy PC. (1982) Assessing interactional competencies: the early social-communication scale. *Inf Mental Hlth J* 3: 244–258.

Seidenberg M, Berent S. (1992) Childhood epilepsy and the role of psychology. *Am Psychol* 47(9): 1130–1133.

Seidenberg M, Beck N, Geisser M, Giordani B, Sackellares JC, Berent S, Dreifuss FE, Boll TJ. (1986) Academic achievement of children with epilepsy. *Epilepsia* 27: 753–759.

Seri S, Cerquiglini A, Pisani F. (1998) Spike-induced interference in auditory sensory processing in Landau–Kleffner syndrome. *Electroencephalogr Clin Neurophysiol* 108(5): 506–510.

Shafrir Y, Prensky AL. (1995) Acquired epileptiform opercular syndrome: a second case report, review of the literature, and comparison to the Landau–Kleffner syndrome. *Epilepsia* 36(10): 1050–1057.

Shewmon DA, Erwin RJ. (1988) Focal spike-induced cerebral dysfunction is related to the after-coming slow wave. *Ann Neurol* 23: 131–137.

Shewmon DA, Erwin RJ. (1989) Transient visual impairment of visual perception induced by simple interictal occipital spikes. *J Clin Exp Neuropsychol* 4(5): 675–691.

Shinnar S, Rapin I, Tuchman RF, Shulman L, Ballaban-Gilk, Maw M, Deuel RK, Volkmar FR. (2001) Language regression in childhood. *Pediatr Neurol* 24(3): 183–189.

Sidenvall R, Forsgren L, Heijbel J. (1996) Prevalence and characteristics of epilepsy in children in northern Sweden. *Seizure* 5(2): 139–146.

Signoret JL. (1991) *Batterie d'efficience mnésique (BEM 144).* Paris: Elsevier.

Sillanpää M. (1992) Epilepsy in children: prevalence, disability, and handicap. *Epilepsia* 33(3): 444–449.

Sillanpää M. (2000) Long-term outcome of epilepsy. *Epileptic Disord* 2(2): 79–88.

Sillanpää M, Jalava M, Kaleva O, Shinnar S. (1998) Long-term prognosis of seizures with onset in childhood. *New Engl J Med* 338: 1715–1722.

Sisodiya SM, Free SL, Stevens JM, Fish DR, Shorvon SD. (1995) Widespread cerebral structural changes in patients with cortical dysgenesis and epilepsy. *Brain* 118: 1039–1050.
Sjenowski TJ, Destexhe A. (2000) Why do we sleep? *Brain Res* 866(1–2): 208–223.
Smith ML, Vriezen ER. (1997) Everyday memory in children with epilepsy. *Epilepsia* 38 Suppl 8: 165. (Abstract.)
Snyder PJ. (1997) Epilepsy as a natural laboratory for the study of human memory. *Brain Cognition* 35(1): 1–4.
Solomon GE, Carson D, Pavlakis S, Fraser R, Labar D. (1993) Intracranial EEG monitoring in Landau–Kleffner associated with left temporal astrocytoma. *Epilepsia* 94(3): 557–560.
Soulayrol R. (1999) *L'enfant foudroyé. Comprendre l'enfant épileptique*. Paris: Editions Odile Jacob.
Staden UE, Isaacs E, Boyd SG, Brandl U, Neville BGR. (1998) Language dysfunction in children with rolandic epilepsy. *Neuropediatrics* 29: 242–248.
Stefanatos GA, Grover W, Geller E. (1995) Case study: Corticosteroid treatment of language regression in pervasive developmental disorder. *J Am Acad Child Adolesc Psychiatry* 34: 1107–1111.
Steriade M, Contreras D. (1998) Spike-wave complexes and fast components of cortically generated seizures. I. Role of neocortex and thalamus. *J Neurophysiol* 80: 1439–1455.
Stiles J. (2000) Neural plasticity and cognitive development. *Dev Neuropsychol* 18(2): 237–272.
Stores G. (2001) *Sleep Disturbance in Children and Adolescents with Disorders of Development: Its Significance and Management*. Cambridge: Cambridge University Press, pp 97–106.
Stores G, Hart J, Piran N. (1978) Inattentiveness in school children with epilepsy. *Epilepsia* 19: 169–175.
Szabò CA, Wyllie E, Stanford LD, Geckler C, Kotagal P, Comair YG, Thornton AE. (1998) Neuropsychological effect of temporal lobe resection in preadolescent children with epilepsy. *Epilepsia* 39(8): 814–819.
Szabò CA, Wyllie E, Dolske M, Stanford LD, Kotagal P, Comair YG. (1999) Epilepsy surgery in children with pervasive developmental disorder. *Pediatr Neurol* 20(5): 349–353.
Szabò CA, Rothner AD, Kotagal P, Erenberg G, Dinner DS, Wyllie E. (2001) Symptomatic of cryptogenic partial epilepsy of childhood onset: fourteen-year follow-up. *Pediatr Neurol* 24: 264–269.
Taft LT, Cohen HJ. (1971) Hypsarrhythmia and infantile autism: a clinical report. *J Autism Child Schizophr* 1(3): 327–336.
Tassinari CA, Rubbioli G, Volpi L, Meletti S, dOrsi G, Franca M, Sabetta AR, Riguzzi P, Gardetta E, Zaniboni A, Michenucci R. (2000) ESES: encephalopathy related to electrical status epilepticus during slow sleep. Review. *Clinical Neurophysiology* Suppl 2: S94–S102.
Taylor DC, Falconer MA. (1971) Focal dysplasia of the cerebral cortex in epilepsy. *J Neurol Neurosurg Psychiatry* 34: 369–387.
Taylor DC, Lochery M. (1991) Behavioral consequences of epilepsy in children. Developing a psychosocial vocabulary. In: Smith D, Treiman D, Trimble M, editors. *Advances in Neurology* 55. New York: Raven Press, pp 153–162.
Taylor DC, Neville BGR, Cross JH. (1999) Autistic spectrum disorders in childhood epilepsy surgery candidates. *Eur Child Adolesc Psychiatry* 8: 189–192.
Temple CM. (1997) *Developmental Cognitive Neuropsychology*. Hove: Psychology Press.
Thomas P, Zifkin B, Migneco O, Lebrun C, Darcourt J, Andermann F. (1999) Nonconvulsive status epilepticus of frontal origin. *Neurology* 52: 1174–1183.
Trimble MR, Cull C. (1988) Children of school age: the influence of antiepileptic drugs on behavior and intellect. Review. *Epilepsia* 29 Suppl 3: S15–S19.
Trimble M, Schmidt B. (2002) *The Neuropsychiatry of Epilepsy*. Cambridge: Cambridge University Press.
Tuchman R. (1995) Regression in pervasive developmental disorders: is there a relationship with Landau–Kleffner syndrome? *Ann Neurol* 38: 526.
Tuchman R. (2000) Treatment of seizure disorders and EEG abnormalities in children with autism spectrum disorders. *J Autism Dev Disord* 30(5): 485–489.
Tuchman R, Rapin I. (1997) Regression in pervasive developmental disorders: seizures and epileptiform electroencephalographic correlates. *Pediatrics* 99: 560–566.
Tuchman R, Rapin I. (2002) Epilepsy in autism. *Lancet Neurol* 1(6): 352–358.
Tuchman RF, Rapin I, Shinnar S. (1991) Autistic and dysphasic children. II. Epilepsy. *Pediatrics* 88: 1219–1225.
Uldall P, Sahlholdt L, Alving J. (2000) Landau–Kleffner syndrome with onset at 18 months and an initial diagnosis of pervasive developmental disorder. *Eur J Paediatr Neurol* 4: 81–86.
Umbricht D, Degreel G, Barr WB, Lieberman JA, Pollack S, Schaul N. (1995) Postictal and chronic psychoses in patients with temporal lobe epilepsy. *Am J Psychiatry* 152(2): 224–231.

Valenstein E. (1997) Geschwind's influence on the study of disorders of attention. In: Schachter SC, Devinsky O, editors. *Behavioral Neurology and the Legacy of Norman Geschwind*. Philadelphia and New York: Lippincott-Raven, pp 127–141.
Vance M. (1991) Educational and therapeutic approaches used with a child presenting with acquired aphasia with convulsive disorder (Landau–Kleffner syndrome). *Child Lang Teach Ther* 7: 41–60.
Vance M. (2001) Christopher Lumpship: developing phonological representations in a child with auditory processing deficit. In: Chiat S, Law J, Marshall J, editors. *Language Disorders in Children and Adults: Psycholinguistic Approaches to Therapy*. London: Whurr, pp 17–41.
Vanderlinden L, Ceulemans B, Boel M, Van Coster R, Lagae L. (2003) Thalamic lesions and epilepsy with continuous spike-waves during slow sleep: a recognizable syndrome. *Eur J Paediatr Neurol* 7(5): 328.
van Emde Boas W. Parra J, Dekker E. (2003) Weiteres zum dialektischen Prozess von Anfallssemiologie zur Klassifikation: Wie 'generalisiert' sind typische Absencen eigentlich? (video demonstration). *Zeitschrift für Epileptologie* 16: 102.
van Landingham KE, Heinz ER, Cavazos JE, Lewis DV. (1998) Magnetic resonance imaging evidence of hippocampal injury after prolonged focal febrile convulsions. *Ann Neurol* 43(4): 413–426.
Vargha-Khadem F, Mishkin M. (1997) Speech and language outcome after hemispherectomy in childhood. In: Tuxhorn I, Holthausen H, Boenigk H, editors. *Pediatric Epilepsy Syndromes and their Surgical Treatment*. London: John Libbey, pp 774–784.
Vargha-Khadem F, Isaacs E, van der Werf S, Robb S, Wilson J. (1992) Development of intelligence and memory in children with hemiplegic cerebral palsy. *Brain* 115: 315–329.
Vargha-Khadem F, Isaacs E, Muter V. (1994) A review of cognitive outcome after unilateral lesions sustained during childhood. *J Child Neurol* Suppl 2: 67–73.
Vargha-Khadem F, Carr LJ, Isaacs E, Brett E, Adams C, Mishkin M. (1997a) Onset of speech after left hemispherectomy in a nine-year-old boy. *Brain* 120: 159–182.
Vargha-Khadem F, Gadian DG, Watkins KE, Connelly A, Van Paesschen W, Mishkin M. (1997b) Differential effects of early hippocampal pathology on episodic and semantic memory. *Science* 277: 376–380.
Vasconcellos E, Wyllie E, Sullivan S, Stanford L, Bulacio J, Kotagal P, Bingaman W. (2001) Mental retardation in pediatric candidates for epilepsy surgery: the role of early seizure onset. *Epilepsia* 42: 268–274.
Veggiotti P, Beccaria F, Papalia G, Termine C, Piazza F, Lanzi G. (1998) Continuous spikes and waves during sleep in children with shunted hydrocephalus. *Child Nerv Syst* 14: 188–194.
Veggiotti P, Beccaria F, Guerrini R, Capovilla G, Lanzi, G. (1999) Continuous spike-and-wave activity during slow-wave sleep: syndrome or EEG pattern? *Epilepsia* 40(11): 1593–1601.
Veggiotti P, Bova S, Granocchio E, Papalia G, Termine C, Lanzi G. (2001) Acquired epileptic frontal syndrome as long-term outcome in two children with CSWS. *Neurophysiol Clin* 31(6): 387–397.
Verity CM, Greenwood R, Golding J. (1998) Long-term intellectual and behavioral outcomes of children with febrile convulsions. *New Engl J Med* 338: 1723–1728.
Vermeulen J, Aldenkamp AP. (1995) Cognitive side-effects of chronic antiepileptic treatment: a review of 25 years of research. *Epilepsy Res* 22: 65–95.
Villemure JG, Rasmussen T. (1993) Functional hemispherectomy in children. *Neuropediatrics* 24(1): 53–55.
Vining EP, Freeman JM, Pillas DJ, Uematsu S, Carson BS, Brandt J, Boatman D, Pulsifer MB, Zuckerberg A. (1997) Why would you remove half a brain? The outcome of 58 children after hemispherectomy – the Johns Hopkins experience: 1968 to 1996. *Pediatrics* 100(2) Pt 1: 163–171.
Voeller KKS, Rothenberg MB. (1973) Psychosocial aspects of the management of seizures in children. *Pediatrics* 51: 1072–1082.
Volkmar FR, Nelson DS. (1990) Seizure disorder in autism. *J Am Acad Child Adolesc Psychiatry* 29: 127–129.
Vuilleumier P, Despland PA, Regli F. (1996) Failure ro recall (but not to remember): pure transient amnesia during nonconvulsive status epilepticus. *Neurology* 46(4): 1036–1039.
Wallace SJ, Farrell K, editors. (2004) *Epilepsy in Children*, 2nd edition. London: Arnold.
Wechsler D. (1996) *Wechsler Intelligence Scale for Children (Version III)*. French adaptation. Paris: Les Editions du Centre de Psychologie Appliquée.
Weglage J, Demsky A, Pietsch M, Kurlemann G. (1997) Neuropsychological, intellectual, and behavioral findings in patients with centrotemporal spikes with and without seizures. *Dev Med Child Neurol* 39: 646–651.
Weise S, Sargess Karl M, Gross-Selbeck G. (1995) Die sogenannten benignen Partilepilepsien – eignesständige Entitäten oder nur unterschiedliche Verlaufsformen? In: *Aktuelle Neuropädiatrie*. Basel, Switzerland: Ciba-Geigy, pp 431–435.

Weissenberger AA, Dell ML, Liow K, Theodore W, Frattali CM, Hernandez D, Zametkin AJ. (2001) Aggression and psychiatric comorbidity in children with hypothalamic hamartomas and their unaffected siblings. *J Am Acad Chid Adolesc Psychiatry* 40(6): 696–703.

Wennberg R, Arruda F, Quesney LF, Olivier A. (2002) Preeminence of extrahippocampal structures in the generation of mesial temporal seizures: evidence from human depth electrode recordings. *Epilepsia* 43(7): 716–726.

White C. (2001) Doctor referred to GMC after inquiry into epilepsy diagnoses. *BMJ* 323(7325): 1323.

Williams J. (1998) Does short-term antiepileptic drug treatment in children result in cognitive or behavioral changes? *Epilepsia* 39(10): 1064–1069.

Williamson PD, French JA, Thadani VM, Kim JH, Novelly RA, Spencer SS, Spencer DD, Mattson RH. (1993) Characteristics of medial temporal epilepsy: interictal and ictal scalp EEG and surgical results (67 cases). *Ann Neurol* 34: 781.

Yung AWY, Park YD, Cohen MJ, Garrison TN. (2000) Cognitive and behavioral problems in children with centrotemporal spikes. *Pediatr Neurol* 23(5): 391–395.

Zaiwalla Z, Stores G. (1995) Case reports. In: Beaumanoir A, Bureau A, Deonna T, Mira C, Tassinari CA, editors. *Continuous Spikes and Waves during Slow Sleep. Electrical Status Epilepticus during Slow Sleep.* Mariani Foundation Neurology Series: 3. London: John Libbey, pp 196–199.

Zardini G, Molteni B, Nardocci N. (1995) Linguistic development in a patient with Landau–Kleffner syndrome: a nine year follow up. *Neuropediatrics* 26: 19–25.

Zeman AZ, Boniface SJ, Hodges JR. (1998) Transient epileptic amnesia: a description of the clinical and neuropsychological features in 10 cases and a review of the literature. Review. *J Neurol Neurosurg Psychiatry* 64(4): 435–443.

Ziegler AL, Reinberg O, Deonna T. (1994) Epilepsie et accidents. Quel risque chez l'enfant? *Archives françaises de Pédiatrie* 1: 801–805.

LIST OF CASE STUDIES

Chapters in which these cases are discussed are given in brackets.

G.S., boy	Left frontal dysplasia with severe epilepsy. No change in language dominance (direct cortical stimulation) (Chapter 9, p. 116)
M.K., girl	Tuberous sclerosis, epilepsy surgery (Chapter 9, p. 117)
C.R., boy	Partial epilepsy with CSWS due to prenatal middle cerebral artery infarct and frontal syndrome treated by hemispherectomy (Chapter 10, p. 125)
A.G., boy	Intractable epilepsy from early infancy due to cortical dysplasia. Pre- and postoperative developmental study (Chapter 10, pp. 126, 127)
E.S., girl	Rett syndrome with regression and multifocal EEG discharges, with some improvement on antiepileptic drug therapy (Chapter 11, p. 130)
H.L., F.M., Z.L.	Three boys with myoclonic-astatic epilepsy: neuropsychological profiles in active phase (Chapter 11, p. 133)
B.A., girl	Severe polymorphic epilepsy of infancy with hippocampal sclerosis (Chapter 11, p. 134)
M.F., boy	Developmental dysphasia with autistic features and bitemporal EEG spikes (Chapter 12, p. 137)
R.E., girl	Early reversible severe developmental retardation (autistic-like), epileptic (Chapter 12, p. 139)
D.C. and J., two families	Siblings from two families with severe developmental disorder and paroxysmal EEG abnormalities (Chapter 12, p. 142)
D.C.M., girl	Early and late language regression (two episodes). Atypical developmental dysphasia (Chapter 12, pp. 144–146)
D.G.T., boy	Reversible autistic regression with late epileptic spasms (Chapter 12, pp. 152, 153)
B.A., boy	Early complex partial epilepsy with autistic regression (Chapter 12, pp. 157, 158)
F.M., boy	Early prelanguage and autistic regression (Chapter 12, p. 159)
D.A., boy	Behavioural regression as epileptic manifestation (Chapter 12, pp. 160–161)
B.P., boy	Frontal epilepsy with 'epileptic disintegrative psychosis' (Chapter 12, p. 161)
D.V., girl	Early frontal epilepsy with severe behaviour disorder and obsessive-compulsive symptoms (Chapter 15, p. 193)
A.O., boy	Prolonged cognitive arrest with frontal epilepsy (Chapter 16, pp. 199–201)
R.M., boy	Adult follow-up of acquired epileptic aphasia, expressive (Chapter 16, pp. 201–202)

INDEX

Note: page numbers in *italics* refer to figures and tables